First edition

How I scored 900 In UCAT

Introduction

Hello future doctors and dentists! I'm Dr Kunal Dasani, one of the founders of Medic Mind, and I'm thrilled to welcome you to this book, 'How I Scored 900 on the UCAT'. If you're gearing up for the UCAT, you're in the right place. Trust me, I've been in your shoes, and I know how challenging and nerve-racking this journey can be. But here's the good news: you're not alone, and with the right strategies and mindset, you can achieve amazing results.

Let me start by sharing a bit about my journey. I'm incredibly grateful to say that I aced the UCAT, scoring a maximum of 900 in three of the five sections. This achievement opened the doors for me to study Medicine at UCL, an experience that was filled with incredible opportunities and unforgettable moments. I hope your time at your dream university will be even more rewarding!

Now, let's rewind to when I was preparing for the UCAT. Those were some of the most intense months of my life. I remember panicking about the UCAT every single day of that summer. The stress was real, and the pressure was immense. I spent countless hours practising, going through question banks, and seeking help from tutors. In fact, it took me three tutors before I found the right fit! This might sound overwhelming, but finding high-quality resources and the right guidance was crucial for my success.

The Birth of Medic Mind

It was this experience that led me, along with my co-founder, Dr Mohil Shah, to create Medic Mind. We felt that the options available for medical applicants were outdated, expensive, and often inaccessible. We wanted to change that and make the journey to medical and dental school easier for students like you. Together, we've worked tremendously hard, along with the amazing Medic Mind team, to provide top-notch resources and support.

Our mission has always been to make high-quality education accessible to everyone. Over the years, we've helped 12,400 applicants succeed in their university goals, with a 98.9% satisfaction rate. Our students have had over 134,000 hours of high-quality lessons from our expert tutors. We're incredibly proud of these achievements, and we're here to help you too with this book.

My UCAT Journey: Challenges and Triumphs

Preparing for the UCAT was no walk in the park. Each section posed its own unique challenges. For instance, the Verbal Reasoning section required quick reading and comprehension skills, which I initially found quite demanding. On the other hand, the Quantitative Reasoning section, which involves a lot of data interpretation and mathematical calculations under time pressure, was a tough nut to crack.

So, how did I manage to score 900 in three sections? Here are some tips and insights from my own journey:

1. Embrace the Test Format

Understanding the UCAT format is the first step. The test consists of five sections: Verbal Reasoning, Decision Making, Quantitative Reasoning, Abstract Reasoning, and Situational Judgement. Each section tests different skills, and familiarising yourself with the format can reduce a lot of the initial anxiety.

2. Practise with Purpose

Practise is crucial, but it's not just about quantity. Focus on quality practise. I used a combination of UCAT question banks, timed tests, and tutoring sessions. Each practice session was a learning opportunity. Pay attention to the types of questions you struggle with and work on them.

3. Develop a Time Management Strategy

Time management is one of the biggest challenges in the UCAT. Use a stopwatch during your practise sessions to get used to the time constraints. Learn to move on if you get stuck on a question. It's better to guess and move forward than to spend too much time on one question.

4. Find the Right Resources and Support

Finding the right resources was a game-changer for me. After going through three tutors, I finally found one that was a perfect fit. Don't be afraid to switch resource if you feel your current path isn't helping. High-quality resources and the right guidance can make a huge difference. However, beware of too many resources as this can cause your revision to slow as you flick through and watch too many tutorials. Remember, quality over quantity is key here.

5. Maintain a Positive Mindset

Staying positive and motivated is key. The journey is tough, and there will be moments of doubt and frustration. Keep reminding yourself why you're doing this. Visualise your end goal – whether it's wearing that white coat, helping patients, or making a difference in the world.

6. Use Real-Life Scenarios for Situational Judgement

For the Situational Judgement section, think about real-life scenarios. Discussing ethical dilemmas and patient interactions with friends, family, or mentors can give you a broader perspective and help you answer questions more thoughtfully.

7. Incorporate Relaxation Techniques

Managing stress is crucial. Incorporate relaxation techniques like mindfulness, deep breathing exercises, or short walks into your routine. Staying calm and focused will help you perform better.

As you embark on this journey, remember that the UCAT is just one step in your path to becoming a doctor or dentist. It's challenging, but with the right preparation and mindset, you can achieve a score that will make your application stand out. This book is filled with detailed strategies, tips, and example questions and answer explanations that I hope will guide you through each section of the UCAT.

Here's to acing the UCAT and moving one step closer to your dream career!

Good luck, and happy studying!

Dr Kunal Dasani

Verbal Reasoning

Verbal Reasoning Tips

When you're just starting out, UCAT Verbal Reasoning can seem to be one of the more straightforward sections in the UCAT. This section asks you to read a passage of text and then answer questions about what you've read. It can seem quite simple but the difficulty comes in the timing. Timing is particularly tight for this section and the texts can often be quite long. Of course, the exam has been designed this way on purpose! In order to succeed, the examiners are looking for you to be able to cope under stressful, time-limited situations.

At the beginning of your UCAT preparation it is key that you completely understand what each section is testing and have good resources and support in place. In this section, we're going to go through sixteen tips to help you devise your own strategy for tackling UCAT Verbal Reasoning.

1. Use our keyword technique

The passages of text that you're given can be really quite long. Time is tight so the longer you spend reading, the less time you have to answer the questions. That's why the majority of tips in this article will be based around reducing the amount you need to read. The number one tip for UCAT Verbal Reasoning is do not read the whole passage! This might seem intuitive but reading the whole thing would take far too long and you'll run out of time very fast.

Instead, we recommend the keyword technique. To do this, firstly you read just the first two lines of the text to give you an idea of the topic. Then read the question so that you know what you're being asked. From the question you pick a keyword which you use to help you find the relevant information in the text. Scan through the passage looking for that keyword, and then read the sentence containing it, as well as the sentences before and after. This should give you enough information without needing to read the whole passage.

You might be thinking, how do I decide which keyword to choose? You want the keyword to be specific. The more specific the less likely the keyword is to be repeated throughout the text. Ideally you want the keyword to be something that will only appear in the sentence relevant to the question, to minimise the amount you need to read.

So to recap, the keyword technique involves:
1. Read the question and pick a keyword
   Pick a keyword in the question statement. Dates, numbers and capitalised words tend to be good keywords because they're easy to spot and stand out from other words.

2. Search for keyword
   Scan for the keyword in the passage
3. Read around the keyword
   If you find the keyword, then read the 2-3 lines around the keyword and hopefully you should find your answer!

Sometimes you won't find your keyword in the text, or it'll be present far too many times to be useful. In these situations you'll need to select an alternative keyword.

2. Identify extreme language in UCAT Verbal Reasoning

Another key technique to use during the Verbal Reasoning questions is identifying extreme language to make educated guesses. Time is extremely tight in this section and the majority of students don't even manage to answer every question. Near the end of the section, you might find yourself with just a handful of seconds left with several questions still to go. In this circumstance it's best to make quick educated guesses rather than leave all of the remaining questions blank.

In these situations, you can look at the wording of the question and use this to help you predict the correct answer. That way your guess has more chance of being right than just randomly selecting an answer to pick.

Statements with extreme language (never, always, will, most…) are much more likely to indicate a false answer as it is a more definitive statement and doesn't allow for any exceptions. Whereas mild language (may, can, sometimes…) is more likely to be true for the opposite reasons.

This technique is particularly useful with the 'True, False or Can't Tell' questions but can be applied to other types of question too. Why don't you have a go at practising some questions using this technique first, and then try the questions properly by reading the text. If you compare how many you get right you'll probably find that using extreme language is more accurate than you might have thought, and can be done in a matter of seconds!

3. Don't miss out True, False, Can't Tell Questions in UCAT Verbal Reasoning

The 'True, False, Can't Tell' questions are normally the quickest to answer compared to the questions where you have to evaluate several statements at once. You definitely don't want to miss out on any of the 'True, False, Can't Tell' questions as they're typically the ones where you can score the most points in the quickest amount of time.
Sometimes these questions can be hidden at the end, meaning that people who spend too long on earlier questions miss them out when they run out of time.

4. But, don't skip through looking for True, False, Can't Tell Questions

However, don't be tempted to skip back and forth looking for the 'True, False, Can't Tell' questions straight away. This will completely mess up your timing and you'll spend too long navigating the exam interface. For example, if you're on question 28 and have 15 minutes left it's hard to work out how long you have left to answer the remaining questions as there's no way to see how many you've skipped at the start.

The best thing to do is to answer the questions in the order they're presented to you, but as you get close to the end of the time, keep in mind there may be some quicker questions at the end of the test. For example, if you've got 3 minutes left and still have two passages to get through, it might be worth making educated guesses on a longer passage and spending the majority of your time left on a 'True, False, Can't Tell' set.

5. For Author questions, look at the conclusion first for the author opinion

We've already spoken about 'True, False' Can't Tell' but there are several different question types in the Verbal Reasoning section of the UCAT. It is worth practising each different type of question ahead of your test and developing a technique for each of them. This will allow for you to be familiar with each one, with a rough idea of how long they all take you to do.

One of the types of questions in the UCAT Verbal Reasoning section is author or writer questions. These questions ask you to evaluate the passage based on someone else's opinion. They can be long and it can be hard to find the author's conclusion or overall opinion without reading the entire text. We've already seen that reading all of the passage in one go is a bad idea so the best bet for author questions is to look in the final paragraph first. The final paragraph usually holds the overall conclusion or closing argument which sums up the entire tone of the article without you needing to read the whole thing.

6. You may want to guess some author questions

Author questions can be long winded and require lots of reading, especially if the conclusion isn't in the final few sentences. So when it comes to deciding which questions you are going to guess, these are probably a good choice.

The tricky part with UCAT Verbal Reasoning is not so much the difficulty of the questions, but trying to answer all of them in the time limit. Remember to be realistic as it is pretty much impossible to answer every single question. This means you're going to need to guess some of them, and should get into the practice of doing so. By making good choices at which questions to guess, you can maximise your score.

7. Watch out for 'strongest opinion' author questions

Sometimes a question may ask for the author's strongest opinion. These questions are particularly difficult as there can be multiple 'correct' answers. The exam is looking for you to select the 'most correct' answer, meaning the statement the author is most likely to agree with.

It is hard to eliminate answers for this type of question, and it can take a long time to work out the answer as you'll need to read a lot of the passage to understand the authors complete point of view. So again, this might be one to guess and skip or save for the end of a set when you're more familiar with the passage.

8. Watch out for negative questions!

Sometimes you'll get negative questions which can easily throw you off when you're under a time pressure. For example, the statement will say 'which of these is NOT true'. Make sure you can spot the negative turn to these questions so you know exactly what you're looking for in the text.

9. Don't spend too long checking

In UCAT Verbal Reasoning, time is precious. So be smart and don't double check your answers. This might feel unnatural as this exam holds a lot of weight on your medical school application. So naturally you'll want to check you haven't made mistakes. But if you check your answers you will definitely run out of time and end up losing more marks than if you accidentally make one or two mistakes.

It's particularly important in the the statement type of question. Here you're given four statements to evaluate. Once you've found the correct answer, there isn't any need to evaluate the remaining statements. Unless you have any big doubts, there's no point and it will save you valuable seconds to spend on other questions that you otherwise might have to blindly guess.

10. Practise in a library

So many students practise the UCAT, but don't practise full two-hour mocks in test conditions. The test environment is likely to be different to any exam you've sat before. There are only very short breaks, it's in a hot stuffy room with other people moving around and it'll be on an old desktop computer.

Your local library will probably be quite similar to this, so we recommend practising at least one mock exam in these conditions. You might be surprised how distracting it can be to have someone sitting down or moving around next to you while you're trying to focus. If you simulate the exam beforehand, you should have fewer surprises on the real day!

11. Work onscreen

During practise you should try and replicate the exam format as much as possible. The exam will be on a computer screen so if you are using books, for example, try not to highlight the text because this won't be an option when you're sitting the real exam. Try to practise on a screen wherever possible. Your eyes can get tired reading passages on a screen, but this is all part of the challenge.

12. Don't fall for time traps!

Sometimes certain questions are made deliberately difficult to try and throw you off! The best candidates are able to identify these questions are going to take too long before they start, and will simply make an educated guess and move on without wasting their time.

This is purposely done and is one of the skills you're being tested on. If you've done work experience in a A&E department you might have noticed doctors triaging, and this is essentially the same skill albeit with questions rather than patients! If you can work out which questions are going to take too long, you can forfeit one mark but save a lot of time and potentially pick up more marks by spending this time on easier questions.

13. Prepare yourself mentally

UCAT Verbal Reasoning is the first section of the exam, so go in and be prepared for it. Remember that the majority of people don't finish this section. Even if you don't answer all the questions you can still score very highly. Many students are unprepared for this reality and feel disheartened when they finish this section. Even if you feel it went badly, don't let it have a knock-on effect for the rest of the exam. The UCAT have put this section first to test your resilience – can you bounce back after not finishing, or do you give up and let it bring down the rest of your exam?

14. Work on skim reading

To do well in the Verbal Reasoning section, you have to skim read the text to find the keyword you're looking for. This is a skill which you will develop over time, and practise helps. Some people say it's good to read newspapers to practise this. But to be honest, if you're going to spend time practising, it's probably more efficient to just do more VR questions. This is where having access to a large question bank or book will really help you.

15. Use the flagging function

In the UCAT you can flag questions and come back to them later. If you're unsure about an answer or simply don't know, it's worth flagging in case you have some time left over.

But you should be cautious doing this! Remember most people don't finish the section so it's unlikely you'll have time to come back to anything. Always put an answer down, even if it's a random guess, before flagging and moving on.

16. Consider your operational time

Sometimes students develop their own techniques for each section. This is great and you should always do what works best for you, but don't waste precious time doing extra things as this really adds up. There have been students in the past who always write down the keyword on their whiteboard, for example, in case they come back to the question. If it would take 5 seconds to do this for every question, by the time you wrote things down and looked back up, which is 220 seconds across 44 questions. This is just under 4 minutes, nearly 20% of your time!

17. Take time to figure out where you went wrong

Whilst doing practice questions, review the answers you get wrong and spend time thinking how you could have got to the right answer. It's very easy to just look at the right answer and think that it seems obvious now, but really take a moment to see if there were any key mistakes you made that caused you to get the answer wrong. A very common mistake is people skim reading too fast, which may seem surprising as the whole point of skim reading is speed. However, if you skim read too fast you may miss details that cause you to choose the wrong answer. Try to identify the common mistakes you make and write these down as a checklist. Then before you practise questions, read over this checklist to serve as a reminder of things to avoid doing.

18. Read the question carefully

As mentioned above, you do want to skim read to use your time effectively. However, one thing you don't want to skim read is the question; ensure you read the question carefully so you don't make mistakes. This could be a mistake such as skim-reading a question as asking you to select a statement that is true, where in fact you should be looking for a statement that is NOT true.

19. Only use the information given

Your answers should be based solely on the information given in the passage, don't use your prior knowledge as this may contradict what is written in the passage and this could lead you down the wrong path. A lot of the topics given in the passages are very niche and can be quite complex, so don't be overwhelmed if you're not familiar with the information presented.

Bonus: UCAT Verbal Reasoning needs confidence

The final tip for the Verbal Reasoning section is to have confidence in yourself. The answers to these questions may not appear as black and white as the other sections, as often there is a degree of inference required to get to the answer. So, here more than ever, trust your gut instinct when you you can't find the answer exactly. You can always come back and review if you have time at the end, but trusting in yourself in that moment could save you lots of time that could make a large difference over the course of the test. Especially when you're making those educated guesses.

Remember, as with every UCAT section, there is no negative marking so make sure you do not leave any question blank. Even if you have absolutely no idea there is still a 25% chance you may guess correctly and pick up an extra mark.

Verbal Reasoning Mock

Question Set 1

Sales at Gucci are expected to fall by 20% in the first quarter due to a slowdown in Asia, according to its Paris-based owner Kering. The warning contrasts with rivals LVMH and Hermès whose sales have remained resilient.

The luxury market has grown in the past decade but sales have not been as impressive in recent years. Gucci is estimated to get more than a third of its sales from China, whose economy has been struggling. Kering said in a statement that the profit warning "reflects a steeper sales drop at Gucci, notably in the Asia-Pacific region". The firm is scheduled to report its financial results on 23 April. Gucci accounted for two-thirds of group operating income last year. Kering's other brands include Yves Saint Laurent, Balenciaga and Bottega Veneta. Last month, Kering reported that its net profit last year fell by 17%. Its shares have fallen by more than 23% over the past year.

In comparison, its bigger rival LVMH, which owns Louis Vuitton, Moët & Chandon and Hennessy, posted higher-than-expected sales for 2023. Hermes also celebrated its record annual sales last year with plans to reward all employees worldwide with a bonus. While their results showed resilience in the luxury market, Gucci is known to target younger, aspirational shoppers who are more vulnerable to economic pressures.

Last year, Kering changed Gucci's top management by appointing Jean-François Palus as its chief executive officer and Sabato De Sarno as its creative director. The first items of his Ancora collection were made available in mid-February. The collection has been met with a "highly favourable reception," Kering's statement said.

Adapted from www.bbc.com.

1. Which of the following is a reason for Gucci's recent decline in sales, according to the passage?

   a. Rising competition from other brands such as Bottega Veneta and Balenciaga.
   b. Gucci have an older target market, who in turn, have little disposable income.
   c. The Chinese economy has been struggling recently.
   d. There has been a recent change in ownership of the company to a Parisian based operation.

2. Which of the following brands are under the same ownership as Gucci?
   a. Louis Vuitton
   b. Moët & Chandon
   c. Yves Saint Laurent
   d. Hennessy

3. Which of the following can be inferred from the passage?

    a. In the first quarter, Gucci sales are expected to fall by 1/3.
    b. Gucci does not give their workers any annual bonuses.
    c. Hermès has a higher net worth as a brand than Gucci.
    d. Net profit of Kering fell by less than 1/5th last year.

4. Which of the following statements are true, according to the passage?

    a. The biggest rival to Kering is the company LMVH.
    b. Jean-François Palus was recently appointed as Kering's creative director.
    c. The release of Ancora collection was most likely not a profitable endeavour.
    d. The financial results of Kering will be published in the fourth month of the year.

Question Set 2

Children with gender dysphoria will no longer receive puberty-suppressing hormones, also known as puberty blockers, as routine practice after an NHS England review concluded there was insufficient evidence for their safety and effectiveness. Under the new policy, the hormones will be only available for children with gender dysphoria through clinical trials intended to fill gaps in medical knowledge, though provision is expected to be made in exceptional circumstances on a case-by-case basis. Treatment for young people already receiving the hormones will not be affected.

Therapies to suppress puberty arose from work in the 1960s and 70s, when researchers discovered what has been called "the conductor of the reproductive system". In work that involved the dissection of hundreds of thousands of pig and lamb brains, Andrew Schally and Roger Guillemin extracted and determined the structure of gonadotropin-releasing hormone (GnRH) work that earned them the 1977 Nobel prize for medicine. GnRH is produced in the brain's hypothalamus. When released, it triggers the pituitary gland to secrete further substances, namely follicle-stimulating hormone and luteinizing hormone, which drive puberty and sexual development. In men, the hormones tell the testicles to make testosterone. In women, they make the ovaries produce oestrogen and progesterone.

What researchers found remarkable as they came to understand GnRH was that while pulses of the hormone stimulate the pituitary to churn out other puberty-driving hormones, a continuous dose effectively shuts down production of follicle-stimulating hormone and luteinizing hormone, putting puberty on ice.

Today, synthetic analogues of GnRH such as triptorelin are given for prostate cancer and endometriosis, and they are also approved for children with precocious puberty, a condition that affects more girls than boys. Affected girls can start puberty as toddlers, but hormone therapy applies the brakes. When children come off the drugs, they go through puberty as normal. "It's been very beneficial in these children," says Ashley Grossman, a professor of endocrinology at the University of Oxford.

Adapted from www.theguardian.com.

5. Children will no longer be able to access puberty blockers in the UK as routine practice under this new policy.

   a. True
   b. False
   c. Can't tell

6. GnRH triggers the release of follicle-stimulating hormone from the hypothalamus.

   a. True
   b. False
   c. Can't tell

7. Triptorelin is prescribed to more females than males, as precocious puberty affects females in more cases than males.

   a. True
   b. False
   c. Can't tell

8. Andrew Schally and Roger Guillemin won the Nobel prize for medicine for discovering the existence of the gonadotropin-releasing hormone through human brain dissection.

   a. True
   b. False
   c. Can't tell

Question Set 3

When used correctly, there's nothing to worry about in terms of your microwave's radiation, according to the World Health Organization. But other concerns are less clear – including whether microwaving food causes nutrient loss, or whether heating food in plastic can trigger hormone disruption.

Some research has shown that vegetables lose some of their nutritional value in the microwave. For example, microwaving has been found to remove 97% of the flavonoids – plant compounds with anti-inflammatory benefits – in broccoli. That's a third more damage than done by boiling. But the conventional oven may be a stronger competitor for the microwave. A 2020 study compared the nutritional levels of a frozen ready meal cooked in the microwave, and the same meal cooked in a conventional oven. The researchers found that the only difference between the two cooked meals was that the microwaved one retained "slightly" more vitamin C. But the researchers didn't explain why this might be.

We often microwave foods in plastic containers and wrapping, but some scientists warn of the risk of ingesting phthalates. When exposed to heat, these plastic additives can break down and leach into food.

"Some plastic isn't designed for microwaves because it has polymers inside to make it soft and flexible, which melt at a lower temperature and may leach out during the microwave process if it goes beyond 100C (212F)," says Juming Tang, professor of food engineering at Washington State University. In a 2011 study, researchers purchased more than 400 plastic containers designed to contain food, and found that the majority leaked chemical that disrupt hormones.

Phthalates are one of the most commonly used plasticisers, added to make plastic more flexible and often found in takeaway containers, plastic wrap and water bottles. They have been found to disrupt hormones and our metabolic system. In children, phthalates can increase blood pressure and insulin resistance, which can increase the risk of metabolic disorders such as diabetes and hypertension. Exposure also has been linked to fertility issues, asthma and ADHD.

Adapted from www.bbc.com.

9. Which of the following is not a concern related to microwaving food within the passage?

   a. The possibility of nutrient loss from microwaving food.
   b. Hormone disruption related to heating food in a microwave.
   c. The potential of cancer development from the microwaving of food.
   d. The issue of polymers leaking into food when microwaved.

10 Which of the following statements cannot be inferred from the passage?

   a. Approximately 3% of flavonoids remain in broccoli with microwaving.
   b. Boiling broccoli preserves increased levels of flavonoids, as opposed to microwaving.
   c. Flavonoids are anti-inflammatory compounds found within plant material.
   d. Microwaves preserve higher levels of vitamin C within food than boiling.

11. Which of the following is untrue regarding phthalates?

   a. Phthalates are commonly found within takeaway containers.
   b. Phthalates improve the strength of plastic substances.
   c. Phthalates can leak out into food when heated above 100 degrees celsius.
   d. Phthalates are a form of hormone disruptors.

12. Which of the following conditions are not linked with phthalate exposure, according to the text?

   a. Attention deficit disorders
   b. Hypotension
   c. Metabolic disorders
   d. Asthma

Question Set 4

Live music fans are losing out because of an array of "sneaky" fees that can add up to 25% to the cost of concert and festival tickets, research from the consumer body Which? has found. Its report comes days after the Labour leader, Keir Starmer, said his party would cap the resale prices of tickets and strengthen the regulation of resale platforms if it wins the next general election.

The Which? research looked at the fees imposed by five leading "primary" ticket agencies: Ticketmaster, See Tickets, AXS, Eventim and the ticketing app Dice. Ticket sites often include some fees in the upfront price, and mention that other charges will be added, but the final price is often not revealed until later in the checkout process. This practice is known as "drip pricing".

When they looked at a show by the singer-songwriter Anne-Marie at Cardiff's Utilita Arena last November, the Which? researchers found tickets with a face value of £45 on Eventim and Ticketmaster – but in both cases, extra fees bumped up the final price to more than £55. Eventim charged a £1.50 processing fee, a £2.50 delivery and transaction fee, a £5.62 booking fee and a £1.75 venue levy, pushing up the overall cost of the ticket to £56.37. Ticketmaster charged a £6.10 service charge, a £1.75 facility charge and a £2.75 order processing fee, which meant the final cost was £55.60.

Rocio Concha, the director of policy and advocacy at Which?, criticised "these sneaky drip pricing tactics", adding: "It's no surprise that music fans sometimes feel like they are being taken for a ride." However, the organisation said forthcoming legislation would give people more clarity. The digital markets, competition and consumers bill – poised to get royal assent in the coming weeks – should ensure that any charges consumers would "necessarily incur" would need to be made clear as part of the upfront total price.

Adapted from www.theguardian.com

13. Which of the following statements is Keir Starmer most likely to agree with based on this article?

    a. Current ticket resale pricing strategies are fair and reflect the means of current music fans.
    b. Drip pricing is an unfair and misleading method of pricing music tickets.
    c. A major issue with ticket sales currently is the lack of variety of ticketing sites.
    d. Resale prices of tickets are already well regulated by the main ticketing agencies.

14. Which of the following is the most accurate description of 'drip pricing' from the text?

    a. A method of payment where customers can pay for their tickets in smaller monthly amounts with interest.
    b. A means of pricing where all fees are given upfront and added to the initial cost at the end of the payment process.
    c. A pricing method where fees can be settled with no initial payment, and the total cost is paid a certain number of months after the initial transaction.
    d. A method of ticket sales where fees are slowly added to the initial ticket cost throughout the payment process and the final cost is revealed at the end.

15. Which of the following statements is the most accurate summary of Rocio Concha's views on ticket pricing?

    a. Drip feeding is a deceptive method of charging fans for tickets and it is understandable why music fans may feel conned by this.
    b. Legislation surrounding ticket pricing will change soon to make buying tickets more straightforward for customers.
    c. Keir Starmer's proposed changes to the way in which tickets are sold will be a positive alteration to the current methods.
    d. Concert and live event prices are currently too expensive at face value.

16. Which of the following ticketing companies are described as having the highest processing fee within the text?

    a. Eventim
    b. See Tickets
    c. AXS
    d. Ticketmaster

Question Set 5

Delhi was the most polluted capital city in the world in 2023, a Swiss-based air-quality monitoring group has found. India, of which Delhi is the capital, was also ranked as the world's third-most polluted country after neighbours Bangladesh and Pakistan, IQAir said. The country's air has worsened since 2022, when it was the eighth most polluted country, it added. Air pollution is a serious problem in several Indian cities. Experts say that rapid industrialisation coupled with weak enforcement of environmental laws have played a role in increasing pollution in the country.

India has seen a lot of development in the past few decades, but poor industrial regulation means that factories do not follow pollution-control measures. Rapid construction has also contributed to rising levels of pollution. The report by IQAir said that India's average level of PM2.5 - fine particulate matter that can clog lungs and cause a host of diseases - was 54.4 micrograms per cubic metre.

Globally, air that has 12 to 15 micrograms per cubic metre of PM2.5 is considered safe to breathe, while air with values above 35 micrograms per cubic metre is considered unhealthy. Delhi's air quality was worse than India's overall air quality with the city having a PM2.5 reading of 92.7 micrograms per cubic metre.

Delhi struggles with bad air around the year, but the air gets particularly toxic during winter. This happens due to various factors, including burning of crop remains by farmers in nearby states, industrial and vehicular emissions, low wind speeds and bursting of firecrackers during festivals. Last year, the government shut schools and colleges for several days in a row due to the toxic air. Meanwhile, the northern Indian city of Beguserai and the northeastern city of Guwahati were ranked as the two most polluted cities in the world. Only seven countries met the World Health Organization (WHO)'s annual PM2.5 guideline, which is an annual average of 5 micrograms per cubic metre or less. These include Australia, New Zealand, Iceland and Finland.

Adapted from www.bbc.com.

17. Which of the following is not a reason for worsening air pollution within India?

    a. Poor law enforcement regarding environmental laws affecting pollution levels.
    b. Increasing levels of construction within the country.
    c. Indian factories are breaking national laws surrounding pollution.
    d. Rapid levels of industrialisation within the nation.

18. Which of the following can be inferred from the text?

    a. The air in India is 39.4 micrograms per cubic metre over the safe limit in terms of fine particulate matter.
    b. The majority of people living in India have clogged lungs as a result of the low air quality within the country.
    c. Icelandic and Finnish residents don't suffer from diseases related to polluted air due to their PM2.5 level being extremely low.
    d. The United Kingdom has safe levels of fine particulate matter within the air as the nation has strict pollution laws.

19. Which of the following is not a reason for the worsening of air within Delhi in winter?

    a. Emissions released from vehicular travel.
    b. Decreased levels of wind speeds.
    c. Fires affecting crop remains.
    d. Fireworks being lit during national holidays.

20. Which of the following options is most likely to be the most polluted country in the world, in terms of air quality, according to the text?

    a. Guwahati
    b. India
    c. Beguserai
    d. Bangladesh

Question Set 6

Lithium batteries are very difficult to recycle and require huge amounts of water and energy to produce. Emerging alternatives could be cheaper and greener. In Australia's Yarra Valley, new battery technology is helping power the country's residential buildings and commercial ventures – without using lithium. These batteries rely on sodium – an element found in table salt – and they could be another step in the quest for a truly sustainable battery.

The global demand for batteries is surging as the world looks to rapidly electrify vehicles and store renewable energy. Companies are frantically looking for more sustainable alternatives that can help power the world's transition to green energy. "Sodium is a much more sustainable source for batteries [than lithium]," says James Quinn, chief executive of Faradion, the UK-based battery technology company that manufactures the sodium-ion batteries for Yarra Valley utility company Nation Energie.
"It's widely available around the world, meaning it's cheaper to source, and less water intensive to extract," says Quinn. "It takes 682 times more water to extract one tonne of lithium versus one tonne of sodium. That is a significant amount."

Faradion's sodium-ion batteries are already being used by energy companies around the world to store renewable electricity. And they are just one alternative to our heavy and growing reliance on lithium, which was listed by the European Union as a "critical raw material" in 2020. The market size for the lithium battery is predicted to grow from $57bn (£45bn) in 2023, to $187bn (£150bn) by 2032. To find promising alternatives to lithium batteries, it helps to consider what has made the lithium battery so popular in the first place. Some of the factors that make a good battery are lifespan, power, energy density, safety and affordability. The downsides are also plentiful: at the end of their lifespan, recycling these batteries is still a complicated process. Extracting individual metals in the battery for recycling involves shedding the metal, then separating them in liquid to extract the desired metal. Studies show that contaminants may be released into the environment during the evaporation process, potentially affecting nearby communities.

Adapted from www.bbc.com.

21. Which of the following statements is not a downside of using lithium batteries stated within the text?

   a. Lithium batteries require huge amounts of water in their manufacturing process.
   b. They are expensive to produce.
   c. It is a lengthy process to recycle these batteries.
   d. Recycling lithium batteries can cause environmental pollution.

22. Which of the following statements can be inferred from the text?

   a. Sodium-ion batteries are the most sustainable commercially available battery.
   b. The main component of sodium-ion batteries is salt, making this battery type very environmentally friendly.
   c. Sodium-ion batteries are cheaper to produce than lithium batteries.
   d. Sodium-ion batteries are easy to recycle.

23. Which of the following is not a current use for sodium-ion batteries according to the text?

   a. The storage of renewable electricity.
   b. Acting as an energy source in residential buildings.
   c. Powering electric vehicles, such as cars.
   d. Acting as an energy source for factories.

24. Which of the following is not a positive characteristic of lithium batteries mentioned within the passage?

   a. They are very affordable to produce.
   b. Lithium batteries are very strong and resistant to damage due to their density.
   c. They are safe batteries to use which makes them favourable.
   d. Lithium batteries are powerful.

Question Set 7

Doctors have developed an artificial intelligence tool that can predict which breast cancer patients are more at risk of side-effects after treatment. Worldwide, 2 million women are diagnosed every year with the disease, which is the most common cancer in females in most countries.

Greater awareness, earlier detection and a wider range of treatment options have improved survival rates in recent years, but many patients will experience often debilitating side-effects after treatment. An international team of medics, scientists and researchers have designed an AI tool that can indicate how likely a patient is to experience problems after surgery and radiotherapy. The technology, being trialled in the UK, France and the Netherlands, could help patients access more personalised care.

"That's why we are developing an AI tool to inform doctors and patients about the risk of chronic arm swelling after surgery and radiotherapy for breast cancer. We hope this will assist doctors and patients in choosing options for radiation treatment and reduce side-effects for all patients," said Dr Tim Rattay. "Side effects include skin changes, scarring, lymphoedema, which is a painful swelling of the arm, and even heart damage from radiation treatment."

The AI tool was trained to predict lymphoedema up to three years after surgery and radiotherapy using data from 6,361 breast cancer patients. Patients found to be at a higher risk of arm swelling could be offered alternative treatments or additional support during and after treatments. "Patients identified at higher risk of arm swelling could be offered additional supportive measures, such as wearing an arm compression sleeve during treatment, which has been shown to reduce arm swelling in the long term," said Rattay. "Clinicians may also use this information to discuss options for lymph node irradiation in patients, where its benefit may be fairly borderline."

Adapted from www.theguardian.com.

25. Which of the following statements can be inferred from the passage?

    a. Breast cancer is the most common cancer affecting females within the UK.
    b. Wearing an arm compression sleeve is a treatment offered to all patients at risk of arm swelling.
    c. Arm swelling is a common side effect of receiving treatment for breast cancer.
    d. As the AI tool is being trialled within the UK, the tool will soon be commonplace within NHS hospital settings.

26. Which of the following measures have not improved breast cancer survival rates in recent years?

    a. Prediction of possible side effects of cancer treatment.
    b. An increased variety of treatment options for patients.
    c. Detecting cancer earlier in patients.
    d. Further public awareness of breast cancer.

27. Which of the following statements best describes a common side effect faced by those receiving treatment for breast cancer?

    a. Breast cancer treatment can cause a host of varied side effects.
    b. Wearing an arm compression sleeve can help reduce long term chronic lymphoedema.
    c. Chronic lymphoedema is a form of swelling which can affect the arms after receiving treatment for breast cancer.
    d. The AI tool can predict side effects of treatment for up to three years after it is received.

28. Which of the following is not a side effect of breast cancer treatment, according to the passage?

    a. Chronic arm swelling.
    b. Lymph node irradiation.
    c. Damage to the heart.
    d. Changes to the skin.

Question Set 8

The first flying taxi could take off in the UK by 2026 and become a regular sight in our skies two years later, if a government announcement goes to plan. The Future of Flight action plan, developed with the aerospace industry, also says drones and other flying vehicles will become more autonomous. It predicts that the first pilotless flying taxi will take off in 2030. But experts say hurdles such as infrastructure and public acceptance need to be overcome first. There are a number of different models, but most flying taxis look like a futuristic helicopter and can usually carry about five people.

They are part of a family of vehicles called "eVTOLs" - which stands for electric vertical take-off and landing aircraft. The technology for them exists now, but it is likely that the aircraft will start off as exclusive modes of transport - replacing expensive journeys currently done by helicopters. The Department for Transport also plans to allow drones to fly beyond visual line of sight - meaning the person controlling the drone cannot see it in the air. Some of the uses of unmanned drones include transporting medical supplies, delivering post in rural areas and tracking down criminals on the run. Their use is still in early stages, but the plan suggests drone deliveries would be commonplace by 2027.

The biggest obstacles to getting flying taxis into the air are infrastructure and public perception, says Craig Roberts, head of drones, at consultancy firm PwC. Last year, he co-authored a report on the topic, in collaboration with the government, on the viability of the technology. "It's challenging, but possible," he says of the 2026 target. Mr Roberts thinks that the most efficient use of the technology is in "longer distance, higher occupancy cases".

Adapted from www.bbc.com.

29. Which of the following statements are true, based upon the passage?

    a. Pilotless flying taxis may exist in the UK by 2026.
    b. Funding is a key issue to overcome to enable flying taxis to operate.
    c. Most flying taxis will be similar in appearance to helicopters, rather than cars.
    d. eVTOLs is an acronym which stands for 'electric vehicle take-off and landing aircraft.'

30. Which of the following is a clear barrier to the introduction of flying taxis, as explained within the passage?

    a. Flying vehicles are generally used for long haul journeys as opposed to shorter ones.
    b. Only five people can be carried in most flying taxis.
    c. Unmanned drones will only be used in rural areas.
    d. The current public perception of flying taxis is not ideal.

31. Which of the following statements are untrue regarding the introduction of flying taxis?

    a. The technology will be challenging to introduce into British society.
    b. Longer journeys, carrying larger numbers of people would most likely be the best use of flying taxi technology.
    c. Pilotless taxis will fly beyond the visual line of sight.
    d. The current infrastructure within the UK is unsuitable for introducing flying taxis.

32. Which of the following is not a potential use of unmanned drones?

    a. Transportation of medical supplies.
    b. Replacing expensive journeys made usually by helicopters.
    c. Replacing services usually carried out by postmen and women.
    d. Aiding the police with identifying criminals.

Question Set 9

Companies selling super green supplements claim a scoop of their magic powder, mixed with water, is all you need to improve your health. Many promise a long list of potential benefits, such as stronger hair and nails, increased energy and decreased bloating. The clean, often green packaging advertises a list of ingredients such as pre and probiotics, antioxidants and vitamins.

Rheal Superfoods, which was featured on BBC programme Dragon's Den in 2021, claims its daily super greens blend supports digestive health, immune system and "overall wellness from within". Free Soul's FS Greens blend also makes similar claims, promising to offer digestion and immunity support through key ingredients such as ashwagandha, golden kiwi and maca.

Miss Hill says she feels that these products, which count as ultra-processed because they have a complicated manufacturing process, "are playing on our health anxieties".
She says from her experience as a dietitian that "younger generations are becoming increasingly health-conscious" but is concerned "people are being misled into spending money for a perceived health benefit that's not really there".

Miss Hill says that while these supplements may not have the science behind them to back up their claims, "they're not harmful, so people can try them if they want to".

There is also another aspect that Ms Hope considers, that "for some people, they can put you in a healthy mindset". Ms Hope also considers that for people who are perhaps time-poor, there might be a benefit. "There really isn't a one size fits all - if you take an individual with a highly stressful job, this could help them get closer to an adequate amount of nutrients," she adds. She says they can also help people with dietary restrictions that prevent them from consuming some types of fruit and vegetables.

Adapted from www.bbc.com.

33. Which of the following is not a believed benefit of green supplements mentioned in the text?

   a. Strengthening nails and hair.
   b. Improving digestive conditions.
   c. Increasing energy levels.
   d. Decreasing gas bloat.

34. Which of the following can be inferred from the passage?

   a. Super green supplements can be harmful in large quantities.
   b. These supplements can help you achieve your required vitamin needs when taken on a daily basis.
   c. These supplements are intended for those with some dietary restrictions.
   d. There hasn't been much research into the effects of these green supplements.

35. Which of the following statements is a statement that Miss Hill would likely agree with, based upon the text?

   a. People are likely to buy these green supplements as they are being deceived into believing that they will drastically improve their health.
   b. Having a multivitamin daily is a great alternative to these supplements.
   c. Younger generations are more anxious nowadays.
   d. Ultra-processed foods are always unhealthy.

36. Which of the following statements sum up Ms Hope's views on the green supplements mentioned in the passage?

   a. All individuals with stressful jobs should include these supplements in their diet.
   b. These supplements do not have any scientific grounding and should therefore be avoided.
   c. Green supplements may be beneficial for some individuals who struggle to attain the correct nutritional levels.
   d. The most important feature of these supplements is the ability to reduce bloating.

Question Set 10

Scotland has become the 'worst country in Europe' for unqualified beauticians injecting customers with cosmetic treatments, healthcare professionals have warned. They said people in the UK are coming to harm because there is no legislation to prevent anyone advertising on social media offering beauty treatments such as dermal fillers. And in Scotland there is no also ban on under-18s receiving these treatments. The British Association of Cosmetic Nurses (BACN) said most other countries have regulations that only allow trained health professionals to carry out procedures.

Tens of thousands of people now get dermal filler treatment across Scotland each year. It is usually an injection into the face which helps to fill wrinkles and add volume to tissue. But as its popularity increases so do the complications which include the risk of infection, blocked arteries, necrosis, blindness and stroke.

Ms Partridge said social media had become a "catalyst" for people falling into unsafe hands. She said the rise of social media as an advertising platform had led to more procedures, with "absolutely no regard for patient safety or accountability". Ms Partridge also said there had been a surge in "unlicensed, counterfeit and unsafe" products being passed off as botulinum toxin (Botox) in the non-medical sector.

Botox injections are anti-wrinkle treatments used to relax the muscles predominantly in the forehead, between the eyebrows and around the eyes, that last between three and six months. Botox is classed as a prescription-only medicine in the UK, meaning it can only be prescribed and given to a patient by a qualified medical professional. However, doctors and nurses say beauticians are finding unlicensed Botox online and injecting patients in high street salons and in their homes. They say there is no way to know what is actually inside these products and little enforcement action to stop them.

Adapted from www.bbc.com.

37. No current legislation exists in the United Kingdom to regulate the administration and distribution of Botox.

    a. True
    b. False
    c. Can't Tell

38. Dermal filler is the most commonly injected beauty treatment in Scotland.

    a. True
    b. False
    c. Can't Tell

39. Complications related to Botox injections can be fatal. (True, False, Can't Tell)

    a. True
    b. False
    c. Can't Tell

40. Ms Partridge would likely support the introduction of legislation which further regulates the administration of Botox injections.

    a. True
    b. False
    c. Can't Tell

Question Set 11

When Lisa Melrose's daughter Evie fell ill in October 2022, it was like no illness the mum-of-three had ever seen. Calpol and Nurofen were having no effect and the six-year-old was displaying worrying symptoms. Lisa said: "I'd never seen a child hallucinate before or become sort of listless and so incredibly lethargic. "We've been through sickness bugs, tonsillitis and broken bones but none of these compared with what happened with Evie. "It was very frightening."

Evie, from Dundee, was diagnosed with Strep A - a bacteria that can cause a variety of illnesses. Symptoms include nausea and vomiting, a rash, sore throat and flu-like symptoms. Scientists at Dundee University are now leading a £2.3m project to develop the world's first vaccine for Strep A. At the time Evie fell ill, the UK was in the grip of an outbreak which claimed the lives of dozens of children - including three in Scotland.

After she was diagnosed, Evie was prescribed antibiotics and took a few days to recover. Her mum Lisa works as a baby sensory teacher, with 200 youngsters across her classes. She found that her experience was a common one. She said: "I asked each class to put their hands up if they had had experience of a baby or a young child in their house who had had Strep A. "I had 35 parents or carers say they'd had that within their household. "Their little ones were very ill and some ended up having to go to out-of-hours or hospital."

Dr Helge Dorfmueller is leading the Dundee University collaboration. He said it was "very challenging" to find a vaccine that protected patients from outbreaks in different countries because they could involve very different bacteria. But he said the project was identifying "key components of vaccine development" which could make it successful.

Adapted from www.bbc.com.

41. Which of the following can be inferred from the passage?

    a. Evie has never had a broken bone.
    b. Strep A is not a common infection which is the reason for the absence of a vaccine.
    c. Calpol is not recommended to alleviate symptoms of a Strep A infection.
    d. Strep A can be a fatal infection.

42. Which of the following cannot be reasonably inferred from the passage?

    a. Strep A infections can cause children to hallucinate.
    b. Antibiotics are used to treat Strep A infections.
    c. Children are more susceptible to becoming infected with Strep A.
    d. Over 10% of parents and carers of children from Lisa's classes know of people who have been infected with Strep A.

43. Which of the following is not a symptom of Strep A infections, according to the text?

    a. A rash.
    b. Sickness and diarrhoea.
    c. Unusual hallucinations.
    d. Sore throats.

44. Which of the following statements accurately summarise Dr Dorfmueller's opinion regarding the Strep A vaccine?

    a. A Strep A vaccine would be very time consuming and costly to engineer.
    b. Finding a singular vaccine to suit a global population is likely difficult.
    c. Key components of vaccine development include identifying Strep A bacteria in patients.
    d. Dundee University has its own dedicated vaccine development hub.

Answers: Verbal Reasoning Mock

Question Set 1

Question 1: C

Statement C is correct as the passage discusses how Gucci's sales have been declining recently partly due to struggles within the Chinese economy, a country where Gucci usually receives a third of their sales.

Statement A is incorrect as the text does not describe the decline in sales as being due to competition from Bottega Veneta and Balenciaga. The text only mentions that the owner of Gucci also owns these other brands.

Statement B is incorrect as the passage states that Gucci have a younger target market which could be contributing to their decline in sales, not an older target market.

Statement D is incorrect as there is no mention of a change of ownership within the text.

Question 2: C

Answer C is correct because Yves Saint Laurent is owned by Kering, who also owns the brand Gucci.

Answers A, B and D are all under ownership by the company LVMH.

Question 3: D

Statement D can be inferred from the passage as the net profit of Kering fell by 17% last year, which is less than 1/5. This is because 1/5 is equal to 20%, and 17% is a lesser figure than this.

Statement A cannot be inferred from the passage as the text states that sales are expected to fall by 20%, whereas 1/3 is equal to 33.3%.

Statement B cannot be inferred from the passage. Although the text states that Hermès plans to reward its employees with a bonus, there is no mention of Gucci not giving out any bonuses.

Statement C cannot be inferred as there are no descriptions in the text specifically stating that Hermès has a higher net worth than Gucci, despite the fact that Hermès sales have been steadier recently.

Question 4: D

Statement D is true, as the text states that the financial results of Kering will be published in April, which is the fourth month of the year.

Statement A is false, as LMVH is described as one of Kering's 'bigger' rivals, but not necessarily the biggest.

Statement B is false, as Jean-François Palus was recently appointed as the company's CEO, and not their creative director.

Statement C cannot be inferred from the passage, as the release of the Ancora collection was described as having a "highly favourable reception". This therefore implies that the collection was probably profitable, rather than the opposite.

Question Set 2

Question 5: C

This is because the article only describes this new policy being set out in NHS England and does not clarify whether this policy will be implemented in other countries within the United Kingdom.

Question 6: B

The article explains that the GnRH is released from the hypothalamus which then triggers the release of follicle-stimulating hormone from the pituitary gland, not the hypothalamus.

Question 7: C

Although the passage states that triptorelin is prescribed for cases of precocious puberty which is explained as affecting more girls than boys, we do not know explicitly if triptorelin is prescribed more to females. Therefore, the answer is C) Can't tell.

Question 8: B

This is because Andrew Schally and Roger Guillemin won the Nobel prize through their research dissecting pig and lamb brains, not human brains.

Examiner's Tip: In most instances, the answers to True, False, Can't tell question types are false or can't tell, as opposed to true. However, there are sometimes exceptions to the rule, so do not assume this is always the case. Instead, just attempt to rule out true firstly to try and work through the questions quickly.

Question Set 3

Question 9: C

Although the passage states that certain health issues are associated with the microwaving of food, cancer is not mentioned within the passage, meaning Statement C is the correct answer.

Statement A is a concern mentioned within the text as nutrient loss is listed as a concern within the first paragraph.

Statement B is a concern also mentioned within the first paragraph.

Statement D is a concern which is listed within the third paragraph.

Question 10: D

The passage reveals that microwaved meals preserved slightly more vitamin C than those cooked in an oven within a certain experiment but does not mention the effect of boiling food on vitamin C levels specifically. Therefore, **Statement D** is the correct answer for this question.

Statement A can be inferred from the passage as the text states that 97% of flavonoids are removed from food by microwaving, meaning 3% of these remain.

Statement B can be inferred from the passage as the text reveals that boiling broccoli preserves a third more flavonoids than microwaving, in paragraph two.

Statement C can be inferred from the passage as the definition of flavonoids are described as "plant compounds with anti-inflammatory benefits" in the second paragraph.

Question 11: B

Statement B is untrue as phthalates improve the flexibility of plastic, as opposed to the strength.

Statement A is true, as phthalates are commonly found with takeaway containers as described in paragraph four.

Statement C is true as paragraph three mentions that phthalates can leach into food above 100C.

Statement D is true as paragraph three states that phthalates can disrupt hormones.

Top Tip: For type 1 questions, read the first two sentences of the passage and then identify a keyword within the question stem. For this question, the best keyword to pick would be 'phthalates.' Locate this within the passage, read the sentence surrounding the keyword, and then work through each of the statements to find the correct answer.

Question 12: B

Hypertension, not hypotension, is listed as being linked to phthalate exposure in paragraph four. Therefore, B is the correct answer.

Answers A, C and D are all listed as being linked to phthalate exposure within the final paragraph and are therefore not the correct answers to this question.

Question Set 4

Question 13: B

Statement B is likely to be one that Keir Starmer agrees with, as he explained that he will attempt to change the current laws around unfair ticket sales if he is to win the next general election. This implies that he does not agree with the current drip pricing methods imposed by ticket companies.

Statement A is incorrect as Starmer wants to change the way tickets are resold, implying he doesn't believe the current strategies are fair.

Statement C is incorrect as Starmer does not allude to the variety of ticketing sites available in the text.

Statement D is incorrect as Keir Starmer wishes to tighten regulations around ticket sales.

Question 14: D

Statement D is correct as the text states that drip pricing is when "Ticket sites often include some fees in the upfront price, and mention that other charges will be added, but the final price is often not revealed until later in the checkout process".

Statement A, B and C are incorrect as they are not an accurate summary of drip pricing.

Question 15: A

Statement A most accurately summarises how Rocio Concha feels about the current way in which tickets for events are sold. They state in the text that drip feeding tactics are "sneaky" and that is understandable why customers feel like they are being taken advantage of.

Statement B is incorrect. Although the text states that 'Which?' believes that upcoming legislation will give customers more clarity, Concha does not allude to this specific statement themselves.

Statement C is incorrect as Rocio does not make any reference to their views on Keir Starmer's proposed laws.

Statement D is incorrect as Rocio doesn't describe any issue they have with the *face value* of tickets, only the way in which tickets are drip priced.

Question 16: D

The reason D is the correct answer is because the text explains that Ticketmaster charges £2.75 as an order processing fee.

A is the incorrect answer as they charge £1.50 in order processing fees.

B and C are incorrect as their order processing charges are not stated within the text.

Question Set 5

Question 17: C

Answer C is not a reason for worsening air pollution in India. Although the text mentions that factories are not following pollution control measures, this is not because they are breaking laws. It is instead because there is a lack of industrial regulation regarding the levels of pollution factories can emit.

Answer A is a reason for increased Indian pollution as stated in paragraph one; "weak enforcement of environmental laws have played a role in increasing pollution in the country". Increased construction is listed in paragraph two as being a reason for increased pollution so Answer B is also correct.

Answer D (industrialisation) is listed in paragraph one as a reason for increased levels of pollution.

Question 18: A

Statement A is correct as the PM2.5 in India on average is 54.4, which is 39.4 micrograms higher than the safe level of 15 micrograms.

Statement B is incorrect as the text does not state the levels of those suffering with health conditions in India related to air pollution.

Statement C is incorrect as the passage doesn't elaborate on the health of Icelandic and Finnish people. The text only describes the low levels of air pollution found within the country.

Statement D is incorrect as the United Kingdom is not mentioned within the text.

Question 19: D

Firecrackers being lit during festivals, not fireworks on national holidays are a reason for air pollution in Delhi and therefore the correct answer is D.

Emissions from vehicles, decreased wind speeds and crop fires are all reasons for worsened air pollution in winter which are described in paragraph four and therefore answers A, B and C are incorrect.

Question 20: D

The text lists Pakistan and Bangladesh as being the most polluted countries in the world, with India being the third most polluted, meaning the answer must be Pakistan or Bangladesh. Pakistan is not an answer option, so therefore, the answer is D.

Option A and C are cities which are listed in the text meaning these answers must be incorrect, as the question asks for a <u>country</u>.

Option B is incorrect as the text explains that India is the third most polluted country globally in terms of air quality.

Question Set 6

Question 21: B

Statement B is not a downside of lithium battery usage as the final paragraph states that they are affordable.

Statement A is the incorrect answer as it is stated multiple times in the text that large amounts of water usage is a massive downside of manufacturing lithium batteries.

Statement C is incorrect as the first and final paragraph discuss the issues surrounding the lengthy recycling process.

Statement D is incorrect as the final sentence in the text explains how lithium battery recycling can pollute the environment.

Question 22: C

The reason that Statement C is correct is because paragraph two discusses the advantages sodium batteries have over lithium batteries. One of the advantages stated is the wide availability of the sodium battery which makes it cheaper to source than lithium batteries.

Statement A is incorrect. Although the text states that sodium-ion batteries are more sustainable than the lithium alternative, it does not say whether they are the <u>most</u> sustainable. The text also does not mention whether they are commercially available. Therefore, this statement is incorrect.

Statement B is incorrect as the text doesn't explain what the composition of sodium-ion batteries are, meaning we cannot infer this.

Statement D is incorrect as there is no reference to the recycling process for sodium-ion batteries within the text.

Question 23: D

The usage of sodium-ion batteries within a factory setting is not discussed within the text, so D is the correct answer to this question.

Answer A is a use of sodium batteries discussed within the final paragraph.
Answer B is a use of sodium batteries which is discussed within the first paragraph.
Answer C is a use of sodium-ion batteries which is stated in paragraph two.

Question 24: B

Answer B is correct. This is because the text states that lithium batteries are energy dense, not physically dense meaning their strength is not a positive characteristic mentioned.

Answer A, C and D are incorrect as their affordability, safety and powerful nature are mentioned as positive characteristics of lithium batteries in the final paragraph.

Question Set 7

Question 25: C

Statement C is correct as the passage explains that "patients will experience often debilitating side-effects after treatment". Because the AI tool focuses mostly on predicting the instance of lymphoedema occurring in patients receiving therapy for breast cancer, we can safely assume that arm swelling is a common side effect.

Statement A is incorrect as we cannot be sure that breast cancer is the most common cancer affecting females within the UK, as the passage only states that it is the most common cancer in females in most countries, not specifically the UK.

Statement B is incorrect as the passage states that patients could be offered this supportive measure if they are at higher risk, but the text does not mention whether this is given to all patients.

Statement D is incorrect as the passage does not mention if the tool will be launched within NHS hospitals, only that the tool is "being trialled in the UK".

Question 26: A

Answer A is the correct answer as the text does not state whether the prediction of treatment related side effects have specifically improved survival rates. The text only suggests that this new AI technology has the potential to "help patients access more personalised care," rather than improve survival rates.

Answer B, C and D are the incorrect answers to this question as the text states in passage two that "Greater awareness, earlier detection and a wider range of treatment options have improved survival rates in recent years."

Question 27: C

Statement C correctly describes the side effect described in detail within the passage, as the text states that a common side effect is lymphoedema, which is a form of "chronic arm swelling after surgery."

Statements A, B and D are incorrect as they do not correctly define the side effect of cancer treatment explained within the passage, despite the content of the statements being correct.

Question 28: B

Answer B is correct as lymph node irradiation is a form of treatment for cancer as described in the final passage, and not a side effect.

Answers A, C and D are not correct as Dr Tim Rattay explains within the passage that "Side effects," (of breast cancer treatment) "include skin changes, scarring, lymphoedema, which is a painful swelling of the arm, and even heart damage from radiation treatment."

Question Set 8

Question 29: C

Statement C correctly summarises a sentence in the first paragraph which states, "most flying taxis look like a futuristic helicopter."

Statement A is a false statement as the text explains that "the first pilotless flying taxi will take off in 2030," as opposed to 2026. Although the first sentence states that the first flying taxi could take off by 2026, this does not specify that it would be pilotless.

Statement B is incorrect as there are no issues with the funding of this project mentioned within the text.

Statement D is also incorrect as eVOTLs stands for "electric vertical take-off and landing aircraft," rather than electric vehicle.

Top Tip: Type 2 questions do not have a specific keyword to look for in their question stem. They instead have a generalised question which requires you to read each statement individually. For these questions, it is helpful to identify keywords in each statement and then locate these within the passage. For example, the best keyword to select for statement C would be 'helicopters'. Once this word is located within the text, you can read around it and then identify it as the correct answer.

Question 30: D

Answer D is correct as the text states that "hurdles such as infrastructure and public acceptance need to be overcome first," implying that public perception of these taxis are less than ideal currently.

Answer A is incorrect as the passage does not describe any barrier related to journey time of the taxis, except for the fact that it will probably be more <u>efficient</u> to take longer journeys which is not necessarily a <u>barrier</u>.

Answer B is incorrect as the number of people carried within the taxis is not explained as an issue.

Answer C is incorrect as the question does not ask about unmanned drones.

Question 31: C

Statement C is the untrue statement as the passage explains that <u>unmanned drones</u> will be able to "fly beyond visual line of sight," rather than <u>pilotless taxis.</u>
Statement A is true as Mr Roberts states within the passage that "It's challenging, but possible," to introduce flying taxis.

Statement B is true as the passage states that "the most efficient use of the technology is in "longer distance, higher occupancy cases"."

Statement D is also true as one of the key issues identified with introducing flying taxis is the lack of infrastructure currently to support this project.

Question 32: B

Answer B is not a potential use of unmanned drones, it is instead a potential use of flying helicopters.

Answers A, C and D are potential uses of unmanned drones as the passage states that "uses of unmanned drones include transporting medical supplies, delivering post in rural areas and tracking down criminals on the run."

Question Set 9

Question 33: B

Although the text mentions that these supplements can "support digestive health," the passage does not elaborate on whether they can actually improve digestive health conditions, so **Answer B** is therefore not a believed benefit of these supplements.

Answers A, C and D are correct as the text states that "Many," (supplements) "promise a long list of potential benefits, such as stronger hair and nails, increased energy and decreased bloating."

Question 34: D

Answer D can be inferred from the passage as Miss Hill states that "these supplements may not have the science behind them to back up their claims," implying that these supplements have not been heavily researched.

Answer A cannot be inferred from the passage as there is no information in the passage regarding which quantities the supplement can be harmful, other than the fact that a 'scoop' of the supplement is recommended.

Answer B cannot be inferred from the passage as the passage states that "this could help them get closer to an adequate amount of nutrients," implying that you cannot achieve an adequate level of nutrition from these supplements alone.

Answer C cannot be inferred as the text does not mention who the target audience for these supplements are.

Question 35: A

Statement A correctly summarises her views upon these green supplements, as she states that "people are being misled into spending money for a perceived health benefit that's not really there."

Statement B is incorrect as Miss Hill does not make reference to multivitamins within the text.

Statement C is incorrect as she states that (these products) "are playing on our health anxieties." She does not specifically refer to young peoples' anxiety levels within the text.

Statement D is incorrect as Miss Hill only explains that these products are ultra-processed, not that ultra-processed products are "always unhealthy."

Question 36: C

Statement C accurately sums up Ms Hope's views on these supplements, as she states in the passage that "this could help them," (those with stressful jobs) "get closer to an adequate amount of nutrients," and that "they can also help people with dietary restrictions."

Statement A is incorrect as Ms Hope only suggests that some people with high stress jobs may benefit from these supplements, not all people in this category.

Statement B is incorrect as it is Miss Hill that states that "these supplements may not have the science behind them to back up their claims,", not Ms Hope.

Statement D is incorrect as Ms Hope makes no reference to the decreased bloating levels attributed to these supplements.

Question Set 10

Question 37: B

Although the passage states that there is no legislation to ban under-18s from receiving these treatments, or to prevent the advertisement of these treatments on social media, the passage states that "Botox is classed as a prescription-only medicine in the UK," meaning there is existing legislation regulating the distribution of Botox.

Question 38: C

We cannot tell whether dermal filler is the most popular of this treatment type, despite the passage stating that "Tens of thousands of people now get dermal filler treatment across Scotland each year." Therefore, C is the correct answer.

Question 39: C

Although the text states that "complications include the risk of infection, blocked arteries, necrosis, blindness and stroke," we cannot infer that these complications may lead to death from this statement alone, so the answer is C.

Question 40: A

This is because she states in the text that "social media had become a "catalyst" for people falling into unsafe hands.", referring to the ease of accessibility to these injections. This therefore infers that she would support tightened regulations for Botox administration.

Question Set 11

Question 41: D

Answer D is correct because the text states that "an outbreak" (of Strep A) "claimed the lives of dozens of children - including three in Scotland," implying that the condition can be fatal.

Answer A is incorrect as the text doesn't specifically state which of Lisa's children had suffered with broken bones, meaning Evie could have potentially had a broken bone in the past.

Answer B is incorrect as the passage does not state the specific reason for the absence of a Strep A vaccine.

Answer C is incorrect as there is no guidance within the passage which recommends against using Calpol for a Strep A infection, despite the fact that this medicine had "no effect" on Evie's condition.

Question 42: C

We cannot reasonably infer that children are more susceptible to becoming infected with Strep A, as there is no specific evidence to support this statement within the passage. Therefore, the correct answer to question two is C.

Answer A is incorrect as the passage states that "I'd never seen a child hallucinate" which implies that the infection can cause children to hallucinate.

Answer B is incorrect as the passage states that "Evie was prescribed antibiotics" after she was diagnosed.

Answer D is incorrect as the passage states that 35 out of 200 from Lisa's classes know of people who have been infected, which is over 10% of 200 (which is 20).

Question 43: B

This is because the text states that "Symptoms include nausea and vomiting, a rash, sore throat and flu-like symptoms." This therefore does not include sickness and diarrhoea, meaning B is the correct answer and answers A, C and D are incorrect.

Question 44: B

This is because Dr Dorfmueller states in the passage that "it was "very challenging" to find a vaccine that protected patients from outbreaks in different countries because they could involve very different bacteria."

Statement A is incorrect as Dr Dorfmueller does not mention any constraints related to time or cost impacting vaccine development.

Statement C is incorrect as he does not mention what the key components of vaccine development are in the passage.

Statement D is incorrect as the doctor doesn't allude to the University having its own vaccine development hub.

1:1 UCAT TUTORING

 Delivered by UCAT experts, who scored in the top 10% of the exam

 A personalised 1:1 approach, tailored to your unique needs

 Proven success, with Medic Mind students achieving an average score of 2810 (top 10% nationally)

Book your FREE consultation now

Visit the link or scan the QR code below for more information:
www.medicmind.co.uk/ucat-tutoring

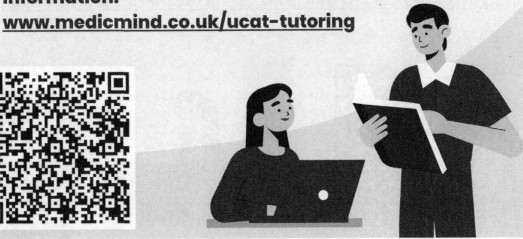

UCAT ONLINE COURSE

 100+ tutorials, designed by our UCAT experts, to guide you through every section of the exam

 Access to our UCAT Question Bank, with 8,000+ practice questions to use in your revision

 Invites to regular UCAT webinars, live classes and interactive sessions

Buy Now!

Visit the link or scan the QR code below for more information:
https://www.medicmind.co.uk/ucat-online-course/

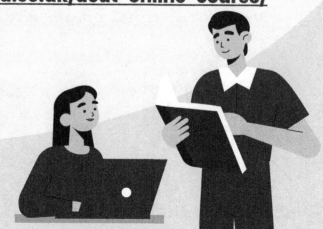

1:1 MEDICINE INTERVIEW TUTORING

 Delivered by Medicine Interview experts, who scored in the top 10% of the exam

 A personalised 1:1 approach, tailored to your unique needs

 Proven success, with Medic Mind students acing their Medicine Interview.

Book your FREE consultation now

**Visit the link or scan the QR code below for more information:
www.medicmind.co.uk/interview-tutoring/**

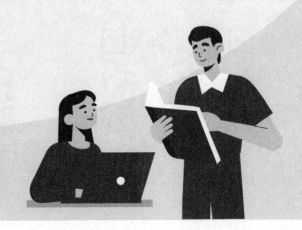

MEDICINE INTERVIEW ONLINE COURSE

 100+ tutorials, and 200+ MMI stations , designed by our Medicine interview experts

 Learn how to answer questions on motivation for Medicine, personal skills, work experience, hot topics, and more

 A range of packages available, including a live day of teaching and 1:1 tutoring

Buy Now!

Visit the link or scan the QR code below for more information:
www.medicmind.co.uk/interview-online-course/

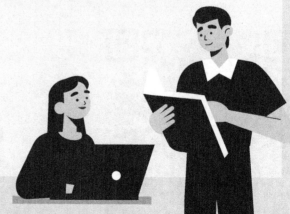

Decision Making

Decision Making Tips

Decision making is the newest section of the UCAT. It was introduced in 2017 to replace an older similarly named section called "decision analysis". The skills tested remain broadly the same, but the question style and timings have changed. This section outlines 10 keys tips for overcoming this challenging and acing this section for UCAT success.

1. Decision making technique is key

The decision making question format can seem complicated. However by systemically applying specific techniques to each question type, you can break the section down into something more manageable. Decision making has a large number of different question types including syllogisms, probability and Venn diagram questions among others. Make sure you have nailed your technique for each of these question types so that you have a set procedure to follow.

For example, syllogism questions can seem like a jumble of confusing words at first. We recommend using a Venn diagram technique to visualise the statements and produce a clear diagram from which you can confidently select the correct answer.

2. Balance decision making question types

There are six different question types in this UCAT section. Therefore, it is important that you have spent time practising each type. Each question type has different techniques and also timing tips linked to them. You need to have spent time on each one to learn these.

- Syllogisms
  You are given two or more statements and have to use logical reasoning to decide what conclusions follow. You will be given 5 conclusions to evaluate.
- Venn Diagrams
  You may be presented with a set of statements or a set of different Venn diagrams as response options.
- Probabilistic Reasoning
  Select best possible response for a question relating to probability.
- Logical Puzzles
  Given a series of statements and facts and need to infer information from this.
- Interpreting Information
  Find which conclusion best follows an argument.
- Recognising Assumptions
  Tests your ability to evaluate how strong an argument is in support for or against a solution to a particular problem.

Decision making is one of the least time pressured subsections; however, timing is still tight! Some question types will tend to take longer than others. By practising each question you will get a feel of how long you should be spending on each type in order to complete the section in a good amount of time.

This also means that there will be no surprises on test day. If you find a particular question type you struggle with you can dedicate time to practising it.

3. Make note of your mistakes

When practising UCAT decision making, make sure to compile a list of all the different question types you encounter. Not only will this allow you to make sure you have covered each type equally, but as you go through you can tally how many times you make mistakes on each question type.

UCAT decision-making has many sub-topics and this is a useful way to begin to structure your revision. It allows you to identify and focus on your weaker areas. Remember not to neglect the questions you find particularly hard as this is the area you can work to improve!

4. Practise Venn diagrams

Venn diagrams are an important part of UCAT decision-making. They are key for both the syllogism and Venn diagram question types. Practising drawing them will get you used to how they work and make sure you can confidently apply them to these two different question types.

When it comes to the test day, even though it might require more time initially, it will mean that you can come to conclusions about the syllogism statements quickly and accurately. Be sure to keep an eye on the clock when practising as you need to have a rough idea of how long it is taking you so as not to run out of time.

5. Avoid making assumptions

Don't infer or fill in gaps with your own personal knowledge for interpreting information questions. Ensure the conclusion you pick is only based on what the text has given you versus what you personally assume. If it isn't explicitly stated in the text given, then don't factor that into your final conclusion.

6. Read the question slowly

Avoid rushing through the question and just picking out keywords as you may do in other UCAT sections. In Decision Making often words such as "must" and "or" are used in the question, which you may miss if you read too fast. So take your time to ensure your pick the right answer.

7. Organise your thoughts on paper

In Decision Making questions, you will often be given a lot of information with many things mentioned e.g names, colours, places. Trying to sort out all these pieces of information in your head can be quite overwhelming and make it easy to forgot key pieces of information. You have time in this section to organise your thoughts on paper to ensure that you can get to the right answer. Ensure you write your thought process out neatly so you follow it easily so you can check your work.

8. Ensure to be strict with timing

Decision making requires you to move through the questions at a rate of about one question per minute. This may seem generous compared to the other sections, but it is very easy to fall into the trap of getting caught up in a question. You have 29 questions that need to be answered in 31 minutes so keep an eye on the clock when answering questions.

Some of the questions are interesting and trying to figure your way through the problems can be quite satisfying. But be careful; this can result in you wasting too much time on one question and may prevent you from finishing. In fact, some of the logical puzzles are designed to be unsolvable on purpose! This has been done to penalise students who spend longer trying to solve the complete puzzle, even after they've worked out the correct answer to the statement. So overall, it is critical to be strict with yourself during this section.

9. Spatial equations

Spatial equations are another question type that can be simplified. If you treat each shape as a letter it will allow you to work out and solve this type of questions much more efficiently. Think about some of the basic algebra manipulation you learnt at secondary school and how you might apply this to work out some unknown values in the statements. You can then utilise the time saved on this question type on some of the more complex time consuming ones.

10. Try not to flag too much

While it is important not to get caught up on tricky questions and to move on when you get stuck, it is also important not to leave any questions unanswered when you flag them. Remember that the UCAT is not negatively marked so there is no harm in guessing if you don't know the answer.

Decision Making is one scenario per question, unlike Verbal Reasoning for example where a set of multiple questions will all relate to the same passage. Therefore, it is quite difficult to come back at the end and re-accustom yourself with the question. So, try to answer the question once and for all when you're actually doing it.

Decision Making Mock

Question 1

Antioxidant supplements, often referred to as "free-radical scavengers," were originally developed to support general health and wellbeing. These supplements are now widely marketed, claiming to combat ageing and enhance physical endurance. Yet, this trend has sparked a debate regarding self-prescribing without a thorough understanding of the potential risks and benefits. Notably, while professionals exposed to high oxidative stress, such as athletes or firefighters, might find theoretical justification for their use, the widespread adoption by the general population, including many teenagers, is harder to support.

Place "Yes" if the conclusion does follow. Place "No" if the conclusion does not follow.

    a. No antioxidant supplement companies recommend consulting a healthcare provider before use.
    b. Firefighters are regularly taking antioxidant supplements to improve their performance.
    c. Antioxidant supplements were not originally produced to enhance physical endurance.
    d. The passage suggests that teenagers may not have a solid justification for using antioxidant supplements regularly.
    e. The main concern regarding the use of antioxidant supplements is their potential to disrupt natural metabolic processes.

Question 2

Samantha gathered some data indicating which fruits 210 people preferred eating during summer.

- *60 people did not prefer any of the fruits listed but the rest preferred at least one of the fruits: apples, bananas, or oranges*
- *55 people preferred only bananas*
- *40 people preferred only oranges*
- *35 people preferred both apples and oranges, and of these 15 had a preference for all three fruits*
- *80 people preferred apples*
- *55 people preferred bananas*
- *75 people preferred oranges*

How many people preferred apples but not bananas or oranges?
    a. 5
    b. 10
    c. 25
    d. 35

Question 3

At a company team-building event, all employees who participated in the treasure hunt also took part in the rock-climbing activity. All participants at the event were employees from the downtown office. No employee enjoyed the vegan wraps. Several employees enjoyed the paddle boarding, while all the participants liked the team quiz.

Place "Yes" if the conclusion does follow. Place "No" if the conclusion does not follow.

a. All the employees from the downtown office were present at the team building event.
b. All the employees at the event enjoyed the team quiz.
c. If the employees from the sales department enjoyed the yoga session, then they were present at the event.
d. All the employees at the event who enjoyed the team quiz also participated in the treasure hunt.
e. The employees at the event who participated in the treasure hunt also enjoyed paddle boarding.

Question 4

At a book club meeting, four avid readers (Ethan, Sarah, Daniel, and Rachel) discuss their favourite genres. Each person has two top genres out of Science Fiction, Romance, Mystery, and Historical Fiction. The readers hail from Canada, Australia, Ireland, and the UK (not in any particular order).

The reader from Canada chose Mystery
Historical Fiction receives 3 votes and Romance received 1 vote
The reader from the UK and Ethan are fans of Science Fiction
The two genres chosen by Sarah did not receive any votes from Daniel and the reader from Ireland
All readers chose Historical Fiction except for the reader from Australia

Who is from Ireland?
a. Ethan
b. Sarah
c. Daniel
d. Rachel

Question 5

In a garden, some flowers are roses. All roses have thorns. Most flowers with thorns are either perennials or have red petals.

Place "Yes" if the conclusion does follow. Place "No" if the conclusion does not follow.

a. All roses are either perennials or have red petals
b. Most perennial flowers are roses
c. Thorned flowers are always roses
d. Some flowers have thorns and are not perennials
e. All flowers have thorns

Question 6

In a small village, all the main roads are lit by streetlights, but these street lights only operate on weekdays. Emily and James both have electric cars that they can charge at the village's single charging station. The charging station operates 24 hours a day but is not powered by streetlight electricity. Emily charges her car on weekdays only, and James charges his car on days when the streetlights are not operating. Emily is only out of the village on weekends, while James never leaves the village.

Place "Yes" if the conclusion does follow. Place "No" if the conclusion does not follow.

   a.   James charges his car whilst Emily is out of the village.
   b.   James does his grocery shopping in the village during the night.
   c.   When Emily is charging her car, the streetlights are on.
   d.   Emily and James can sometimes charge their cars at the same time.
   e.   The charging station closes on weekends.

Question 7

The chart below shows the number of participants in Cooking, Garden and Pottery classes in a community. Some of these classes are held at the library, and some are held at the recreation centre.

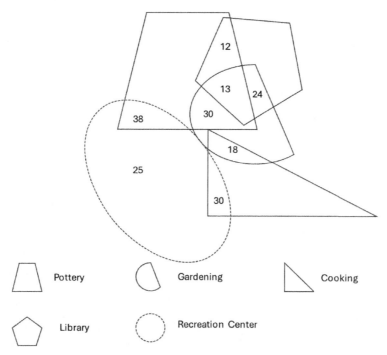

Which of the following statements is true?

   a.   The gardening class was more popular than the pottery class.
   b.   The number of people who did cooking classes is less than half the number of people who did gardening classes.
   c.   44 more people did classes at the recreation centre compared to the library.
   d.   The number of people who did cooking, garden and pottery is 15.

Question 8

The image below depicts four parking spaces in a row at a grocery store. Each space is for a different type of vehicle, and each has a different number of vehicles parked in it throughout the day. No space is ever empty, and none has more than three vehicles parked in it at any time.

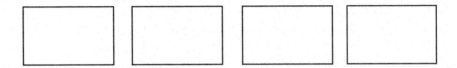

The space for electric vehicles (EVs) is next to both the space for compact cars and the space for motorcycles.
The leftmost space has three vehicles.
The space for bicycles is not in the rightmost spot.
The space with the fewest vehicles is immediately to the right of the compact cars.

Which of the following must be true?

    a.   There are more motorcycles than EVs
    b.   There are fewer bicycles than compact cars
    c.   There are more compact cars than motorcycles
    d.   There are fewer bicycles than EVs

Question 9

Alex, Jordan, and Taylor are competing in a swimming race. Each athlete finishes at different times.

- *Alex is younger than Taylor*
- *Taylor is neither the fastest swimmer among the three nor the youngest.*
- *Taylor's lap time is shorter than Jordan's.*
- *The fastest swimmer is not the youngest.*

Which of the following is true?

    a.   Alex has the fastest lap time and Jordan is the youngest.
    b.   Taylor has the slowest lap time and is the oldest.
    c.   Jordan has the fastest lap time and is the youngest.
    d.   Jordan is the youngest and Alex has the fastest lap time.

Question 10

Community gardening refers to the collective cultivation of a garden space in an urban area where individuals or groups engage in growing plants. Such gardens are often on land that is not exclusively reserved for gardening purposes. Community gardens can encompass a variety of plant types, from flowers to vegetables. They are spaces that foster community interaction and connection to nature. There are two key motivators behind the creation of community gardens: social engagement and urban beautification.

Place "Yes" if the conclusion does follow. Place "No" if the conclusion does not follow.

a. Mia decides to plant sunflowers in the community garden to contribute to the neighbourhood's beautification. As she is doing it with the community's aesthetic in mind, her actions are an example of community gardening.
b. Community gardening is usually not a solitary activity nor solely focused on individual benefit but rather community involvement where it takes place.
c. Planting vegetables in the community garden for the exclusive use of one's restaurant is not an example of community gardening.
d. A community garden initiative is only considered successful if the initiative transforms an unused plot of land into a cultivated garden space.
e. Individuals should engage in community gardening only in designated areas that were intended for such use.

Question 11

I roll two six-sided dice at the same time (a 'double roll'). Each die has an equal probability of landing on any of its faces, numbered one through six. On the first roll, one die shows six, the other a four. I roll the dice again, both at the same time.

The probability that at least one of the double rolls will result in both dice showing the same number is 1/6.

Which of the following is true?

a. Yes, if you do the double roll twice in a row, then the odds are that you will get a pair of the same number on at least one of those rolls.
b. Yes, there are thirty-six possible outcomes for the second double roll, and six of these outcomes would result in both dice showing the same number.
c. No, the probability of both dice showing the same number on one roll is 1/36.
d. No, the probability of both dice showing different numbers on one roll is 5/6.

Question 12

Four chefs – Lucas, Marie, Owen, and Nora – each prepared a different dish for a cooking competition: a salad, a dessert, a soup, and a pasta dish. The time taken to prepare each dish was 45 minutes, 60 minutes, 30 minutes, and 75 minutes (in no particular order).

- *Lucas either made the salad or the dessert*
- *Marie's dish took the longest time to prepare*
- *Owen took fifteen minutes less to prepare his dish compared to Nora, and he made the soup*
- *The pasta dish was the second quickest to prepare*

Which of the following statements is true?

a. Lucas took 60 minutes to complete his dish of making a salad
b. Owen took 75 minutes to complete her dish of making a soup
c. Nora took 45 minutes to complete her dish of making pasta
d. Marie took 75 minutes to complete her dish of making a dessert

Question 13

A school is organising an extracurricular activity day, and students can sign up for chess, basketball, or a pottery class. In total, 150 students have signed up to participate. 80 students will play basketball, 70 will attend the pottery class and 50 will play chess. There are 40 students who will play both chess and basketball, and 20 of these will also attend the pottery class.

Which of the following diagrams best represents the above data?

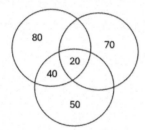

a.

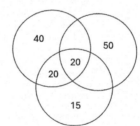

c.

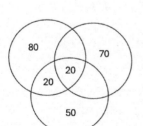

b.

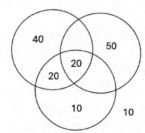

d.

Question 14

In Jack's orchard, all trees bear either apples, oranges, or pears. All pear trees have green leaves, and the leaves on apple trees can be of any colour. Jack will prune all "overgrowths" which in his view are trees he did not plant that bear orange fruit.

Place "Yes" if the conclusion does follow. Place "No" if the conclusion does not follow.

a. Jack will prune all orange trees from the orchard.
b. Some apple trees in the orchard are overgrowths.
c. Jack did not plant any coniferous trees, which means that he will prune all coniferous trees from the orchard.
d. All trees in Jack's orchard which do not have green leaves bear apples or oranges.
e. The peach trees in Jack's orchard are overgrowths.

Question 15

Marco and Eva are playing a game with two spinner wheels. Marco's spinner has eight equal sections numbered 1 through 8. Eva's spinner has sections numbered 1 through 10.

- *Marco wins if he spins an even number*
- *Eva wins if she spins a multiple of 3*
- *Marco and Eva have an equal chance of winning.*

Which of the following statements is true?

a. Yes, because there are eight sections on Marco's spinner and ten on Eva's spinner.
b. Yes, there are four even numbers between 1 and 8 and three multiples of 3 between 1 and 10.
c. No, Eva has a higher chance of winning because she can spin a 9, which is greater than 8.
d. No, there are more even numbers than multiples of 3 between 1 and 8.

Question 16

All of Jasper's cars are electric and some are hatchbacks. None of Claudia's cars are blue, but some are convertibles. If a car is electric, it must not have a diesel engine.

Place "Yes" if the conclusion does follow. Place "No" if the conclusion does not follow.

a. A white electric car could be Jasper's or Claudia's.
b. If a car belongs to Jasper, it must be a hatchback electric car.
c. If a car is blue and a convertible, it is neither Claudia's nor Jasper's.
d. There are no cars that are diesel-powered.
e. If there is a car that is a convertible, it must belong to Claudia.

Question 17

The following graphs compare the annual sales volumes of two different book genres at a bookstore over a 5-year period.

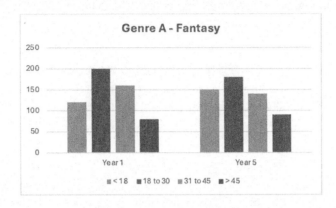

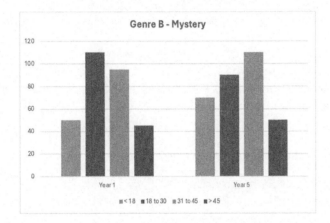

Place "Yes" if the conclusion does follow. Place "No" if the conclusion does not follow.

a. Both genres saw an increase in sales for the youngest age category from Year 1 to Year 5.
b. In Genre A, the total number of books sold to people aged 31 to 45 decreased over this 5-year period.
c. For Genres A and B combined, fewer people over the age of 45 purchased books in Year 5 compared to Year 1.
d. In Year 1, the under 18 age group was the smallest demographic for Genre B.
e. In Year 5, the "18 to 30" group was the largest demographic across both genres.

Question 18

In the solar system, some planets have rings. However, all gas giants in the solar system have more than one moon. No terrestrial planets have rings, except for Earth and Mars.

Place "Yes" if the conclusion does follow. Place "No" if the conclusion does not follow.

   a. Some of the planets in the solar system with more than one moon could be terrestrial or gas giants.
   b. All gas giants in the solar system have more than one moon and can have rings.
   c. All planets with rings in the solar system have more than one moon.
   d. Terrestrial planets are smaller than gas giants, and none have more than one moon.
   e. If a planet in the solar system has more than 1 moon and isn't a gas giant, it must be Earth.

Question 19

A special election was held this week in Warwick to fill a recently vacated Member of Parliament seat. Each of the four applicants received different votes (8500, 9000, 9500, 10,000) and they all came from various occupations including doctor, academic, engineer and architect,

   - *The politician who received 10,000 votes was either the architect or Ida*
   - *The engineer finished an unknown number of votes ahead of the doctor.*
   - *Of the candidates who received 9000 votes and the academic, one was Jed and the other was Gilda.*
   - *Ida finished 500 votes behind Kelly and 1000 votes ahead of Jed.*

Which of the following statements must be true?

   a. Gilda worked as a doctor and received 9500 votes
   b. Ida, the engineer, received the lowest number of votes.
   c. Jed, who is an architect, received 8500 votes
   d. Kelly won the election with 10,000 votes

Question 20

Capacitors of different capacitances are connected to circuits with resistors and inductors by an electrical engineer to study their charge and discharge behaviours. Upon connection, capacitors above 500 microfarads (µF) will discharge in a simple RC circuit within 5 minutes. Those below 500 µF will take longer unless they are connected in a circuit with a specific resistor value of less than 200 ohms.

Place "Yes" if the conclusion does follow. Place "No" if the conclusion does not follow.

   a. A 750uF capacitor requires only a standard resistor to discharge within five minutes.
   b. A 450uF capacitor needs to be connected to a resistor less than 200 ohms to discharge within 5 minutes.
   c. The only way to discharge a capacitor below 500 µF within 5 minutes is to connect in a circuit with a resistor less than 200 ohms
   d. Capacitors above 500µF can discharge under 5 minutes regardless of the resistor value in the circuit
   e. If a 300uF capacitor is connected in a circuit with a 150-ohm resistor, it will discharge in less than 5 minutes

Question 21

Four of Mr. Morris' European History students each gave an oral presentation today on different UK Prime Ministers which included Atlee, Blair, Eden and Grey. Each of the students took either 6,8, 10 or 12 minutes (in no particular order).

- Blake spoke for 4 minutes longer than Zachary
- Lucy spoke for somewhat longer than the presenter who gave the presentation on Prime Minister Atlee
- The presenter who spoke for 12 minutes talked about Prime Minister Eden
- Of Wesley and the student who spoke for 8 minutes, one talked about Prime Minister Grey and the other talked about Prime Minister Eden

Which of the following statements must be incorrect?

a. Wesley delivered the longest oral presentation
b. Blake and Zachary took 10 and 6 minutes respectively, and Zachary presented on Prime Minister Atlee
c. Lucy presented for 8 minutes on Prime Minister Blair
d. Lucy and Zachary combined spoke for 14 minutes.

Question 22

Should the UK increase funding for renewable energy research?

Select the strongest argument from the statements below

a. Yes, it is essential for the UK to be self-sufficient in energy and to lead globally in green technology innovation
b. Yes, advancing renewable energy technology is critical for reducing carbon emissions and combating climate change
c. No, the UK should prioritise immediate economic challenges over long-term investment in renewable energy research
d. No, the current renewable technology is sufficient, and additional fundings should be directed to more immediate public services

Question 23

Elena has only one bookstore. In her bookstore, Elena stocks a variety of fiction and non-fiction books but she does not stock horror novels or magazines.

Place "Yes" if the conclusion does follow. Place "No" if the conclusion does not follow.

a. Elena does not stock cooking magazines in her bookstore.
b. Elena stocks at least two science fiction books in her bookstore.
c. All books in Elena's bookstore are either fiction or non-fiction.
d. No books in Elena's bookstore are less than 100 pages long.
e. If a store stocks only books on history, that store is not Elena's.

Question 24

A garden has tulips, roses, and daisies. Most of the daisies in the garden have wilted. Any unwilted flowers in the garden are either pink or yellow.

Place "Yes" if the conclusion does follow. Place "No" if the conclusion does not follow.

   a. There is at least one unwilted pink tulip in the garden.
   b. Some yellow flowers in the garden are roses.
   c. All wilted flowers in the garden must be daisies.
   d. It may not be the case that all tulips in the garden are either pink or yellow.
   e. Any daisy in the garden that is not wilted, or pink must be yellow.

Question 25

Should the government increase the budget for public transportation to reduce traffic congestion?

Select the strongest argument from the statements below

   a. No, the high cost of upgrading public transport infrastructure could outweigh the benefits, and the money might be better spent on road improvements.
   b. No, increasing the public transport budget could lead to higher taxes and not all citizens would benefit from the service enhancements.
   c. Yes, improved public transport will encourage more people to commute via these systems, which is environmentally beneficial and reduces traffic.
   d. Yes, investment in public transportation has been shown to significantly reduce the number of vehicles on the road, leading to less congestion.

Question 26

Should the government increase tax on sugary drinks to improve public health?

Select the strongest argument from the statements below

   a. No, such taxes are regressive and disproportionately affect lower-income households, which could lead to increased financial strain.
   b. No, there is insufficient evidence to suggest that increasing taxes on sugary drinks would significantly improve public health outcomes.
   c. Yes, higher taxes on sugary drinks would discourage consumption, leading to lower rates of obesity and related health issues.
   d. Yes, the revenue generated from these taxes could be invested in healthcare and public health campaigns.

Question 27

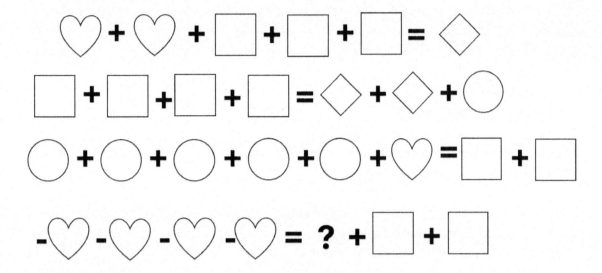

Which of the following shapes completes the equation?

    a. Heart
    b. Square
    c. Diamond
    d. Circle

Question 28

There is a 40% chance of rain and a 40% chance of sunshine. Both cannot occur.

What is the chance of either occurring?

    a. 80% because 0.4 + 0.4 = 0.8
    b. 16% because 0.4 x 0.4 = 0.16
    c. 36% because 0.6 x 0.6 = 0.36
    d. 64% because 1 - (0.6 x 0.6) = 0.64

Question 29

Observatory X and Observatory Y have the same number of telescopes, used to view distant galaxies.
Every day, 30% of the telescopes in Observatory Y are defective, whilst 70% are fully functional in Observatory X.
On any given day, the probability that a telescope will collapse is one-third in Observatory X, and two in nine in Observatory Y.

When considering only the functionality and likelihood of collapse, is Observatory Y the better choice to view distant galaxies?

   a. Yes, both observatories have the same numbers of telescopes, but Observatory Y has a lower chance of telescope collapse.
   b. Yes, Observatory Y has more telescopes.
   c. No, both observatories have the same numbers of telescopes, and the same chances of telescope collapse.
   d. No, Observatory Y has a higher chance of telescope collapse.

Answers: Decision Making Mock

Question 1

a. **No** - No antioxidant supplement companies recommend consulting a healthcare provider before use. The passage does not mention whether companies recommend consultant health providers before usage so no conclusion can be made. This statement does not follow.

b. **No** - Firefighters are regularly taking antioxidant supplements to improve their performance. While firefighters might find justification for their use, the passage does not confirm that they are regularly taking these supplements. This statement does not follow.

c. **Yes** - Antioxidant supplements were not originally produced to enhance physical endurance. The passage suggests that the original development of antioxidant supplements was for general health and not specifically for physical endurance. This statement does follow.

d. **Yes** - The passage suggests that teenagers may not have a solid justification for using antioxidant supplements regularly. The widespread adoption by teenagers is described as harder to support, implying a lack of solid justification. This statement does follow.

e. **No** - The main concern regarding the use of antioxidant supplements is their potential to disrupt natural metabolic processes. The passage discusses the debate around potential risks and benefits but does not specify that disrupting natural metabolic processes is the principal concern. This statement does not follow.

Question 2: D

This is a **Text to Venn Question** that is best solved by drawing out a Venn Diagram to represent the information.

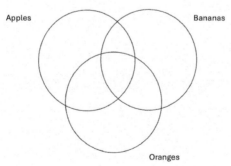

60 people did not prefer any of the fruits. 30 people preferred only bananas while 40 people preferred only oranges.

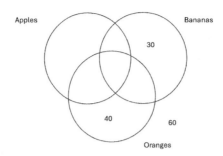

35 people preferred both apples and oranges, and of these 15 preferred all three fruits.

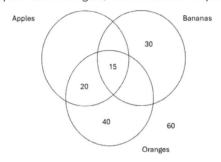

75 people preferred oranges and 55 people preferred bananas

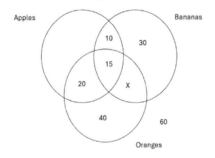

The orange circle in the Venn Diagram already adds up to 75 so there are 0 people who preferred oranges and bananas and not apples.
The banana circle currently adds up to 45, which means there are 10 people who like apples and bananas and not oranges.

80 people preferred apples

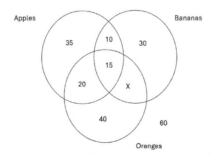

The apple circle in the Venn Diagram currently adds up to 45 which means that there are 35 people who like apples only.

Question 3

a. **No** - All the employees from the downtown office were present at the team building event. We know that all the participants present at the event were from the downtown office however, we do not know if the reverse is also true. This statement does not follow.

b. **Yes** - All the employees at the event enjoyed the team quiz. The passage states that all the participants liked the team quiz. This statement does follow.

c. **No** - If the employees from the sales department enjoyed the yoga session, then they were present at the event. The passage does not mention any information either about employees from the sales department or a yoga session, therefore we cannot conclude this. This statement does not follow.

d. **No** - All the employees at the event who enjoyed the team quiz also participated in the treasure hunt. The passage does not mention any connection between the employees who participated in the quiz and those who took part in the treasure hunt. This statement does not follow.

e. **No** - The employees at the event who participated in the treasure hunt also enjoyed paddle boarding. While the question tells us that the employees who participated in the treasure hunt also did rock-climbing, we cannot conclude if they also did paddle boarding. This statement does not follow.

Question 4: A

Begin by creating a table which we can use to fill in as we work through the statements

Country	Canada	Australia	Ireland	UK
Person				
Genre 1				
Genre 2				

The reader from Canada chose Mystery. All readers chose Historical Fiction except for the reader from Australia.

Country	Canada	Australia	Ireland	UK
Person				
Genre 1	Mystery			
Genre 2	Historical Fiction		Historical Fiction	Historical Fiction

The reader from the UK and Ethan are fans of Science Fiction

Country	Canada	Australia	Ireland	UK
Person		E	E	
Genre 1	Mystery			Science Fiction
Genre 2	Historical Fiction		Historical Fiction	Historical Fiction

We can also infer that Ethan could either be from Australia or Ireland

The two genres chosen by Sarah did not receive any votes from Daniel and the reader from Ireland.

Country	Canada	Australia	Ireland	UK
Person		Sarah	Ethan	
Genre 1	Mystery			Science Fiction
Genre 2	Historical Fiction		Historical Fiction	Historical Fiction

As the genres chosen by Sarah did not receive any votes from two other people, she could not have picked Historical Fiction, therefore she must be from Australia, which would mean **Ethan is from Ireland.**

Question 5

a. **No** - All roses are either perennials or have red petals. Whilst the question does mention that all roses have thorns, only most flowers with thorns are either perennials or have red petals. This statement does not follow.

b. **No** - Most perennial flowers are roses. The passage does not provide any information about the number of perennial flowers that are also roses. This statement does not follow.

c. **No** - Thorned flowers are always roses. The passage states that all roses have thorns. We cannot assume the reverse is also true and that all thorned flowers are roses. This statement does not follow.

d. **Yes** - Some flowers have thorns and are not perennials. The question states that most thorned flowers are either perennials or have red plants. This implies that there are some thorned flowers that may not be perennials. This statement does follow.

e. **No** - All flowers have thorns. The passage only tells us that all roses have thorns so we cannot generalise this for all flowers. This statement does not follow.

Question 6

a. **Yes** - James charges his car whilst Emily is out of the village. Emily is out of the village on weekends and James charges his car when the streetlights are not operating, which is on weekends. This statement does follow.

b. **No** - James does his grocery shopping in the village during the night. The question does not provide any information about when James does his grocery shopping. This statement does not follow.

c. **Yes** - When Emily is charging her car, the streetlights are on. The question states that Emily charges her car on weekends and the streetlights operate on weekdays. This statement does follow.

d. **Yes** - Emily and James can sometimes charge their cars at the same time. As the charging stations operate 24/7, it is possible for Emily and James to charge their cars at the same time. This statement does follow.

e. **No** - The charging station closes on weekends. The question states that the charging station operates 24/7, which means that it does not close on weekends. This statement does not follow.

Question 7: C

Use the Venn Diagram to evaluate each of the given statements.

Option A: The gardening class was more popular than the pottery class.

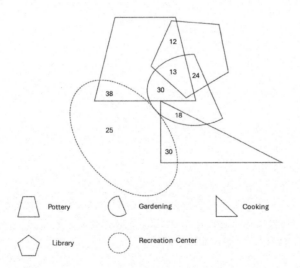

Total number of people taking a gardening class = 18 + 30 + 13 + 24 = 85
Total number of people taking a pottery class = 38 + 30 + 13 + 12 = 93
Therefore, this statement is incorrect as the number of people taking a pottery class is higher than those taking gardening.
Option B: The number of people who did cooking classes is less than half the number of people who did gardening classes.

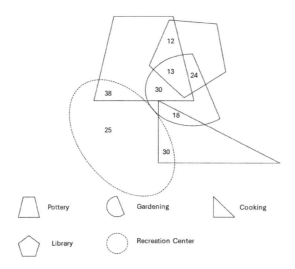

Total number of people taking a gardening class = 85
Total number of people taking a cooking class = 30 + 18 = 48
Half of 85 = 85 ÷ 2 = 42.5 and 48 is greater than 42.5, therefore this statement is incorrect.

Option C: 44 more people did classes at the recreation centre compared to the library.

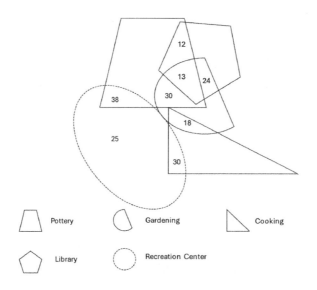

Number of people taking classes at the recreation centre = 38 + 25 + 30 = 93
Number of people taking classes at the library = 12 + 13 + 24 = 49
The difference can be calculated as 93 − 49 = 44
This statement is correct.

Question 8: A

The space for electric vehicles is next to both the space for compact cars and the space for motorcycles.
This means that the electric vehicles could either be in the second or third spot.

	EV	EV	

The space for bicycles is not in the rightmost spot.
The bicycles could either be in the first, second or third spot. However, if the bicycles were in Position 2 or 3, the EVs will no longer be in the middle of the compact cars and motorcycles.

B		EVs	

The leftmost space has three vehicles. The space with the fewest vehicles is immediately to the right of the compact cars.

B	C	EVs	M
3		1	

(a) Option A is correct as since the electric vehicles have the fewest number of vehicles, there will be more motorcycles than EVs.
(b) Option B is incorrect as we do not know the number of compact cars so we cannot make a comparison.
(c) Option C is incorrect as we do not know the number of compact cars or motorcycles so we cannot make a comparison.
(d) Option D is incorrect as there are 3 bicycles and 1 electronic vehicle.

Question 9: A

Begin by creating a table to represent the ages and lap times of the three boys.

Age (Youngest to Oldest)	Lap Time (Fastest to Slowest)

If Alex is younger than Taylor, Alex could either be the youngest with Taylor being in the middle or Alex could be in the middle, making Taylor the oldest

Age (Youngest to Oldest)	Lap Time (Fastest to Slowest)
Alex	
Taylor / Alex	
Taylor	

Taylor is neither the fastest swimmer among the three nor the youngest. Taylor's lap time is shorter than Jordan's

Age (Youngest to Oldest)	Lap Time (Fastest to Slowest)
Alex	Alex
Taylor / Alex	Taylor
Taylor	Jordan

The fastest swimmer is not the youngest. Therefore, Alex cannot be the youngest.

Age (Youngest to Oldest)	Lap Time (Fastest to Slowest)
Jordan	Alex
Alex	Taylor
Taylor	Jordan

Question 10

a. **Yes** - Mia decides to plant sunflowers in the community garden to contribute to the neighbourhood's beautification. As she is doing it with the community's aesthetic in mind, her actions are an example of community gardening. Mia's actions align with the main purposes of community gardening, which include urban beautification and community involvement. This statement does follow.

b. **Yes** - Community gardening is usually not a solitary activity nor solely focused on individual benefit but rather community involvement where it takes place. While the question states that community gardening can be done in an individual setting, they are spaces that foster community interaction and improvement to the look of the community. This statement does follow.

c. **Yes** - Planting vegetables in the community garden for the exclusive use of one's restaurant is not an example of community gardening. This action goes against the community aspect of gardening, as it is for individual benefit rather than community involvement. This statement does follow.

d. **No** - A community garden initiative is only considered successful if the initiative transforms an unused plot of land into a cultivated garden space. The question does not mention any criteria to determine the success of a community garden initiative, so we cannot conclude this. This statement does not follow.

e. **No** - Individuals should engage in community gardening only in designated areas that were intended for such use. The question states that community gardens are often on land not exclusively reserved for gardening. This statement does not follow.

Question 11: B

When rolling two fair six-sided dices, there is a total of 36 possible outcomes that can occur. 6 of those outcomes will result in both dice showing the same number [(1,1) (2,2) (3,3) (4,4) (5,5) (6,6)].

P (getting the same number on both dice) = $\dfrac{6}{36} = \dfrac{1}{6}$

Question 12: C

Begin by creating a table that you can use to fill in as you work through each of the statements.

	Lucas	Marie	Owen	Nora
Dish				
Time				

Marie's dish took the longest time to prepare.
This would mean that Marie's dish takes 75 minutes to make.

	Lucas	Marie	Owen	Nora
Dish				
Time		75 minutes		

Owen took fifteen minutes less to prepare his dish compared to Nora, and he made the soup.
As 75 minutes has already been allocated, Owen and Nora could either take 30 and 45 minutes respectively or take 45 and 60 minutes respectively.

	Lucas	Marie	Owen	Nora
Dish			Soup	
Time		75 minutes		

Lucas either made the salad or the dessert. The pasta dish was the second quickest to prepare.
Lucas and Owen do not prepare the soup and since Marie takes 75 minutes, this would mean Nora prepares the pasta and it took 45 minutes.

	Lucas	Marie	Owen	Nora
Dish			Soup	Pasta
Time		75 minutes		45 minutes

As Owen takes 15 minutes less than Nora, he would therefore take 30 minutes to prepare the soup.

	Lucas	Marie	Owen	Nora
Dish			Soup	Pasta
Time	60 minutes	75 minutes	30 minutes	45 minutes

Question 13: D

Option **A** is incorrect as the total of the Venn Diagram is >150. It fails to consider that the number of students playing the sport represents the entire circle adding up that number rather than the number of students solely playing the sport.

Option **B** is incorrect as the total of the Venn Diagram is >150 and the individual numbers have incorrectly represented as the number of people playing ONLY that sport.

Option **C** is incorrect as the sum of the total circle which represents chess adds up to 55 instead of 50.

Option **D** is correct as it correctly allocates the numbers into the Venn Diagram based on the statement. It also ensures the total of the Venn Diagram is 150 by placing 10 students outside the diagram.

Question 14

a. **No** - Jack will prune all orange trees from the orchard. The question states that Jack will only prove those trees that he did not plant that produced orange fruit. It could be possible that Jack plants orange trees. This statement does not follow.

b. **No** - Some apple trees in the orchard are overgrowths. The question defines overgrowths as trees bearing oranges that he did not plant. This statement does not follow.

c. **No** - Jack did not plant any coniferous trees, which means that he will prune all coniferous trees from the orchard. The question does not provide any information about coniferous trees; it only discusses fruit trees. Therefore, we cannot conclude this. This statement does not follow.

d. **Yes** - All trees in Jack's orchard which do not have green leaves bear apples or oranges. The question mentions that pear trees have solely green trees, so any trees that do not have green leaves in Jack's orchard would have to be either apple or orange trees. This statement does follow.

e. **No** - The peach trees in Jack's orchard are overgrowths. Peach trees are not mentioned in the information given, so we cannot conclude whether Jack planted them or considers them overgrowths. This statement does not follow.

Question 15: D

Calculate Marco's probability of winning:
His spinner has 8 equal sections, numbered 1 through 8. For Marco to win, he needs to spin an even number.
There are 4 outcomes (2,4,6 or 8) that will allow this so Marco's Probability = 4/8 = ½ = 5/10

Calculate Eva's probability of winning:
Her spinner has 10 equal sections, numbered 1 through 10. For Eva to win, he needs to spin a multiple of 3.
There are 3 outcomes (3,6 or 9) that will allow this so Eva's Probability = 3/10
Therefore, Marco's probability is higher than Eva's probability.

Question 16

a. **Yes** - A white electric car could be Jasper's or Claudia's. The question states that all of Jasper's cars are electric. No information has been given about Claudia's cars so it could be electric too. This statement does follow.

b. **No** - If a car belongs to Jasper, it must be a hatchback electric car. While all of Jasper's cars are electric, only some of the cars are hatchbacks so we cannot conclude that every car is both an electric and a hatchback. This statement does not follow.

c. **No** - If a car is blue and a convertible, it is neither Claudia's nor Jasper's. The question does tell us that Claudia does not have any blue cars so the car cannot belong to her. However, we do not have any information about whether Jasper has any blue cars so we cannot conclude this. This statement does not follow.

d. **No** - There are no cars that are diesel-powered. The question only tells us that electric cars do not have diesel engines. There is no information provided about the existence of diesel cars in general. This statement does not follow.

e. **No** - If there is a car that is a convertible, it must belong to Claudia. The question tells us that only some of Claudia's cars are convertibles and does not make any links between Jasper's cars and convertibles. This statement does not follow.

Question 17

a. **Yes** - Both genres saw an increase in sales for the youngest age category from Year 1 to Year 5. For Genre A, in the <18 category, 120 books were sold in Y1, and this increased to 150 in Y5. For Genre B, in the <18 category, 50 books were sold in Y1, and this increased to 70 in Y5. This statement does follow.

b. **Yes** - In Genre A, the total number of books sold to people aged 31 to 45 decreased over this 5-year period. In Genre A, the number of books sold to people aged 31 to 45 in Year 1 = 160 This decreased to approximately 140 in Year 5. This statement does follow.

c. **No** - For Genres A and B combined, fewer people over the age of 45 purchased books in Year 5 compared to Year 1. In Year 1, the number of people >45 who purchased books = 80+45= 125 In Year 5, the number of people >45 who purchased books 90+ 50 = 140. This statement does not follow.

d. **No** - In Year 1, the under 18 age group was the smallest demographic for Genre B. For Genre B, the smallest demographic was the over 45 category with approximately 45 books. This statement does not follow.

e. **No** - In Year 5, the "18 to 30" group was the largest demographic across both genres. In Year 5, the largest demographic was 18-30 for Genre A and 31 to 45 for Genre B. This statement does not follow.

Question 18

a. **No** - Some of the planets in the solar system with more than one moon could be terrestrial or gas giants. The question states that all gas giants in the solar system have more than one moon but no connection is drawn between terrestrial planets and the number of moons. This statement does not follow.

b. **No** - All gas giants in the solar system have more than one moon and can have rings. While we have been told that all gas giants in the solar system have more than one ring, we do not have any information about whether they have rings as well. This statement does not follow.

c. **No** - All planets with rings in the solar system have more than one moon. No connections have been drawn between planets with rings and planets with moons. This statement does not follow.

d. **No** - Terrestrial planets are smaller than gas giants, and none have more than one moon. The question does not provide any information about the size of terrestrial planets or gas giants so we cannot make a comparison. This statement does not follow.

e. **No** - If a planet in the solar system has more than one moon and is not a gas giant, it must be Earth. Mars is another example of a planet that is not a gas giant and also has one moon, so the planet could either be Earth or Mars. This statement does not follow.

Question 19: D

Begin by creating a table that you can fill in as you work through the statements.

	Gilda	Ida	Jed	Kelly
Votes				
Occupation				

Ida finished 500 votes behind Kelly and 1000 votes ahead of Jed.
If Ida is finishing behind someone, she could not have received the highest amount of votes and likewise if she is finishing ahead of someone, she cannot have received the lowest number of votes. Ida either receives 9000 or 9500 votes. As she needs to be 1000 votes ahead of Jed, she will therefore receive 9500 votes.

	Gilda	Ida	Jed	Kelly
Votes		9500	8500	
Occupation				

Of the candidate who received 9000 votes and the academic, one was Jed, and the other was Gilda.

As we know that Jed is already receiving 8500 votes, therefore he must be the academic and Gilda receives 9000 votes.

	Gilda	Ida	Jed	Kelly
Votes	9000	9500	8500	10,000
Occupation			Academic	

The politician who received 10,000 votes was either the architect or Ida.
We know that Ida does not receive 10,000 votes so Kelly must be the architect.

	Gilda	Ida	Jed	Kelly
Votes	9000	9500	8500	10,000
Occupation			Academic	Architect

The engineer finished an unknown number of votes ahead of the doctor.
We can conclude that Ida must be the engineer and Gilda is the doctor.

	Gilda	Ida	Jed	Kelly
Votes	9000	9500	8500	10,000
Occupation	Doctor	Engineer	Academic	Architect

Question 20

a. **No** - A 750uF capacitor requires only a standard resistor to discharge within five minutes. While the question does state that capacitors above 500μF are able to discharge within 5 minutes, we do not know if they require a resistor or not to discharge. This statement does not follow.

b. **Yes** - A 450uF capacitor needs to be connected to a resistor less than 200 ohms to discharge within 5 minutes. As the capacitor is below 500μF, it will require a resistor less than 200 ohms to discharge within the required time frame. This statement does follow.

c. **Yes** - The only way to discharge a capacitor below 500 μF within 5 minutes is to connect in a circuit with a resistor less than 200 ohms. The question states that a capacitor below 500μF will not be able to discharge in 5 mins UNLESS they are connected to a resistor less than 200 ohms. This statement does follow.

d. **Yes** - Capacitors above 500μF can discharge under 5 minutes regardless of the resistor value in the circuit. The question does specify that capacitors above 500uF are able to discharge within 5 minutes. This statement does follow.

e. **Yes** - If a 300uF capacitor is connected in a circuit with a 150-ohm resistor, it will discharge in less than 5 minutes. As the capacitor is below 500μF and it is connected to a resistor less than 200-ohms, it will be able to discharge within 5 minutes. This statement does follow.

Question 21: C

Begin by creating a table that you can fill in as you work through each of the statements.

	Blake	Lucy	Zachary	Wesley
Time				
Prime Minister				

The presenter who spoke for 12 minutes talked about Prime Minister Eden.
Of Wesley and the student who spoke for 8 minutes, one talked about Prime Minister Grey and the other talked about Prime Minister Eden.

	Blake	Lucy	Zachary	Wesley
Time				12 minutes
Prime Minister				Eden

Since the person who spoke for 12 minutes talked about Prime Minister Eden, using Statement 4, PM Eden's speech could not have been 8 minutes so therefore it would have to be allocated to Wesley.

Blake spoke for 4 minutes longer than Zachary.

	Blake	Lucy	Zachary	Wesley
Time	10 minutes	8 minutes	6 minutes	12 minutes
Prime Minister		Grey		Eden

As Blake and Zachary's timings need to be 4 minutes apart, the only two options available for this are 6 and 10 minutes. This would mean Lucy speaks for 8 minutes and also speaks about PM Grey.

Lucy spoke for somewhat longer than the presenter who talked about PM Atlee

	Blake	Lucy	Zachary	Wesley
Time	10 minutes	8 minutes	6 minutes	12 minutes
Prime Minister	Blair	Grey	Atlee	Eden

Question 22: B

a. Option A is not the strongest argument because it does not directly address the overarching global issue of climate change which can be seen as a more important concern. Green technology may not provide an immediate solution to the current environmental challenges being faced.

b. Option B is the strongest argument because it focuses on the urgent global issue of clinical change. The argument goes above to even mention potential benefits from renewable energy such as carbon emissions.

c. Option C is not the strongest argument because it fails to consider the long-term benefits of renewable energy research such as climate change, economic growth, and job creation in new sectors.

d. Option D is not the strongest argument as it assumes that the current technology is sufficient. This argument also does not specify what public services require more immediate attention.

Question 23

a. **Yes.** The question states that Elena does not stock any magazines in her bookstore so she would not stock any cooking magazines. This statement does follow.

b. **No.** While the question does tell us that Elena stocks fiction books in her bookstore, we are not told any further details about the genre of the fiction books, so we cannot confirm if there are any science fiction books or their amount. This statement does not follow.

c. **No.** The question does state that Elena stocks a variety of fiction and non-fiction books, but it does not explicitly state that she only stocks these two types of books. This statement does not follow.

d. **No.** No information has been provided about the length of the books in Elena's bookstore or the number of pages they contain. This statement does not follow.

e. **Yes.** Elena's bookstore does contain a variety of both non-fiction and fiction books so a bookstore contain only history books cannot be Elena's. This statement does follow.

Question 24

a. **No.** The question only states that most of the daisies are wilted. We cannot conclude this statement based on the information given. This statement does not follow.

b. **No.** While the question does state that all unwilted flowers are either pink or yellow, we cannot be sure that there are yellow roses. All the yellow unwilted flowers may be tulips and daisies. This statement does not follow.

c. **No.** The question states that most of the daisies have wilted not that all wilted flowers are daisies. This statement does not follow.

d. **Yes.** It could be possible that there are some wilted tulips and therefore, they may not be pink or yellow in colour. This statement does follow.

e. **Yes.** If the daisies are not wilted, they must be either pink or yellow. If they are not pink, then by elimination, they would have to be yellow. This statement does follow.

Question 25: D

a. Option A is not the strongest argument as it presumes that the cost of upgrading public transport will not be justified by the benefits. It also suggests that road-improvements are more cost-effective than increasing the budget for public transport.

b. Option B is not the strongest argument as it fails to address the central issue of reducing traffic congestion and instead introduces another issue of tax. The argument does not consider the overall positive impact on society.

c. Option C is not the strongest argument as it assumes that improvements in public transportation will automatically lead to a change in commuting habits. The effectiveness of this argument relies heavily on whether the public is willing to shift their transportation mode.

d. Option D is the strongest argument as it directly addresses investment in public transportation with reducing traffic congestion. The statement claims that there is historical success with previous initiatives.

Question 26: C

a. Option A is not the strongest argument as it is primarily concerns with the socio-economic impact of increasing tax on sugary drinks rather than the public health outcomes that the policy intends to improve.

b. Option B is not the strongest argument as it lacks a definitive stance and it does not propose a clear link between the tax and health outcomes.

c. Option C is the strongest answer because the argument directly links the action of taxing sugary drinks to a significant public health goal – reducing obesity rates. Reducing the consumption of sugary drinks can also have wider health benefits beyond just obesity which aligns with the policy's aim of improving public health.

d. Option D is not the strongest answer because it relies on the assumption that the funds will be used effectively and specifically for health improvement initiatives. It fails to address whether the tax would actually lead to better health outcomes.

Question 27: D

Begin by rewriting the equations replacing each shape with its corresponding answer option variable

Equation 1: $2a + 3b = c$
Equation 2: $4b = 2c + d$
Equation 3: $5d + a = 2b$

Test Question
$-4a - 2b = x$

Use Equation 1 and rearrange it to make '**a**' as the subject
2a + 3b = c
2a = c - 3b
4a = 2 x (c - 3b)
4a = 2c - 6b
-4a = -2c + 6b

Substitute the value of **-4a** into the original test equation.
-4a – 2b = x
-2c + 6b – 2b = x
4b – 2c = x

Using Equation 2:
4b – 2c = d
The value of 'x' is d which means the missing shape is a **Circle**

Question 28: A

This is a situation with the probability of two events when both cannot occur and so we add the probabilities together to find the probability of either.

Question 29: A

70% of the telescopes in Observatory Y are fully functional – the same as those in Observatory X.

The chance of telescope collapse is 1/3 for Observatory X, which is higher than the 2/9 chance for Observatory Y. Therefore, Observatory Y is the better choice, since it has a lower chance of telescope collapse.

Quantitative Reasoning

Quantitative Reasoning Tips

Quantitative Reasoning is one of the most divisive UCAT sections. Those that love maths enjoy it, those that don't find it a challenge. But with careful planning and preparation anyone can be successful.

Even if you love maths, familiarising yourself with the questions is still a must. So regardless of your level or confidence in maths you can find our top 10 tips below.

1. Practise each UCAT quantitative reasoning topic

Like every other section of the UCAT, there are multiple different question types in the quantitative reasoning section. These include questions focusing on ratios, percentages, graphs, both simple and complex calculation. You may find some of these easy, but others more challenging. Regardless, it is important that you practise every type so you know what to expect and identify the questions you're most likely to struggle with.

Many students find it useful to keep a list of the different type of questions or topics they come across during their preparation. This helps you take note of any areas you're struggling with and also lets you see which topics are most common. Some of the common types of questions that come up in the UCAT quantitative reasoning section are:

- **Percentages** – calculating percentage increases/decreases
- **Rates** – calculating speed, distance and time and converting between rates
- **Graph reading** – being able to pull data from a graph for calculations
- **Ratios** – calculating ratios of given quantities
- **Averages** – calculating mode, medians and means
- **Perimeters, areas and volumes** – being familiar with the formulas to carry out these

2. Find appropriate practice material

There are many different resources on the market for practising UCAT quantitative reasoning. But, be careful with the ones you choose.

For example, the ISC 1250 book is often found to be more difficult than the actual test. Choose carefully so that you have appropriate questions to practise, but also so as not to overwhelm yourself.

3. Master the calculator

Being proficient in using the on-screen calculator has a massive impact on both your speed and accuracy for this section. It is key that you practise with it prior to the test so you know how to use it effectively.

But as many of you will find when practising with this calculator, it is slow and awkward to use. The onscreen calculator is designed to impede your ability to answer questions. This is why mastering it is key to both speed and success.

4. Know your strengths (and weaknesses)

Some people struggle with maths more than others. If you find maths challenging, make sure you do not neglect this section, no matter how tricky it might be to start with. Just a few hours of carefully structured practise revising GCSE topics and looking at the basics such as ratios, percentages and strengthening your mental maths skills will make a huge difference.

5. Use mental maths

Just as important as knowing when to use the calculator, is knowing when not to use it. Using mental maths for a suitable calculation will save you from having to input all of the numbers into the calculator, saving you time on that question. When this happens over several questions, the time saved will add up and could even be the difference between you finishing the section or not.

6. Know your units

Another way to save time during the UCAT quantitative reasoning section is to have memorised unit conversions. Below are a few conversions worth remembering:

Unit	Conversion
Distance	
1 kilometre	1000 metres
1 metre	100 centimetres
1 centimetre	10 millimetres
Weight	
1 kilogram	1000 grams
1 gram	1000 milligrams
Volume	
1 litre	1000 millilitres

7. Write down intermediate steps

The UCAT calculator does not have the answer function you might be used to on a scientific calculator, so it is easy to lose numbers during longer and more complex calculations. To avoid this happening, it can be worth making a quick note of the mid-step numbers on your white board, so they're available for you to use later on.

8. Use the flagging function

If you are struggling with a particular question, don't get caught up with it and waste lots of time trying to arrive at the answer. Here it would be a good idea to make use of the flagging function, which marks the question so it's easier for you to come back to it later. Try not to rely too heavily on this though as timing is tight and it's unlikely you'll have much (if any) time left at the end to review the flagged questions.

9. Know when to estimate

The timing in quantitative reasoning can often be a greater struggle than carrying out the calculation. To maximise your time, it can sometimes be appropriate to estimate. Depending on the question it may be appropriate to round numbers to the nearest 10 or 100, to make it easier to do mental maths and avoid wasting time using the calculator.

As the UCAT quantitative reasoning section is multiple-choice, this means you can compare your estimated answer to the given choices to make an educated guess. It is important that you leave no question unanswered as the UCAT is not negatively marked, even if it is just a guess, as you still have a chance of selecting the correct answer.

10. Practise under timed conditions

Timing is one of the greatest challenges throughout the UCAT. In the quantitative reasoning section, you will have 24 minutes to answer 36 questions. Initially when practising, get used to doing the questions and carrying out calculations using the UCAT calculator so you become comfortable. Then start to practise under timed conditions to ensure that you're able to work both accurately and with speed.

Quantitative Reasoning Mock

Question Set 1

To grow carrots, a chef uses a 40m by 8m rectangular garden. On average, each carrot plant produces 7 carrots. Each carrot harvested weighs around 100 grams on average.

1. To the nearest percent, what percentage of the garden does the chef need to cover to grow 200 carrot plants?
   a. 14%
   b. 15%
   c. 16%
   d. 17%
   e. 18%

2. If the chef plants carrots on 80% of the garden, how many carrots could be harvested, assuming each plant yields the same average?
   a. 7162 carrots
   b. 7164 carrots
   c. 7166 carrots
   d. 7168 carrots
   e. 7170 carrots

3. If production costs are 30p and selling price is 80p per kilogram of carrots, calculate the profit in pounds when the garden is fully used for carrot cultivation.
   a. £444
   b. £446
   c. £448
   d. £450
   e. £452

4. A 15% crop tax is applied to the yield. If the chef wants to harvest 3000 carrots for himself, what percentage of his vegetable garden should he allocate to plant and grow carrots?
   a. 39.2%
   b. 39.4%
   c. 39.6%
   d. 39.8%
   e. 40.0%

Question Set 2

The table below shows the amount of fibre, protein and carbohydrates for different breakfast cereals.

Each serving contains 40 grams and each cereal box contains 12 servings.

Product Name	Amount of Fibre per Serving (g)	Amount of Protein per Serving (g)	Amount of Carbohydrates per Serving (g)
Bran Flakes	5.2	3.6	22
Muesli	3.0	4.2	30
Cornflakes	1.5	2.0	26
Rice Crispies	0.2	2.5	33
Oat Porridge	4.0	5.0	20

5. How many times greater is the amount of fibre in a box of Bran Flakes than the amount of fibre in a box of Cornflakes?
   a. 3.41
   b. 3.43
   c. 3.45
   d. 3.47
   e. 3.49

6. If a fitness enthusiast aims to maximise their protein intake for breakfast and decides to mix two servings of Muesli with one serving of Oat Porridge, how many grams of protein will they consume in total?
   a. 8.2 grams
   b. 9.2 grams
   c. 10.2 grams
   d. 11.2 grams
   e. 12.2 grams

7. Given the nutritional information in the table for various breakfast cereals, consider a situation where a nutritionist is planning a diet schedule for a week (7 days). The diet plan includes a rotation of different cereals for breakfast, ensuring a variety of nutrient intake. The nutritionist recommends:

   1 serving of Bran Flakes on Monday, Wednesday, and Friday.
   Muesli on Tuesday and Saturday.
   Oat Porridge on Thursday and Sunday.

How much Oat Porridge (in grams) should be consumed on Thursday and Sunday if the total grams of carbohydrates for these two days from the Oat Porridge should equal the total grams of carbohydrates consumed from Bran Flakes over its three days?

a. 130g
b. 132g
c. 134g
d. 136g
e. 138g

8. A dietician is creating a meal plan for a client who has specific nutritional goals. The client needs to consume exactly 20 grams of protein and no more than 200 grams of carbohydrates from cereals over the course of three days. The dietician decides to use only two types of cereal for this plan: Rice Crispies and Muesli.

Given the nutritional content per serving listed in the table, if the dietician includes one serving of Muesli each day, how many whole number servings of Rice Crispies should the client consume in total over the three days to meet their protein goal without exceeding their carbohydrate limit?

a. 1
b. 2
c. 3
d. 4
e. None of the Above

Question Set 3

Blossom Elegance Events is a boutique event planning company that specialises in floral arrangements and event accessories. Their rates are shown in the table below.

Floral Arrangements

Arrangement	Price (per arrangement)
Roses and Peonies	£45
Tulips and Daisies	£30
Orchids and Lilies	£55
Sunflowers and Baby's Breath	£35
Lavender and Hydrangea	£40
Wildflower Medley	£50

Event Accessories

Accessory	Price (per item)
Handmade table runners	£15
Vintage lanterns	£10
Crystal vases	£20
Fairy lights (10m)	£8
Silk chair sashes	£2

Delivery Fee: £50 flat rate
Setup and arrangement: 15% of the total flower order
Event day support staff: £100 flat rate

9. A couple orders 12 arrangements of Wildflower Medley, 7 arrangements of Orchids and Lilies, and 3 arrangements of Lavender and Hydrangea. If they require delivery and setup of the floral arrangements, what would be the total cost?
   a. 1318.75
   b. 1319.75
   c. 1320.75
   d. 1321.75
   e. 1322.75

10. For a small private event, a customer orders 7 Lavender and Hydrangea arrangements and hires 7 crystal vases. If Blossom Elegance Events provides a 10% discount on the accessories, what is the total cost?
   a. 400
   b. 402
   c. 404
   d. 406
   e. 408

11. Blossom Elegance Events offers a special package that costs £450 for any 15 arrangements of flowers. What is the maximum amount someone could save from the special package compared to buying the arrangements individually?
   a. 300
   b. 325
   c. 350
   d. 375
   e. 400

12. If a client orders two Orchids and Lilies arrangements for each Lavender and Hydrangea arrangement, with a total spend of £660 on flowers, how many of each type have they ordered?

    a. 3 Orchids and Lilies and 6 Lavender and Hydrangea arrangements
    b. 6 Orchids and Lilies and 3 Lavender and Hydrangea arrangements
    c. 4 Orchids and Lilies and 8 Lavender and Hydrangea arrangements
    d. 8 Orchids and Lilies and 4 Lavender and Hydrangea arrangements
    e. 5 Orchids and Lilies and 10 Lavender and Hydrangea arrangements

Question Set 4

Savings Account Options

A customer is comparing three savings account options at a bank, each with different interest rates and conditions as shown below:

Account Type	Interest Rate (for balances up to £10,000)	Interest Rate (for the portion of balance above £10,000)	Other Conditions
Fixed Saver	2.5% per annum	3.0% per annum	No withdrawals in first year
Flexi Saver	1.5% per annum	1.5% per annum	Withdrawal fee = 1% of the amount withdrawn
Super Saver	5% per annum	6% per annum	Annual account maintenance fee = £50; Maximum deposit = £50,000

The Fixed Saver does not allow any withdrawals within the first year.
The Super Saver account imposes an annual account maintenance fee.

13. A customer plans to deposit £20,000 into a new savings account. If the customer chooses the Super Saver account and leaves the deposit untouched for one year, what is the total interest earned at the end of the year after the annual account maintenance fee has been deducted?

    a. 1000
    b. 1050
    c. 1100
    d. 1150
    e. 1200

14. How much more interest can a customer earn by choosing the Super Saver account over the Fixed Saver account for a £15,000 deposit over one year, accounting for any applicable fees?
    a. 250
    b. 300
    c. 350
    d. 400
    e. 450

15. A customer invests £30,000 in a Flexi Saver account. Assuming the customer makes no withdrawals, how much will they have earned after the end of 3 years?
    a. 1330.35
    b. 1340.35
    c. 1350.35
    d. 1360.35
    e. 1370.35

16. A customer deposits £20,000 into the Flexi Saver account for 2 years, then decides to withdraw £5,000 at the start of the third year, incurring a 1% withdrawal fee. Assuming that no other withdrawals are made, how much total interest does the customer earn by the end of the third year?
    a. £838.82
    b. £839.82
    c. £840.82
    d. £841.82
    e. £842.82

Question Set 5

A city's zoning map shows the layout for a new residential area with a scale of 1:15000.
1 hectare = 10,000 m^2 = 2.47 acres

The average market value for these residential plots is £60,000 per hectare.

17. A premium square plot is sold for three times the market value. If the sale price was £810,000, what would be the area of the plot on the map in square centimetres (cm^2)?
    a. 3.5cm²
    b. 4.0cm²
    c. 4.5cm²
    d. 5.0cm²
    e. 5.5cm²

18. A waterfront square plot measuring 2 hectares is sold at one and a half times the standard market value. What is the length of one side of the plot on the map in centimetres (cm)?
    a. 0.91cm
    b. 0.92cm
    c. 0.93cm
    d. 0.94cm
    e. 0.95cm

19. A public garden has an area of 6 hectares. What is the area of the garden on the map in cm²?
    a. 2.63
    b. 2.64
    c. 2.65
    d. 2.66
    e. 2.67

20. The city plans to create a rectangular park that is twice as long as it is wide, covering an area of 4 hectares. What is the perimeter of the park on the map in centimetres (cm)?
    a. 5.64cm
    b. 5.66cm
    c. 5.68cm
    d. 5.70cm
    e. 5.72cm

Question Set 6

Book Sales

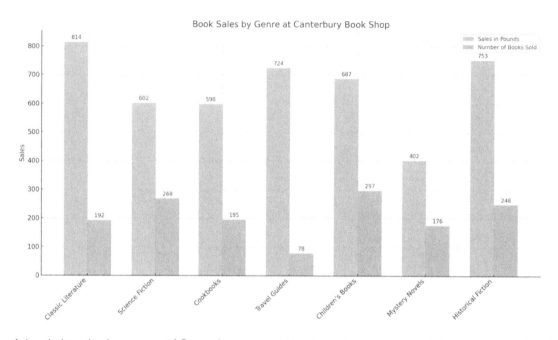

A bookshop in the centre of Canterbury specialises in a diverse range of literary genres. The bar graph below shows the breakdown in sales of seven different genres of books over the past month.

21. Based on the data above. which genre has the lowest average cost per book?
    a. Classic Literature
    b. Science Fiction
    c. Cookbooks
    d. Travel Guides
    e. Children's Books

22. A customer has a budget of £50 to spend on books at the Canterbury Book Shop. She is interested in purchasing books from two genres: Science Fiction and Children's Books. What is the maximum number of books she can purchase if she decides to buy an equal number of Science Fiction and Children's Books?
    a. 20 books (10 each)
    b. 22 books (11 each)
    c. 24 books (12 each)
    d. 26 books (13 each)
    e. 28 books (14 each)

23. Assuming that the average cost of books does not change, if the Canterbury Book Shop wants to increase the sales revenue from Cookbooks to exceed that of Children's Books, by how much does the number of Cookbooks sold need to increase?
    a. 29
    b. 30
    c. 31
    d. 32
    e. 33

24. If the Canterbury Book Shop decides to offer a 10% discount on Cookbooks, Science Fiction, and Classic Literature genre books, how much less revenue will be generated from the discounted sales of these three genres combined?
    a. £201.40
    b. £163.40
    c. £141.20
    d. £128.40
    e. £115.20

Question Set 7

Medical Supply Delivery

25. A delivery truck departs from a central warehouse at 8:00 AM and heads to Hospital A, located 100 km away. If the truck travels at a constant speed of 80 km/h, what is the estimated time of arrival at Hospital A?
    a. 9:05am
    b. 9:15am
    c. 9:25am
    d. 9:35am
    e. 9:45am

26. On a separate delivery, the truck needs to make a detour due to road construction and travel an additional 20 km at a speed of 60 km/h to reach Hospital B. If the original direct route was 50 km and could be travelled at 100 km/h, how much longer does the detour take compared to the direct route?
    a. 20
    b. 30
    c. 40
    d. 50
    e. 60

27. For a delivery to Hospital C, the truck travels the first half of the trip at an average speed of 50 km/h due to traffic, and the second half at 90 km/h on an open highway. If the total trip takes 2 hours, what is the total distance (rounded to the nearest km) to Hospital C?
    a. 125
    b. 126
    c. 127
    d. 128
    e. 129

28. The truck is scheduled to leave for Hospital D at 3:00 PM and must cover a distance of 120 km. If the truck leaves 30 minutes late and has to maintain an average speed that is 20 km/h faster than originally planned to arrive at the same scheduled time, what was the truck's new average speed?
    a. 60 km/h
    b. 70 km/h
    c. 80 km/h
    d. 90 km/h
    e. 100 km/h

Question Set 8

29. Calculate the total length of the fencing required to enclose all four plots if each plot is to be fenced separately, including the paths around them.
    a. 300m
    b. 320m
    c. 340m
    d. 360m
    e. 380m

30. Determine the total area available for planting in Plot A and Plot B combined, excluding the area taken up by the paths.
    a. 641m²
    b. 643m²
    c. 645m²
    d. 647m²
    e. 649m²

31. If the group received a donation specifically to cover the cost of the playground surface and an extra £500, calculate the maximum area (to the nearest m) of the playground that can be created without exceeding the total donation.
    a. 400m²
    b. 433m²
    c. 467m²
    d. 500m²
    e. 533m²

32. The group decides to sell a 5m wide strip from the flower plot, running along the entire 40m length, to raise funds. How much profit would they earn from selling this section of the plot at £9 per square metre?
    a. £400
    b. £450
    c. £500
    d. £550
    e. £600

Question Set 9

Charlie has compiled data on his company's sales for the last quarter, segmenting them into different product categories. The pie chart below illustrates the proportion of total sales each category contributes. Below is a pie chart representing his work. The total sales revenue across all product categories for Charlie's company was £500,000 last quarter.

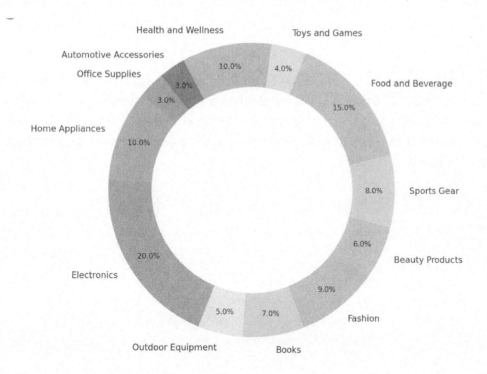

33. Charlie decides to introduce a new product category: Pet Supplies. He aims for this category to represent 5% of the total sales within the next quarter. If the total sales revenue is expected to remain at £500,000, how much sales revenue should the Pet Supplies category generate to meet this goal?
    a. £5,000
    b. £10,000
    c. £15,000
    d. £20,000
    e. £25,000

34. Charlie plans to focus on the two smallest categories by sales, aiming to boost them by 10%. If the combined sales for these two categories currently stand at £25,000, how much additional revenue must be generated to achieve this goal?
    a. £1000
    b. £1500
    c. £2000
    d. £2500
    e. £3000

35. If Charlie observes that each sale in the Food and Beverage category averages £50, how many individual sales transactions occurred in this category during the last quarter?
    a. 500
    b. 1000
    c. 1500
    d. 2000
    e. 2500

36. If the average transaction value in the Food and Beverage category is £50, and Charlie wants to adjust the pricing to make the average transaction value in the Electronics and Home Appliances categories the same as Food and Beverage, how much would the average transaction value have to be if the number of transactions for Electronics and Home Appliances is 1,800?
    a. £40
    b. £41
    c. £42
    d. £43
    e. £44

Answers: Quantitative Reasoning Mock

Question Set 1

Question 1: C

To calculate the percentage of the garden the chef needs to cover to grow 200 carrot plants, we need two things.

1) The area of the vegetable garden.
2) The area taken up by the 200 carrot plants.

Common Trap: Note that we are calculating based on carrot plants and not the number of carrots. Be sure to read carefully what the question is asking for.

Computing area of vegetable garden:

Length of the garden = 40 metres
Width of the garden = 8 metres
Total number of square metres in the garden = Length × Width
Total number of square metres = 40 metres × 8 metres = 320 square metres

Computing area taken up by the 200 carrot plants:
Number of square metres needed for 200 plants = 200 carrot plants ÷ 4 carrot plants/m^2 = 50 square metres

In order to solve the question, we need to divide the area of the vegetable garden by the area taken up by the 200 plants.

Percentage of the garden needed to grow 200 carrot plants = (Area needed / Total area of the garden) × 100

Percentage = (50 square metres / 320 square metres) × 100 = 15.625% ≈ 16%

Therefore, the percentage of the garden the chef needs to cover to grow 200 carrots plants is 16%.

Question 2: D

We first need to compute the number of square metres used for planting, before calculating the number of carrot plants, and finally the potential carrot yield.

Calculate the number of square metres used for planting:

Number of square metres used for planting = 80% of 320 square metres = 0.8 × 320 = 256 square metres

Calculate the number of carrot plants:

Number of carrot plants = (Number of square metres used for planting) × (Number of plants per square metre)

Number of plants = 256 square metres × 4 plants/m² = 1024 plants

Calculate the potential carrot yield:

Potential carrot yield = (Number of plants) × (Number of carrots per plant)

Potential yield = 1024 plants × 7 carrots/plant = 7168 carrots

Top Tip: Keep track of units to avoid making careless mistakes in multi-step questions.

Therefore, the potential carrot yield is 7168 carrots.

Question 3: C

The chef makes a profit of 50 pence per kilogram of carrot based on the production costs and selling price. To find the net profit he gets from harvesting the entire vegetable garden, we have to find the total number of kilograms the farmer can harvest from the vegetable garden and multiply this by the profit per kilogram.

Calculate total number of carrots harvested from vegetable garden:

Number of carrot plants = (Number of square metres used for planting) × (Number of plants per square metre)

Number of plants = 320 square metres × 4 plants/m² = 1280 plants

Potential carrot yield = (Number of plants) × (Number of carrots per plant)

Potential yield = 1280 plants × 7 carrots/plant = 8960 carrots

Timing Tip: Utilising the answer from the previous question, we can simply just do 7168/0.8=8960 to get the total number of carrots harvested from the vegetable garden.

Calculate total number of kilograms harvested from vegetable garden:

Total weight of carrots harvested = (Total number of carrots) × (Average weight per carrot)

Total weight = 8960 carrots × (100 grams / 1000 grams) = 896.0 kg

Calculate net profit:

Total profit = Total weight × Profit per kg

Total revenue = 896.0 kg × £0.50/kg = £448

Therefore, the chef can make a profit of £448 if he harvests his entire vegetable garden.

Timing Tip: Calculate the net profit per kilogram and multiply by total kilograms for a quicker solution.

Question 4: B

We need to first compute the total number of carrots the chef needs to harvest, taking into account the government tax.

Calculate total numbers of carrot that chef needs to harvest:
Total number of carrots to harvest = Desired number of carrots / (1 - Tax rate)
Total carrots = 3000 / (1 - 0.15) = 3000 / 0.85 ≈ 3529.41 (rounded to two decimal places)

With this number, we can then calculate the amount of space needed to harvest this many carrots.

Calculate amount of space needed to harvest carrots:
Amount of space= (Number of carrots needed / (Number of carrot plants per square metre)×(Number of carrots per carrot plant)
Amount of space= 3529.41 / (4×7)=3529.41 / 28≈ 126.05(rounded to two decimal places)

We divide this by the total area of the rectangular garden to calculate the percentage of garden the chef should allocate to plant and grow carrots.

Calculate percentage of space needed to harvest carrots:
Percentage of space=(Amount of space needed / Total area of the garden) × 100
Percentage of space= (126.05/320) × 100≈ 39.4% (rounded to one decimal place)

Top Tip: We should round up as we need the minimum percentage of space needed to plant the desired number of carrots. If we were to use 39.3% this would not be possible.

Therefore, the chef should allocate 39.4% of the vegetable garden to plant and grow carrots.

Question Set 2

Question 5: D

In order to answer this question, we need to compare the amount of Fibre **per box** between Bran Flakes and Cornflakes. This information can be found in the first column of the table, and we start out by calculating the total amount of fibre in a box of Bran Flakes and Cornflakes respectively.

Total Amount of Fibre in a box of Bran Flakes:

Fibre Content per serving × Number of servings in 1 box

$5.2 × 12 = 62.4$

Total Amount of Fibre in a box of Cornflakes:

Fibre Content per serving × Number of servings in 1 box

$1.5 × 12 = 18$

Once we have computed the total amount of Fibre for both cornflake brands, we can compare the two totals and divide the total fibre content in the Bran Flakes box by the total fibre content in the Cornflakes box to find out how many times greater the fibre content is in Bran Flakes compared to Cornflakes.

Comparing Fibre content between both brands:

Total Fibre Content (Bran Flakes) / Total Fibre Content (Cornflakes)

$62.4 / 18 ≈ 3.47$

Timing Tip: Since the serving per box is the same for both brands, instead of calculating the total amount of fibre in a box, we could have simply divided 5.2/1.5 to calculate the fibre content between the two brands.
The answer is 3.47 times.

Question 6: D

In order to answer this question, we need to look for the protein content per serving of Muesli and Oat Porridge respectively in the table, before multiplying and adding the totals together to get the protein content for the fitness enthusiast.

Protein Content of Muesli:

Protein content per serving × Number of servings

$3.6 × 2 = 7.2$

Protein Content of Oat Porridge:

Protein content per serving × Number of servings

$4.0 × 1 = 4.0$

Total Protein Content:

Muesli Protein Content + Oat Porridge Protein Content

$7.2 + 4.0 = 11.2$

The fitness enthusiast will consume 11.2 grams of protein in total.

Question 7: B

Timing Tip: Be sure to read only WHAT the question is asking for, especially when the stimulus statement is very long. In this case, the first paragraph is irrelevant and does not give any supporting information to solve the question, and we should avoid being distracted by it.

Calculate the total grams of carbohydrates consumed from Bran Flakes over three days:
The carbohydrate content per serving of Bran Flakes is 22 grams. Over three days, consuming one serving per day, the total carbohydrates would be:
$$22 \text{ g} \times 3 \text{ days} = 66 \text{ g}.$$

Determine the total grams of carbohydrates that should be consumed from Oat Porridge on Thursday and Sunday:
This needs to match the total carbohydrate intake from Bran Flakes over its three days, which is 66 grams.

Establish how many servings of Oat Porridge are needed to match this carbohydrate intake:
Since each serving of Oat Porridge contains 20 grams of carbohydrates, you would need:
$$66g \ / \ (20g/serving) = 3.3 \text{ servings}$$

Calculate the total grams of Oat Porridge needed for these servings:
Since one serving of Oat Porridge is 40 grams, for 3.3 servings, you would need:
$$3.3 \text{ servings} \times 40 \text{ g/serving} = 132 \text{ g}$$

132 grams of oat porridge should be consumed.

Question 8: C

Since the question mentions that the dietician already includes one serving of Muesli each day, we can work from here to compute the servings of Rice Crispies the client should consume to meet their protein goal without exceeding their carbohydrate limit.

Calculate the total protein provided by Muesli over three days:
If the protein content per serving of Muesli is 4.2 grams, then in three days, the client would consume:
$$4.2 \text{ g/day} \times 3 \text{ days} = 12.6 \text{ g of protein from Muesli.}$$

Determine the remaining amount of protein needed to reach the goal:
The client's protein goal is 20 grams, so they need:
$$20 \text{ g} - 12.6 \text{ g} = 7.4 \text{ g more protein from Rice Crispies.}$$

Calculate the total carbohydrates provided by Muesli over three days:

$$30 \text{ g/day} \times 3 \text{ days} = 90 \text{ g of carbohydrates from Muesli.}$$

Establish the carbohydrate limit for Rice Crispies:
The carbohydrate limit is 150 grams, so the remaining allowance for Rice Crispies is:

$$150 \text{ g} - 90 \text{ g} = 60 \text{ g}$$

Calculate the number of Rice Crispies servings needed to meet the protein requirement without exceeding the carbohydrate limit:
The client needs 7.4 grams of protein from Rice Crispies, and each serving provides 2.5 grams. Thus, they would need:

$$7.4 \text{ g} \div 2.5 \text{ g/serving} \approx 3 \text{ servings}$$

Therefore, the client should consume 3 servings of Rice Crispies in total to meet the meal plan.

Top Tip: Although we are done, we should make sure that the servings of Rice Crispies do not exceed the carbohydrate limit:

Total Carbohydrate Amount:

Rice Crispie Carbohydrate Amount

Number of Servings × Carbohydrate Content

$$3 \text{ servings} \times 33 \text{ g/serving} \approx 99 \text{ g of carbohydrates}$$

Total: Rice Crispie + Muesli

$$99 + 90 = 189$$

Since 189 is less than 200, the servings of Rice Crispies do not exceed the carbohydrate limit, and thus 3 is the correct answer.

Question Set 3

Question 9: C

To calculate the total cost for the couple's order we'll break down the costs step by step:

Calculate the cost of each type of floral arrangement:
- Wildflower Medley: £50 each x 12 arrangements = £600
- Orchids and Lilies: £55 each x 7 arrangements = £385
- Lavender and Hydrangea: £40 each x 3 arrangements = £120

Add up the costs of all floral arrangements:
£600 (Wildflower Medley) + £385 (Orchids and Lilies) + £120 (Lavender and Hydrangea) = £1105

The setup cost is 15% of the total flower order, so we calculate the setup cost **BEFORE** adding the delivery cost.

Calculate the setup cost:
15% of £1105 = 0.15 x £1105 = £165.75

Calculate the total cost:
£1105 (subtotal for arrangements) + £165.75 (setup cost) + £50 (delivery fee) = £1320.75
The total cost for the couple is £1320.75 (option C).

Question 10: D

To calculate the total cost for the order, let us separately calculate the costs for the accessories and flower arrangements, before applying any relevant discounts and finding the total.

Common Trap: Make sure to read the question carefully! Note that the 10% discount applies only on the accessories, which are the 7 crystal vases and NOT the 7 Lavender and Hydrangea arrangements.

Calculate the cost of the Lavender and Hydrangea arrangements:
- Each Lavender and Hydrangea arrangement is priced at £40.
- Total cost for 7 arrangements = 7 * £40 = £280.

Calculate the full price of hiring 7 crystal vases before the discount:
- Each crystal vase is priced at £20.
- Total cost for hiring 7 vases = 7 * £20 = £140.

Calculate the discounted price for the vases:
- The discount is 10% of £140 = 0.10 * £140 = £14.
- £140 (original price for vases) - £14 (discount) = £126.

Timing Tip: A 10% discount is equivalent to paying 90% (100-10) of the original item price. Multiply 0.90 by 140 for a quicker solution.

Calculate the total cost of the order:
- Total cost for floral arrangements = £280.
- Discounted total cost for vases = £126.
- Total cost = £280 (arrangements) + £126 (vases) = £406.

The total cost of the order is £406 (option D).

Question 11: D

To find the maximum savings, we need to identify the costliest arrangement available and compare the costs of buying the aforementioned arrangement individually against the package deal.

From the pricing information, the most expensive floral arrangement was the Orchids and Lilies at £55 each.

Calculate the cost of 15 Orchids and Lilies arrangements if bought individually:
- Cost of one Orchids and Lilies arrangement = £55
- Total cost for 15 arrangements = 15 * £55 = £825

Calculate the savings:
- Savings = Cost if bought individually - Special package cost
- Savings = £825 - £450 = £375

The maximum amount someone could save is £375 (option D).

Question 12. D

In order to solve this question, we can use algebra to craft a series of equations.

Let...
- O=Orchids and Lilies
- L=Lavender and Hydrangea

Based on the information given, we can express the total cost as follows:
$$55O+40L=660$$

And since O=2L (two Orchids and Lilies arrangements for each Lavender and Hydrangea arrangement), we can substitute O in the equation with 2L to get:
$$55(2L)+40L=660$$
Simplifying this gives us:

$$110L+40L=600$$
$$150L=600$$
$$L=4$$

Since L denotes Lavender and Hydrangea arrangements, we know that the client ordered 4 Lavender and Hydrangea arrangements, and 8 Orchids and Lilies arrangements (double of Lavender and Hydrangea arrangements).

Timing Tip: For a quicker solution, consider the alternative solution below that integrates reasoning and elimination strategies through a guess-and-check approach.

Alternative Solution

Knowing that the client orders two times as many Orchids and Lilies arrangements compared to Lavender and Hydrangea arrangements, we can immediately eliminate answer choices A, C, and E because they do NOT follow this pattern (they follow the opposite). This leaves us with option B and D only.

We can then proceed to test these remaining two options to see which one results in a total spend of £660.

Testing option B
- Orchids and Lilies: 6 arrangements at £55 each = £330
- Lavender and Hydrangea: 3 arrangements at £40 each = £120
- Total spend = £330 (Orchids and Lilies) + £120 (Lavender and Hydrangea) = £450

Since option B gives us a total of £490 and not £600 , we can immediately conclude that option D is the correct answer.

For reference, the steps to test option D are included below.

Testing option D
- Orchids and Lilies: 8 arrangements at £55 each = £440
- Lavender and Hydrangea: 4 arrangements at £40 each = £160
- Total spend = £440 (Orchids and Lilies) + £160 (Lavender and Hydrangea) = £600

Question Set 4

Question 13: B

To calculate the total interest earned, we separately calculate the interest for the amount up to £10,000 and above 10,000 respectively, before adding them together and factoring in the annual maintenance fee.

Calculate the interest earned on the first £10,000:
- This portion of the deposit earns interest at a rate of 5% per annum.
- Interest for the first £10,000 = 5% of £10,000 = 0.05 * £10,000 = £500.

Calculate the interest earned on the remaining £10,000:
- The remaining deposit earns interest at a rate of 6% per annum (since it is above the £10,000 threshold).
- Interest for the remaining £10,000 = 6% of £10,000 = 0.06 * £10,000 = £600.

Calculate the total interest earned before fees:
- Total interest = Interest on the first £10,000 + Interest on the remaining £10,000.
- Total interest = £500 + £600 = £1,100.

Subtract the annual account maintenance fee:
- The Super Saver account has an annual maintenance fee of £50.
- Total interest after fees = Total interest - Annual maintenance fee.
- Total interest after fees = £1,100 - £50 = £1,050.

The total interest after fees is £1,050 (option B).

Question 14: The correct answer is C.

To solve this question, we first calculate the interest for both the Fixed Saver and the Super Saver accounts respectively before finding the difference in interest earnings between the two after one year.

Fixed Saver Account:

1. Interest on the first £10,000 at 2.5% per annum: $£10,000 \times 0.025 = £250$
2. Interest on the remaining £5,000 at 3.0% per annum: $£5,000 \times 0.03 = £150$
3. Total interest for the Fixed Saver: $£250 + £150 = £400$
4. There are no fees for the Fixed Saver account.

Super Saver Account:

1. Interest on the first £10,000 at 5% per annum: $£10,000 \times 0.05 = £500$
2. Interest on the remaining £5,000 at 6% per annum: $£5,000 \times 0.06 = £300$
3. Total interest for the Super Saver: $£500 + £300 = £800$
4. Subtract the annual maintenance fee of £50: $£800 - £50 = £750$

The difference in interest earnings between the two accounts is:
$$£750 - £400 = £350$$

A customer can earn £350 interest by choosing the Super Saver account over the Fixed Saver account (option C).

Question 15: E

Year 1 Interest:
- Interest = £30,000 * 1.5% = £450

Year 2 Interest:
- New total = £30,000 + £450 = £30,450
- Interest = £30,450 * 1.5% = £456.75

Year 3 Interest:
- New total = £30,450 + £456.75 = £30,906.75
- Interest = £30,906.75 * 1.5% = £463.60

Total Interest Earned Over 3 Years:
- Year 1 + Year 2 + Year 3
- £450 + £456.75 + £463.60 = £1,370.35

The total interest earned from the Flexi Saver account over 3 years is £1,370.35 (option E).

Timing Tip: Apply the formula for compound interest (shown below) for a quicker solution that involves less steps.

$$A = P(1 + \frac{r}{n})^{nt}$$

A = final amount

P = initial principal balance

r = interest rate

n = number of times interest applied per time period

t = number of time periods elapsed

Substituting the values we know:

A=30,000(1+0.015)^3
A=30,000(1.015)^3
A=31370.35125≈31370.35

Subtracting the final amount from the initial amount:

Interest Earned=Final Amount - Initial Amount
31370.35 - 30000 = 1,370.35

Using the formula for compound interest gives us the solution to the question without having to calculate the interest amount year-by-year.

Question 16: A

Since there is a withdrawal of £5,000 at the start of the third year, we are unable to apply the formula for compound interest and will instead calculate the amounts year-by-year.

Year 1:
Interest = £20,000 * 1.5% = £300.

Year 2:
New total = £20,000 + £300 = £20,300.
Interest = £20,300 * 1.5% = £304.50.

Start of Year 3 (before withdrawal):
New total = £20,300 + £304.50 = £20,604.50.

Withdrawal:
- Withdrawal amount = £5,000.
- Withdrawal fee = £5,000 * 1% = £50.
- Remaining after withdrawal = £20,604.50 - £5,000 = £15,604.50.
- Amount after deducting withdrawal fee = £15,604.50 - £50 = £15,554.50.

Year 3 Interest:
Interest = £15,554.50 * 1.5% = £233.32.

Total Interest Earned Over 3 Years:
Year 1 + Year 2 + Year 3 = £300 + £304.50 + £233.32 = £838.82.

Top Tip: Clearly label and keep track of your interest calculations to avoid calculating the interest for the wrong amount/total.

The total interest earned over 3 years is £838.82 (option A).

Question Set 5

Question 17: C

To solve this question, we first want to calculate the market value of the residential plot, before using this information and a series of conversions to compute the area of the plot on the map in square centimetres (cm^2).

Determine the area of the plot in hectares based on the sale price:
Since the sale price at three times the market value is £810,000, we divide by three times the market value per hectare (£60,000) to find the area: £810,000/ (3×60,000)=4.5 hectares

Calculate the actual area in square metres:
1 hectare = 10,000 m², so:
4.5 hectares = 4.5 × 10,000 m² = 45,000 m²

Convert the actual area into square centimetres:
1 m² = 10,000 cm², therefore:
45,000 m² = 45,000 × 10,000 cm² = 450,000,000 cm²

Scale down the actual area to the area on the map using the map's scale (1:10,000):
The area on the map in cm² = the actual area in cm² / scale²
450,000,000 cm²/ (10,000×10,000)=450,000,000 cm² / 100,000,000 = 4.5 cm²

Common Trap: Make sure to divide by scale² instead of scale because we are dealing with area instead of linear dimensions.

The area of the plot on the map would be 4.5 cm² (option C).

Question 18: D

Timing Tip: Avoid being distracted by the information on market value, as it does not provide any value in helping us answer the question.

The actual area of the waterfront plot is 2 hectares, which is equivalent to:

$$2 \times 10,000 \text{ m}^2 = 20,000 \text{ m}^2$$

To find the length of one side of the square plot in reality, we take the square root of the area:

$$\text{Side length} = \sqrt{20,000 \text{ m}^2}$$
$$\text{Side length} = \sqrt{20,000} \text{ m}$$
$$\text{Side length} \approx 141.42 \text{ m}$$

The map's scale is 1:15000, so to find the length on the map, we divide the real side length by the scale:

$$\text{Map side length} = \frac{141.42 \text{ m}}{15000}$$
$$\text{Map side length} \approx 0.009428 \text{ m}$$
$$\text{Map side length} \approx 0.94 \text{ cm (since 1 m = 100 cm)}$$

The length of one side of the plot on the map is 0.94cm (option D).

Question 19: E

To solve this question, we first convert the area from hectares to square metres, before we find the area on the map using the scale factor.

Convert hectares to square metres:

Since 1 hectare = 10,000 square meters:

$$\text{Actual area in m}^2 = 6 \text{ ha} \times 10,000 \text{ m}^2/\text{ha}$$
$$\text{Actual area in m}^2 = 60,000 \text{ m}^2$$

Convert the actual area to the area on the map:
If the map scale is 1:15000, then 1 cm on the map represents 15000 cm in real life. Since the area is a two-dimensional measurement, we must square the scale factor to convert the actual area to the map area.

$$\text{Area on map in cm}^2 = \frac{\text{Actual area in m}^2 \times 10,000 \text{ cm}^2/\text{m}^2}{(15000 \times 15000)}$$
$$\text{Area on map in cm}^2 = \frac{60,000 \text{ m}^2 \times 10,000 \text{ cm}^2/\text{m}^2}{225,000,000}$$
$$\text{Area on map in cm}^2 = \frac{600,000,000 \text{ cm}^2}{225,000,000}$$
$$\text{Area on map in cm}^2 = 2.67$$

Thus, the area of the garden on the map would be 2.67 cm² (option E)

Question 20: B

To compute the perimeter of the park on the map, we first need to determine the real-life dimensions of the park, before finding the real-life perimeter of the park and finally using the scale factor to find the perimeter of the park on the map.

Find the actual dimensions in metres:
- We know that the area of the park is 4 hectares, which is 40,000 square metres (since 1 hectare = 10,000 square metres).
- If the length is twice the width, we can represent the width as w and the length as 2w.
- The area A=length×width=2w×w=2w²
- We can solve for w² by dividing the area by 2: w²=A/2=40,000/2=20,000m²
- The width w is the square root of 20,000m²,which is approximately 141.42 metres.
- The length is twice the width, so the length is approximately 282.84 metres.

Top Tip: When the answer choices are very close in numerical value, try to avoid rounding till the last step to make sure your answer is accurate. If you do have to round, round to at least 2 decimal points.

The perimeter of the park in reality is:
- 2×(w+2w)
- 2x(141.42 m+282.84 m)
- 2×424.26 m
- 848.52m

Convert the actual dimensions to the map scale:
- Scale is 1:15000, meaning 1 cm on the map represents 15,000 cm or 150m in reality.
- To find the map dimensions, divide the real dimensions by 150.
- 848.52m*1cm/150m=5.6558≈5.66cm

The perimeter of the park on the map is 5.66cm.

Question Set 6

Question 21: B

The average cost per book can be found by dividing the total sales in pounds by the number of books sold for each genre.

Here's the calculation for each genre based on the provided data:
- Classic Literature: £814 / 192 books = £4.24 per book
- Science Fiction: £602 / 268 books = £2.25 per book
- Cookbooks: £598 / 195 books = £3.07 per book
- Travel Guides: £724 / 78 books = £9.28 per book
- Children's Books: £687 / 297 books = £2.31 per book

Upon calculating these averages, it's clear that Science Fiction (option B) has the lowest average cost at approximately £2.25 per book.

Timing Tip: Round the total sales and number of books sold to the nearest hundred before calculating the average cost per book for a quicker solution.

- Classic Literature: £800 / 200 books ≈ £4 per book
- Science Fiction: £600 / 300 books ≈ £2 per book
- Cookbooks: £600 / 200 books ≈ £3 per book
- Travel Guides: £700 / 100 books ≈ £7 per book
- Children's Books: £700 / 300 books ≈ £2.33 per book

We still get the same answer that Science Fiction (option B) has the lowest average cost.

Question 22: A

The customer wants to buy an equal number of Science Fiction and Children's Books with a £50 budget. Using the answers we got from the previous question, the average costs for these books are £2.25 and £2.31 respectively.

Let's quickly work this out. The customer wants to buy an equal number of Science Fiction and Children's Books with a £50 budget. The average costs for these books are £2.25 and £2.31 respectively.

Firstly, we find out the combined cost of buying one book from each genre:
£2.25 (Science Fiction) + £2.31 (Children's Books) = £4.56 for a pair of books.

Now, we'll see how many such pairs she can buy with £50:
£50 / £4.56 per pair ≈ 10.96 pairs.

Since she cannot purchase a fraction of a pair, she can only buy a maximum of 10 pairs of books.

Therefore, with her £50 budget, the customer can purchase 20 books in total (option A).

Question 23: B

To solve this, we need to find the current sales revenue of Children's Books and Cookbooks, as shown on the graph:
- Sales revenue from Children's Books is £687.
- Sales revenue from Cookbooks is £598.
- The difference that needs to be made up is £687 - £598 = £89.

Next, we calculate the average cost of a Cookbook. This is given by the sales revenue divided by the number of Cookbooks sold:
- Cookbooks: £598 / 195 books = £3.06666666667 per book

Common Trap: Do not round to two decimal points here, only round at the end. Instead, use the number given by the calculator for the next few steps.

Now, to find out how many additional Cookbooks need to be sold to match the sales revenue of Children's Books, we divide the sales difference by the average cost of a Cookbook:
- £89 / £3.06666666667 per book ≈ 29.02 books.

Since we can't sell a fraction of a book, we would round up to the next whole book (30 books).

Top Tip: Be able to distinguish when to round up and when to round down. Here, we need to round up instead of rounding to the nearest whole number because we can't sell a fraction of a book.

30 additional Cookbooks (option B) need to be sold to ensure that the revenue from Cookbooks exceeds that of Children's Books.

Question 24: A

To solve this question, calculate the total current revenue of the three genres combined before applying the discount to find the loss in revenue.

Calculate the total revenue from these three genres:
- Current revenue from Cookbooks: £598
- Current revenue from Science Fiction: £602
- Current revenue from Classic Literature: £814
- Total revenue=£598+£602+£814=£2014

Now, apply the 10% discount to the total revenue:
- Discounted revenue=10%×£2014=£201.40

Timing Tip: Calculate the total revenue for all three genres before applying the discount for a quicker solution (instead of applying the discount for each genre and taking the total).

Therefore, with the 10% discount, the revenue will decrease by £201.40 (option A).

Question Set 7

Question 25: The correct answer is B.

To find the estimated time of arrival at Hospital A, we need to calculate the travel time and then add it to the departure time.

The formula for travel time is:
$$Travel\ Time = Distance/Speed$$

Given:
Distance=100km
Speed=80km/h
Travel Time=100km/(80km/h)=1.25 hours

To find the estimated time of arrival, we add the travel time to the departure time of 8:00 AM.

Time of Departure=8:00 AM

Estimated Time of Arrival=8:00 AM+1.25 hours=9:15am

Common Trap: 1.25 hours is NOT equal to 1 hour and 25 minutes. Instead 1.25 hours is equal to 1.25*60=75 minutes, or 1 hour and 15 minutes.

Therefore, option B is the correct answer.

Question 26. C

To determine how much longer the detour takes compared to the direct route, we need to calculate the travel time for both routes and then find the difference.

Direct Route
Given:

- Distance = 50 km
- Speed = 100 km/h
- Travel Time=Distance/Speed=50km/(100km/h)=0.5 hours (30 minutes)

Top Tip: Know how to rearrange the speed/distance formulas for your own calculations. As long as we know two variables in the formula, we can solve for the last one.

Detour Route
Given:

- Original Distance = 50 km
- Additional Distance due to Detour = 20 km
- Total Distance for Detour = 50 km + 20 km
- Speed on Detour = 60 km/h
- Travel Time=Distance/Speed=70km/(60km/h)=1.17 hours (70 minutes)

Let's calculate the travel times for both routes and then find the difference.

The direct route to Hospital B takes 30 minutes, while the detour route takes 70 minutes. Therefore, the detour takes an additional 40 minutes compared to the direct route.

Question 27: E

To find the total distance to Hospital C, we can use the total trip time and the average speeds for each half of the trip.

Let d be the total distance to Hospital C. Since the truck travels the first half of the distance (d/2) at 50 km/h and the second half (d/2) at 90 km/h, and the total trip time is 2 hours, we can set up the equation:

Total Time=Time for First Half+Time for Second Half

Given:
- Total Time = 2 hours
- Speed for First Half = 50 km/h
- Speed for Second Half = 90 km/h

Therefore:
- Time for First Half=Distance/Speed=(d/2)/(50)
- Time for Second Half=Distance/Speed=(d/2)/(90)

Substituting these values in the total time equation gives:
- Total Time=Time for First Half+Time for Second Half
- 2=(d/2)/(50)+(d/2)/(90)
- 2=(d/100)+(d/180)
- 2=(9d/900)+(5d/900)
- 2=(14d/900)
- 1800=14d
- d=128.57≈129

Therefore, the total distance to hospital C is approximately 129 km.

Question 28: C

To find the truck's new average speed, we first need to determine the original travel time based on the assumption that the truck would have arrived on time if it had departed as scheduled. Since the truck leaves 30 minutes late but still needs to arrive at the originally scheduled time, this delay needs to be compensated for by increasing the speed.

Let's denote:
- The original average speed as v km/h.
- The new average speed as v+20 km/h (since it's 20 km/h faster than planned).
- The original travel time as t, and is equal to 120/v (distance/speed)
- The distance to cover is 120 km.

Based on the delay, the truck needs to cover the distance in t−0.5 hours (30 minutes less than the original plan) to compensate for the delay. Therefore, using the speed-distance-time equation and the variables we defined, the equation to solve for the new speed is:
- Time=Distance/Speed
- t-0.5=120/(v+20)
- Substituting the formula we found for t in terms of v, we get:

$$\frac{120}{v} - 0.5 = \frac{120}{v+20}$$

Now, we try and solve for **v**,

The goal is to isolate **v** on one side of the equation. To do this, we first aim to eliminate the denominators by finding a common base or multiplying through by the denominators:

$$\frac{120}{v} - \frac{120}{v+20} = 0.5$$

We multiply each term by $v(v+20)$, the common denominator, to clear the fractions:

$$120(v + 20) - 120v = 0.5 \cdot v(v + 20)$$

$$120v + 2400 - 120v = 0.5v^2 + 10v$$

$$2400 = 0.5v^2 + 10v$$

$$2 \cdot 2400 = v^2 + 20v$$

$$v^2 + 20v - 4800 = 0$$

$$(v + 80)(v - 60) = 0$$

We discard the negative value, meaning that the v (the original speed) is equal to 60 km/h.

Since the question is asking for the truck's new average speed, which is v+20, we add 20 to to 60 to get 80 km/h.

Therefore, if the truck leaves 30 minutes late and has to maintain an average speed that is 20 km/h faster than originally planned to arrive at the same scheduled time, the truck's new average speed is 80 km/h.

Question Set 8

Question 29: D

To calculate the fencing needed for each plot, we must determine the perimeter, which is the total distance around the plot. For a rectangular plot, the perimeter is calculated by adding together the lengths of all four sides. Since the opposite sides of a rectangle are equal in length, the formula for perimeter is simply twice the width plus twice the length, or 2×(width+length). Note that the dimensions given for each plot are inclusive of a path that is 2 metres wide around the plot, but since this path is part of what needs to be enclosed by the fence, we do not need to make any additional calculations.

TOP TIP: Since each plot is to be fenced separately, the perimeter of each plot is calculated separately instead of calculating the entire perimeter of the garden.

Perimeter Calculation for Each Plot:
- Plot A (Vegetables): 2×(20m+30m)=100m
- Plot B (Fruits): 2×(15m+25m)=80m
- Plot C (Flowers): 2×(10m+40m)=100m
- Plot D (Playground): 2×(20m+20m)=80m
- Total=Plot A+Plot B+Plot C+Plot D=100m+80m+100m+80m=360m

Therefore, 360 metres of fencing is needed to enclose all plots.

Question 30: D

Let's draw a simple diagram of plot A to better visualise how the plot looks with the fencing.

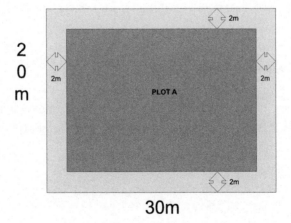

30m

Note that the diagram is not drawn to scale

As we can see in the diagram, the red area represents the actual area of the plot, while the green portion represents the 2m path that surrounds the plot. Therefore, if we want to compute the area of the plot only, we need to subtract the path length (2m) twice from each side length (20m and 30m).

Top Tip: Remember that the plot dimensions given in the stimulus are INCLUSIVE of the 2m path, so we need to factor this in when we want to calculate the area of the plot only (without the path).

Plot A (Vegetables):
The given dimensions are 20m by 30m, including a 2m path around the plot. Subtracting the path from each side gives us the planting dimensions:
$(20m-4m)\times(30m-4m)=16m\times26m=416m^2$

Plot B (Fruits):
The given dimensions are 15m by 25m, including a 2m path around the plot. Subtracting the path from each side gives us the planting dimensions:
$(15m-4m)\times(25m-4m)=11m\times21m=231m^2$

Adding these areas together gives us the total area available for planting:
$416^2+231^2=647m^2$

The combined planting area for plot A and plot B is $647m^2$ (excluding path).

Question 31: B

If we already have the specified dimensions for the playground, which is 20m by 20m, we know its initial area is 400 square metres. The donation is intended to cover the cost of surfacing this area plus an additional £500 that could be used for further surfacing or other purposes.

Common Trap: Remember to factor in the original area of the playground, and also remember that this is already covered by the donation.

Now, we can determine how much the £500 can be used to increase the area based on the £15 per square metre cost. We can do this by dividing the total amount of money available by the cost per square metre to get the area.

Therefore:
£500/(£15 per square metre)=33.33m²

We add this to the original 400m² area of the playground to get:
Maximum Area=400m²+33.33m²=433.33m²

Question 32: A

To calculate the profit (net gain) from selling the flower plot, we need to subtract the cost to acquire this section of the plot from the total funds raised by selling it to find the net gain.

Area of the Section Being Sold:
The section sold is a strip of land that is 5 metres wide and runs along the entire 40 metres length of the plot. To find the area of this section, we multiply the width by the length:
$5m \times 40m = 200m^2$

Common Trap: Note that we are not selling the entire flower top, just a portion of it so we have to calculate the appropriate area.

Total Funds Raised from Selling the Section:
The selling price of the land is £9 per square metre. To find out how much money is raised from selling this 200 square metre section, we multiply the area by the price per square metre:
$200m^2 \times £9/m^2 = £1,800$.

Cost to Acquire the Section Being Sold:
The buying price of the land was £7 per square metre. The cost to originally acquire this section is calculated by multiplying the area by the buying price per square metre:
$200m^2 \times £7/m^2 = £1,400$.

Net Gain from the Sale:
To find the net gain, or the profit, from selling the land, we subtract the cost to acquire the section from the total funds raised: £1,800 (funds raised) - £1,400 (cost to acquire) = £400.

Therefore, a profit of £400 was made from selling the flower plot.

Question Set 9

Question 33: E

The sales of Pet Supplies make up 5% of the total sales revenue. Therefore, we calculate 5% of the total sales revenue to get our answer:

5% of total sales revenue=
5% of £500,000=
0.05*£500,000=
£25,000

Therefore, for the Pet Supplies category to achieve its goal of representing 5% of the total sales, it must generate £25,000 in sales revenue within the next quarter.

Question 34: D

To increase the sales of the two smallest categories by 10%, Charlie would need to generate an additional 10% of their current combined sales of £25,000.

Here's how we can do that:
- Since the current combined sales is £25,000, we calculate 10% of it to determine the increase in sales.
    - £25,000*0.1=£2500
    - This value represents the additional revenue needed to achieve the 10% sales boost.

Timing Tip: Notice that all the information to solve this question is within the question itself. Make sure to read the question first, to know what information you need to look for.

To achieve the goal of boosting sales by 10% in the two smallest categories, Charlie must generate an additional £2,500 in revenue on top of the current £25,000.

Question 35: C

To find the number of individual sales transactions in the Food and Beverage category, we need to calculate the total sales for this category and then divide it by the average sale value.

Here's how we can do this:
- We know the total sales revenue is £500,000.
- The Food and Beverage category accounts for 15% of total sales.
- Therefore, we first calculate the total sales for Food and Beverage by finding 15% of the total sales revenue.
    - 0.15 (15%) * £500,000=£75,000
- Then, we divide the total sales of Food and Beverage by the average sale value of £50 to get the number of transactions.
    - £75,000 / £50 = 1500 transactions

Therefore, there were 1,500 individual sales transactions in the Food and Beverage category during the last quarter.

Question 36: C

In order to solve this question, we need to break the question down into the following steps:

Step 1: Calculate the Total Sales for Food and Beverage
- We use the total sales revenue of £500,000. Since Food and Beverage make up 15% of this, we calculate 15% of £500,000.
- $0.15 * £500,000 = £75,000$
- This gives us the total sales for Food and Beverage, which we found to be £75,000.

Step 2: Calculate the Required Average Transaction Value for Electronics and Home Appliances
- Find the average transaction value required for Electronics and Home Appliances to match the average of the Food and Beverage category under the new condition.
- Since we established the total sales for Food and Beverage at £75,000, the combined sales of Electronics and Home Appliances is also £75,000 (since they are equal)
- We know the combined number of transactions for Electronics and Home Appliances is 1,800. To find the required average transaction value, we divide the combined sales total (£75,000) by this number of transactions.
- $£75,000/1800 = £41.67 \approx £42$

Therefore, the average transaction value needs to be approximately £42 for Electronics and Home Appliances to ensure their sales match the Food and Beverage category in terms of the average transaction value.

Abstract Reasoning

Abstract Reasoning Tips

Abstract Reasoning has long been thought of as one of the hardest and most frustrating UCAT sections. It has a reputation with students for causing confusion and trick questions eating up a lot of precious time. The section can be intimidating at first, as it can look quite different to traditional exam questions you've faced before, but don't let this put you off!

This section, like all the others can be mastered. All it takes is some well-structured practice and an insight into the structure behind the questions. Remember that no matter how random the question shapes appear, there is always a pattern behind them. All you need to do is find that pattern and use it to answer the other questions. Hopefully by following these six key tips you can start your mastery of the UCAT abstract reasoning section.

1. Use UCAT Abstract Reasoning pattern tables

UCAT Abstract Reasoning tests your ability to recognise patterns in what initially appear to be random arrangements of shapes. When you approach this for the first time it can seem completely incomprehensible. Remember that there is always a pattern, and not only that but, there is ultimately only a **finite number of patterns** that can exist within the UCAT Abstract Reasoning section.

When you're preparing you should create a pattern table to list and organise all of the different patterns that you come across. This allows for you to approach each question more systemically and identify the most common patterns.

To begin with this technique may seem laborious but as you begin to memorise the patterns you will be able to speed up. Hopefully over time this will allow you to be move through questions more efficiently and accurately.

There are four different questions types in the UCAT Abstract Reasoning. Knowing these question types well and having set strategies on how to tackle each of them will help in ensuring that you don't get thrown off by difficult questions. The four question types are:

Question Type	Example
Set A, B or Neither	There are two sets of shapes shown as Set A and Set B. You will be shown additional test shapes and need to decide if they belong to Set A, B or neither.
Sequence	Choose the shape that comes next in the sequence based on a sequence of four shapes that change based on a specific pattern.
Finish the statement	A question will be displayed with an incomplete statement: Shape A is to Shape B as Shape X is to Shape ? You need to choose the image to complete this statement.
Set A or B	There are two sets of shapes shown as Set A and Set B. You will be shown to select a shape that belongs to either Set A or Set B.

2. Memorise key triggers

As you prepare for this section you will become more familiar with the different types of question in UCAT Abstract Reasoning. You may also start to see that different patterns will have certain things in common. You can use this to your advantage by noticing these shared characteristics quickly, and focusing your attention to certain categories of pattern first. This will help you find the underlying pattern faster.

What is meant by this, for example, is that if you see crescent moons, this should trigger you to start looking for a pattern based around curved and straight shapes. This is because the number of shapes with curved lines is quite small, so if they're being included it is likely that the curved aspect is central to the pattern.

Another example is if you see lots of overlapping shapes, look for a pattern based on the number of intersections between these shapes.

Once you have begun to recognise triggers you can add these into your pattern table to help remind you of what to look for. This is one of the best tips to help to increase your speed, as from the trigger alone you can already narrow the possible patterns in front of you. Below are a few common patterns that you should keep an eye out for:

- **Shape:** Look out for a particular shape being repeated within the Set or if all the shapes in a Set share a particular feature e.g even number of sides
- **Position:** Try to spot if a particular shape is always in a certain place within the box e.g right upper corner or if it's always placed between two other shapes
- **Rotation:** Consider if a shape is rotating within a set pattern e.g clockwise

3. Choosing appropriate resources

With UCAT Abstract Reasoning practise and becoming familiar with question types is key. This means that you need to have access to some high-quality resources or books to provide you with good practise material.

It's important to note that sometimes these practice questions may be harder than those in the actual UCAT itself. For example, the ISC 1250 book is typically reported to be very difficult. It's useful to bear this mind as while some students may find this good preparation, others may find it overwhelming and off-putting.

4. Abstract Reasoning: Timing Tips

UCAT Abstract Reasoning is the shortest section at just 12 minutes, but it also has the largest number of questions at a whopping 50. It is critical that you know how long (or little!) you have per question and do not lose track of this. If you have not practised extensively ahead of test day, it is very easy to get caught up on the challenging questions and run out of time.

There are several different question types in this section. You need to adjust how long you spend on each question depending on the type.

For example, Type 1 questions have 1 pattern with 5 associated questions. So here you have a minute to spend on the whole question set. Where as for Type 2 questions you just have 1 pattern and 1 question, giving you 14 seconds per pattern. This means you have to adjust how long you spend looking for the pattern accordingly, so as not to get stuck on these lower yield questions.

Type 1 Questions	Type 2 Questions
1 Pattern	1 Pattern
5 questions per set	1 question per set
1 minute per pattern	14 seconds per pattern

5. Know when to move on

UCAT Abstract Reasoning is a challenging section, and it is easy to get carried away trying to solve tricky questions. In the end some of the patterns are just too hard, and they've been designed this way!

Hard questions with very complex intricate patterns are deliberately put into the exam to try and slow students down. Candidates who don't have the ability to quickly identify that a question is beyond their capabilities in the time limit will end up wasting minutes trying to solve the problem. If you find a question like this, put your best guess and move on. Your time will be of better use and yield more marks elsewhere.

Remember, the UCAT is not negatively marked so if you're going to move on there is no harm in guessing. Never leave a question blank on the UCAT, even if it's a guess as you still have a chance of guessing correctly.

6. Always start with the simplest box

Whenever you get presented with two sets of patterns, you should always look at the box in each set with the fewest number of shapes. This will enable you to properly compare each set and keep you from getting distracted.

The simplest box doesn't always have to be the one with the fewest shapes. It can also be:

- the box with fewest colour variations e.g. striped, black etc.
- the box with obvious pattern e.g. a very large shape
- the box with repeating units e.g. 4 triangles

Abstract Reasoning Mock

Question Set 1

Set A   *Set B*

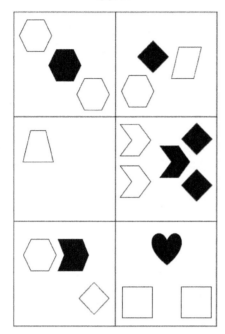
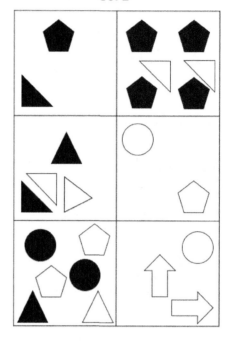

Question 1

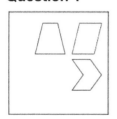

a. Set A
b. Set B
c. Neither

Question 2

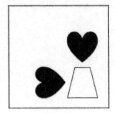

    a. Set A
    b. Set B
    c. Neither

Question 3

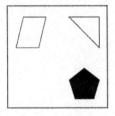

    a. Set A
    b. Set B
    c. Neither

Question 4

    a. Set A
    b. Set B
    c. Neither

Question 5

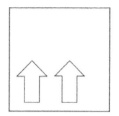

a. Set A
b. Set B
c. Neither

Question Set 2

Set A

Set B

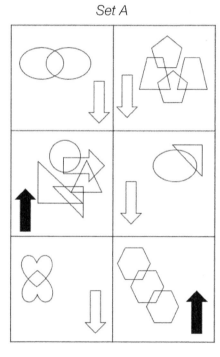

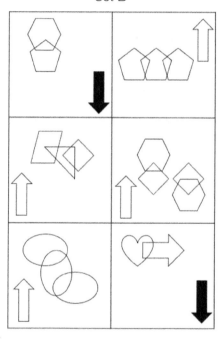

Question 6

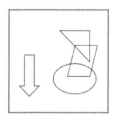

a. Set A
b. Set B
c. Neither

Question 7

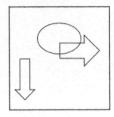

    a. Set A
    b. Set B
    c. Neither

Question 8

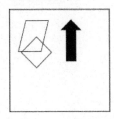

    a. Set A
    b. Set B
    c. Neither

Question 9

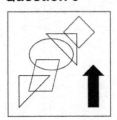

    a. Set A
    b. Set B
    c. Neither

Question 10

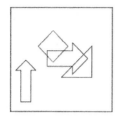

- a. Set A
- b. Set B
- c. Neither

Question Set 3

Set A

Set B

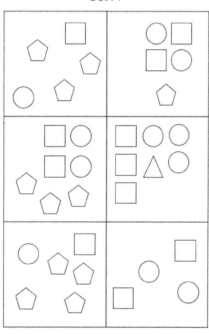
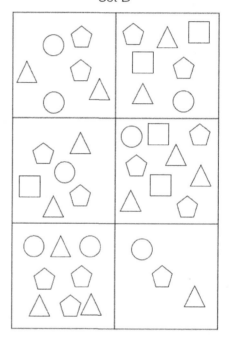

Question 11

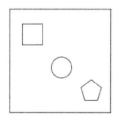

- a. Set A
- b. Set B
- c. Neither

Question 12

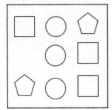

    a. Set A
    b. Set B
    c. Neither

Question 13

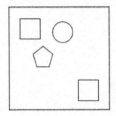

    a. Set A
    b. Set B
    c. Neither

Question 14

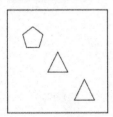

    a. Set A
    b. Set B
    c. Neither

Question 15

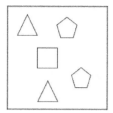

   a. Set A
   b. Set B
   c. Neither

Question Set 4

Set A

Set B

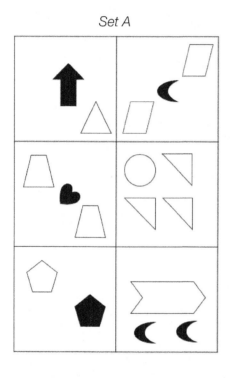
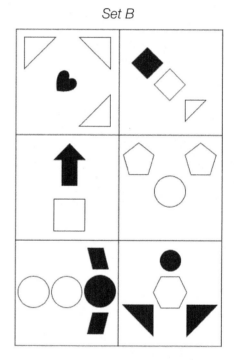

Question 16

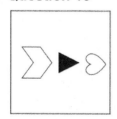

   a. Set A
   b. Set B
   c. Neither

Question 17

a. Set A
b. Set B
c. Neither

Question 18

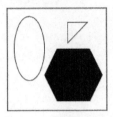

a. Set A
b. Set B
c. Neither

Question 19

a. Set A
b. Set B
c. Neither

Question 20

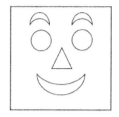

    a.   Set A
    b.   Set B
    c.   Neither

Question Set 5

Set A

Set B

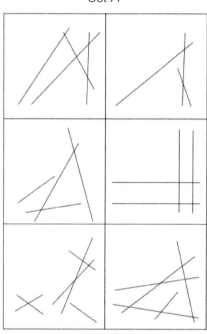
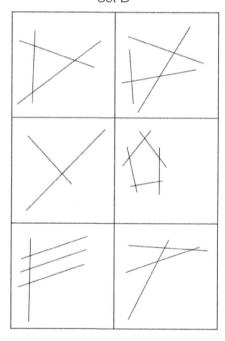

Question 21

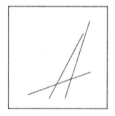

    a.   Set A
    b.   Set B
    c.   Neither

Question 22

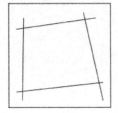

    a.   Set A
    b.   Set B
    c.   Neither

Question 23

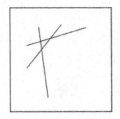

    a.   Set A
    b.   Set B
    c.   Neither

Question 24

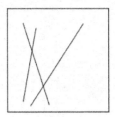

    a.   Set A
    b.   Set B
    c.   Neither

Question 25

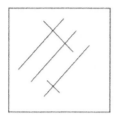

    a. Set A
    b. Set B
    c. Neither

Question Set 6

Set A

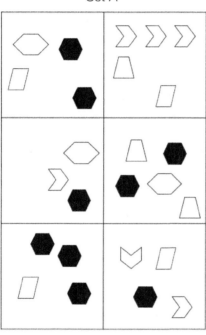

Set B

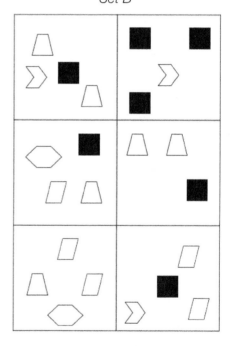

Question 26

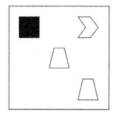

    a. Set A
    b. Set B
    c. Neither

Question 27

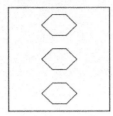

    a.   Set A
    b.   Set B
    c.   Neither

Question 28

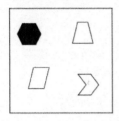

    a.   Set A
    b.   Set B
    c.   Neither

Question 29

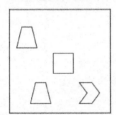

    a.   Set A
    b.   Set B
    c.   Neither

Question 30

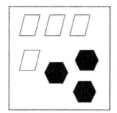

    a. Set A

    b. Set B

    c. Neither

Question Set 7

Set A

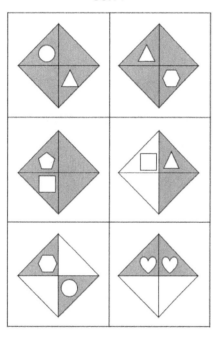

Set B

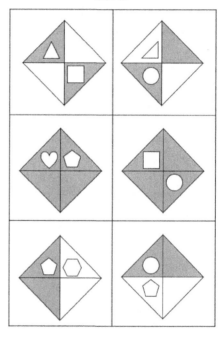

Question 31

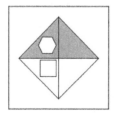

    a. Set A

    b. Set B

    c. Neither

Question 32

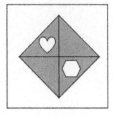

a. Set A
b. Set B
c. Neither

Question 33

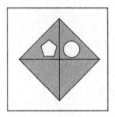

a. Set A
b. Set B
c. Neither

Question 34

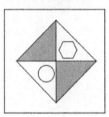

a. Set A
b. Set B
c. Neither

Question 35

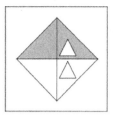

    a. Set A
    b. Set B
    c. Neither

Question Set 8

Set A

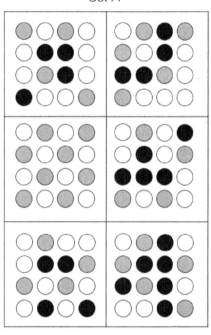

Set B

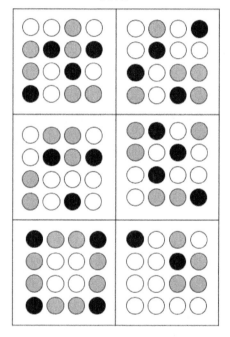

Question 36

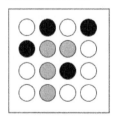

    a. Set A
    b. Set B
    c. Neither

Question 37

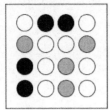

    a.   Set A
    b.   Set B
    c.   Neither

Question 38

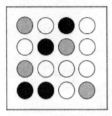

    a.   Set A
    b.   Set B
    c.   Neither

Question 39

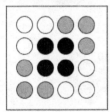

    a.   Set A
    b.   Set B
    c.   Neither

Question 40

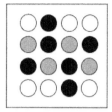

   a. Set A
   b. Set B
   c. Neither

Question Set 9

Set A

Set B

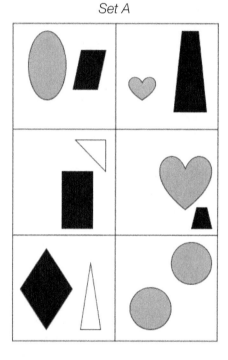
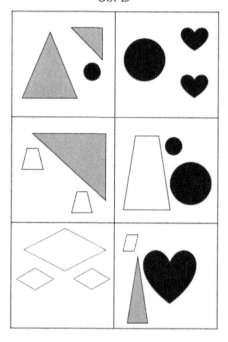

Question 41

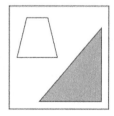

   a. Set A
   b. Set B
   c. Neither

Question 42

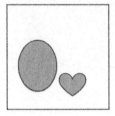

    a. Set A
    b. Set B
    c. Neither

Question 43

    a. Set A
    b. Set B
    c. Neither

Question 44

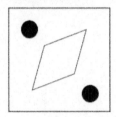

    a. Set A
    b. Set B
    c. Neither

Question 45

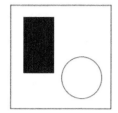

   a. Set A
   b. Set B
   c. Neither

Question Set 10

Set A

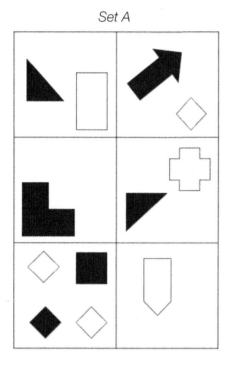

Set B

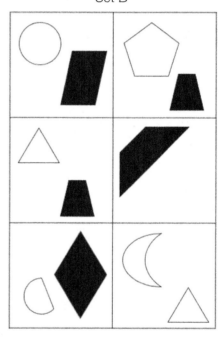

Question 46

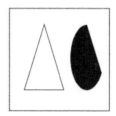

   a. Set A
   b. Set B
   c. Neither

Question 47

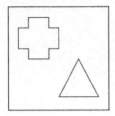

    a. Set A
    b. Set B
    c. Neither

Question 48

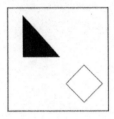

    a. Set A
    b. Set B
    c. Neither

Question 49

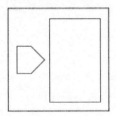

    a. Set A
    b. Set B
    c. Neither

Question 50

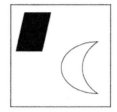

    a. Set A

    b. Set B

    c. Neither

Answers: Abstract Reasoning Mock

Question Set 1

SET A: All shapes have an even number of sides. There is an odd number of these shapes.
SET B: All shapes have an odd number of sides. There is an even number of these shapes.

Question 1: A

All shapes have an even number of sides, and there are three shapes. Therefore, this belongs to set A.

Question 2: A

There are three shapes, and all have an even number of sides, so this belongs to set A.

Question 3: C

Two of the shapes have an odd number of sides, and one has an even number of sides. Therefore, this belongs to neither set.

Question 4: C

The shape has only one side, but there is only one shape. Since both factors cannot be odd, this belongs to neither set.

Question 5: B

Both shapes have an odd number of sides, and there is an even number of shapes. Therefore, this belongs to set B.

Top Tip: Try to work through each of the possible patterns in a systematic way e.g. using SPONCS. This will ensure that you do not miss any key patterns.

Question Set 2

SET A: If the number of overlaps is even, the arrow is shaded. If the number of overlaps is odd, the arrow is white.
SET B: If the number of overlaps is even, the arrow points up. If the number of overlaps is odd, the arrow points down.

Question 6: C

There is an even number of overlaps. However, the arrow is white, so this cannot belong to set A. This cannot belong to set B as the arrow points down. Therefore, this belongs to neither set.

Question 7: A

There is one overlap. There is one white arrow which points down, so this belongs to set A.

Question 8: B

There is one overlap. The only arrow is shaded and points up, so this belongs to set B.

Question 9: A

There are four overlaps and one shaded arrow which points up. Therefore, this belongs to set A.

Question 10: C

There are two overlaps. The arrow is white, so this cannot belong to set A. The arrow points up, so this cannot belong to set B.

Top Tip: Memorise the common triggers. These are aspects of each set which might lead you to look for specific patterns. In this scenario, the presence of arrows should trigger you to think about direction (up/down) and colour as potential patterns.

Question Set 3

SET A: The number of squares is equal to the number of circles.
SET B: The number of triangles is equal to the number of pentagons.

Question 11: A

There is one square and one circle, so this belongs to set A.

Question 12: A

There are three squares and three circles, so this belongs to set A.

Question 13: C

There are two squares and only one circle, so this cannot belong to set A. There are no triangles, so this cannot belong to set B. Therefore, this belongs to neither set.

Question 14: C

There are no squares or circles, so this cannot belong to set A. There are two triangles and one pentagon, so this cannot belong to set B. Therefore, this belongs to neither set.

Question 15: B

There are two pentagons and two triangles, so this belongs to set B.

Top Tip: To work out the pattern, look at the simplest box in each set first. Once you think you have spotted a pattern, check this against the most complicated boxes in the set.

Question Set 4

SET A: The total number of sides is 10. There are no lines of symmetry.
SET B: The total number of sides is 11. There is at least one line of symmetry.

Question 16: B

There are 11 sides in total and one line of symmetry, so this belongs to set B.

Question 17: C

There are 11 sides in total, but there are no lines of symmetry, so this cannot belong to set B. Therefore, this belongs to neither set.

Question 18: A

There are 10 sides in total, and no lines of symmetry, so this belongs to set A.

Question 19: C

There are 10 sides in total, but there is a line of symmetry, so this cannot belong to set A. Therefore, this belongs to neither set.

Question 20: B

There are 11 sides in total and one line of symmetry, so this belongs to set B.

Timing Tip: It is easy to become overwhelmed by the pattern on first glance. Focus on one set first and work out the pattern. For example, once you have worked out the pattern in set A, see whether a similar pattern applies to set B.

Question Set 5

SET A: There are an even number of intersections. The top left corner of each box is blank.
SET B: There are an odd number of intersections. The bottom right corner of each box is blank.

Question 21: A

There are two intersections and the top left of the corner is blank, so this belongs to set A.

Question 22: C

There are four intersections, but the top left of the corner is not blank, so this cannot belong to set A. Therefore, this belongs to neither set.

Question 23: B

There are an odd number of intersections and the bottom right corner is empty. Therefore, this belongs to set B.

Question 24: C

There are two intersections but the top left corner is occupied by the lines, so this cannot belong to set A. Therefore, this belongs to neither set.

Question 25: B

There are three intersections, and the bottom right corner is blank. Therefore, this belongs to set B.

Common Trap: Some candidates will only spot one part of the pattern, for example, the number of intersections. Always work through all the possible pattern types to make sure you do not miss any additional patterns.

Question Set 6

SET A: There are three hexagons in every box. All regular hexagons are shaded black.
SET B: There are three quadrilaterals in every box. All squares are shaded black.

Question 26: B

There are three quadrilaterals in the box. The square is shaded black. Therefore, this belongs to set B.

Question 27: A

There are three hexagons. They are all irregular, and none are shaded, so this belongs to set A.

Question 28: C

There are two hexagons and two quadrilaterals, so this cannot belong to either set.

Question 29: C

There are three quadrilaterals, but the square is unshaded, so this cannot belong to set B. Therefore, this belongs to neither set.

Question 30: A

There are three hexagons. They are all regular and all shaded, so this belongs to set A.

Question Set 7

SET A: If the shape in the top left segment has an even number of sides, two of the segments will be shaded. If the shape in the top left segment has an odd number of sides, all the segments will be shaded.

SET B: If the shape in the top left has an odd number of sides, two of the segments will be shaded. If the shape in the top left segment has an even number of sides, all the segments will be shaded.

Question 31: A

The shape in the top left corner has an even number of sides and there are two shaded segments, so this belongs to set A.

Question 32: B

The shape in the top left corner has an even number of sides and all segments are shaded, so this belongs to set B.

Question 33: A

The shape in the top left corner has an odd number of sides, and all segments are shaded, so this belongs to set B.

Question 34: C

There is no shape in the top left corner, so this cannot belong to either set.

Question 35: C

There is no shape in the top left corner, so this cannot belong to either set.

Timing Tip: Some patterns are intentionally very difficult to spot and are classed as time wasters. Try not to spend more than a minute per pattern; if it is taking too long, flag the questions and come back to them at the end.

Question Set 8

SET A: Grey circles are never horizontally or vertically adjacent.
SET B: Black circles are never horizontally or vertically adjacent.

Question 36: B

The black circles are not horizontally or vertically adjacent, so this belongs to set B.

Question 37: C

The black circles and grey circles are both adjacent to each other, so this cannot belong to either set.

Question 38: A

The grey circles are not horizontally or vertically adjacent, so this belongs to set A.

Question 39: C

The black and grey circles are both adjacent to each other, so this cannot belong to either set.

Question 40: A

The grey circles are not horizontally or vertically adjacent, so this belongs to set A.

Top Tip: Whenever you see grey shapes, think about colour as a potential pattern. In the AR section, black and white are commonly used but grey shapes will often indicate a colour pattern.

Question Set 9

SET A: There are two shapes. All shapes with curved sides are shaded grey. All shapes with four sides are shaded black.
SET B: There are three shapes. All shapes with curved sides are black. All triangles are shaded grey.

Question 41: C

There are two shapes, but the shape with four sides is not shaded black, so this cannot belong to set A. Therefore, this belongs to neither set.

Question 42: A

There are two shapes. Both shapes have curved sides and they are both shaded grey, so this belongs to set A.

Question 43: A

There are two shapes which have four sides. Both shapes are shaded, so this belongs to set A.

Question 44: B

There are three shapes. Both circles are shaded, and the quadrilateral is not, so this belongs to set B.

Question 45: C

There are two shapes, but the shape with curved sides is not shaded. Therefore, this cannot belong to set A.

Top Tip: Think about which patterns are most common. Number patterns are generally uncommon unless there are few shapes in each box.

Question Set 10

SET A: All shapes have right angles. Colour is irrelevant.
SET B: No shapes have right angles. Colour is irrelevant.

Question 46: B

Neither of the shapes have right angles. Therefore, this belongs to set B.

Question 47: C

One shape has right angles and the other does not, so this belongs to neither set.

Question 48: A

Both shapes have right angles, so this belongs to set A.

Question 49: A

Both shapes have right angles, so this belongs to set A.

Question 50: B

Neither shape has a right angle, so this belongs to set B.

Timing Tip: Try to work out how much time each question should take. Remember that there are only 13 minutes for the whole AR section, so each set should take you around a minute.

Situational Judgement Test

Situational Judgement Tips

The Situational Judgement is the final section of the UCAT. It looks at how you would react in certain clinical or professional settings. Despite being the last section, and arguably the least time pressured, do not think that it is any less important. You need to make sure that you do not neglect it so you ensure you are a Band 3 or above as this is a common cut-off for lots of UCAT universities. These ten tips will help you to succeed with your preparation.

1.   Make sure you look at the GMC guidance

Many students tend to learn UCAT Situational Judgement by trial and error. Doing mock questions is great practice however. As with every part of the UCAT, it is best to learn the **theory** first. This will then give you a great foundation for practising this section.

The GMC is the General Medical Council in the UK. Amongst other things, they set the professional standards expected of medical students and doctors in the UK. The UCAT was designed to be used for admission to NHS UK medical schools so a lot of the answers for the Situational Judgement section are based around the GMC's published guidance.

The first thing to do is to read through and got your head around the GMC guidelines. The document is quite long so it may help if you make your own document to summarise them in. This will mean you always have something to refer back to while you are practising. Over time, try to refer less and less to the document when you answer.

The GMC have also published guidance for medical students. This covers the same principles as the original document but is more tailored to situations you may encounter during medical school. A lot of the scenarios given to you will be like this so it's a good addition to your revision.

2.   Understand the options

The difference between the SJT options in the UCAT can be incredibly minute and consequently, very confusing! In order to choose the right answer, you need to understand what the options mean. Here's a guide to one of the most common question types:

- *A very appropriate thing to do* means it addresses the main problem in the stem without negative consequences
- *Appropriate, but not ideal* means that whilst it solves one of the issues in the stem, it isn't the most ideal solution
- *Inappropriate, but not awful* means that it has transient negative consequences

- *A very inappropriate thing to do* means it either doesn't address the problem at all or actively makes the issue worse

3.   Use the 'Rule of 3' when reading the question

The 'rule of 3' comprises the three primary things you need to make a mental note of before attempting the question. These are:

- **Role:** What is your role in this scenario? How a doctor reacts to a situation will be very different to how a medical student may be expected to act. Therefore, note down your role and react accordingly.
- **Setting:** How one responds to a scenario depends on the setting of the problem. For example, it is always best to have personal conversations with a colleague in private and so, doing this in public would be inappropriate.
- **Main problem:** Most scenarios will have more than one issue that needs solving; find the main one and focus on solving it in the most appropriate manner.

4.   Always keep the patient at the forefront of your decision-making

Patient safety is a key factor in decision making in Medicine. This included their health and physical safety, but also safety of their information (i.e. confidentiality). Therefore, options that do not respect these are often inappropriate. Similarly, scenarios where patient safety is at stake, amongst other problems, should prompt recognition that this is the primary issue. It can be helpful to use the four pillars of medical ethics when considering what is best for patients:

- **Beneficence** – "do good", consider if your actions benefit the patient
- **Non-Maleficence** – "do no harm", consider if your actions are causing the patient harm and how to avoid this
- **Autonomy** – allowing the patient to make their own decisions and respecting them
- **Justice** – treat all patients equally and in consideration of the law

5.   Don't neglect the Situational Judgement section

As aforementioned, being the last section, some students neglect this section.

It is important to note that some universities look at Situational Judgement more than others. For some universities, your application will not be considered if you have a poor score but apart from this the section is not considered. Other universities will put a greater emphasis on Situational Judgement by using it as part of the MMI interview process. Make sure to research your chosen universities and find out just how much it is taken into account.

Regardless of how much your chosen Universities consider the SJT section, it is critical that you do not neglect studying for it. As scoring highly in this section will keep as many options as possible open to you when applying.

Additionally, your SJT score is the only score that you cannot hide behind your UCAT average as it is stated as a separate "banding score" alongside your UCAT total or average numerical score.

This section has a different scoring system to the other sections, so it's useful to familiarise yourself with this too.

Band 1	Performed at an excellent level, displaying judgement similar to the majority of the expert panel.
Band 2	Displayed a decent level of performance, often demonstrating appropriate judgement, with several responses corresponding to model answers.
Band 3	Performed at a modest level, displaying appropriate judgement for some questions and significant differences from model responses for other questions.
Band 4	Performed poorly, displaying significantly different judgement than the model response in several cases.

6. Search for resources carefully

Situational Judgement tests are used throughout medical careers for doctors at all stages of training. For example, situational judgement tests are used at university, during Foundation Years and even when you specialise. Therefore, make sure to search for 'Situational Judgement UCAT' if you're looking for the best questions. There is so much out there, you what to make sure the ones you are doing are appropriate, as you don't want to end up doing a Cardiology Speciality test!

Additionally, various resources will argue their own rationales for the problems in the SJT. Therefore, it's important to rely on formal sources and experts to guide you.

7. Analyse the rationale properly

When practising, it is important to understand the reason behind the right answers. This is the case even if you got it right. If a book or question bank doesn't give good explanations for the questions, then it may be an inadequate resource to prepare you. If this is the case, try and reference back to the GMC guidance and see where your particular scenario would fit in.

As you do more scenarios, you'll find that certain themes and rules pop up more than others. Use these as a guide to answer questions! For example, when solving interprofessional issues, always solve them locally (i.e. with the person in question) before escalating unless there is an acute threat to someone's safety.

8. Prepare for the full length of the test

Many students' intellectual energy fades during the Situational Judgement section. They have prepared hard for the other sections and have expended all their energy answering all of the previous questions. This impacts their score in the final section as they run out of steam right at the end. Remember that your score for this section is reported separately – there's no point getting 900 (the maximum score) in all other sections if you have no energy left for situational judgement and get a Band 4!

You need to make sure that this does not happen to you on test day. Make sure you practise mock exams that are the full length of the UCAT, so you will learn the stamina needed to get you all the way through on test day. Remember if you get extra time in the test be sure to add this on to your practise.

9. Timing tips

This section is the least time pressured section. You have the luxury of having time to fully read each question carefully to make sure you don't miss any key details. In the Situational Judgement section you have 26 minutes to answer 69 questions, so ensure you use this time well. Make sure not to rush but think carefully about your answers. Equally, do not become complacent – the test is not finished yet.

Once again this reiterates why it is so important not to neglect this section of the test. Practising and preparing for it will allow you to find a rhythm when answering the questions. And by knowing roughly how long it takes you to answer a question, you will know on test day if you answering too slowly or too quickly.

10. Do not be too indecisive

Sometimes students deliberate too much in Situational Judgement and go back and forth between answer options. You will get a half mark just for getting the right side (a/b or c/d). This does not mean that you should rush, but try not to spend too long deciding between a or b for example.

Practise is something that will help significantly if this is something that you struggle with. It will allow you to get used to the question types and understand the ethics behind the questions. Once you are familiar with both of these things you will be able to **move through the questions confidently and efficiently.**

Situational Judgement Mock

Question Set 1

Dr Green is a GP partner working in a large GP practice. One of her patients is a 19-year-old woman. She tells Dr Green that she regularly smokes cannabis and often takes stronger drugs at parties. Dr Green knows these drugs are illegal and is unsure whether she should report the patient.

How **appropriate** are each of the following responses by **<u>Dr Green</u>** in this situation?

1. Report the patient to the police
   a. A very appropriate thing to do
   b. Appropriate, but not ideal
   c. Inappropriate, but not awful
   d. A very inappropriate thing to do

2. Advise the patient on drug addiction
   a. A very appropriate thing to do
   b. Appropriate, but not ideal
   c. Inappropriate, but not awful
   d. A very inappropriate thing to do

3. Threaten to report the patient unless she stops taking drugs
   a. A very appropriate thing to do
   b. Appropriate, but not ideal
   c. Inappropriate, but not awful
   d. A very inappropriate thing to do

4. Tell the patient's parents about her drug use
   a. A very appropriate thing to do
   b. Appropriate, but not ideal
   c. Inappropriate, but not awful
   d. A very inappropriate thing to do

5. Do nothing
   a. A very appropriate thing to do
   b. Appropriate, but not ideal
   c. Inappropriate, but not awful
   d. A very inappropriate thing to do

Question Set 2

Jack is a fifth-year medical student undertaking his neurosurgery placement. Today, he is shadowing a consultant surgeon called Mr Whitehall. Mr Whitehall is due to perform surgery on his patient to remove a tumour, which is a delicate and complex operation. Whilst Jack is scrubbing into the surgery, he smells alcohol on Mr Whitehall breath and is concerned he may have been drinking before the surgery.

*How **appropriate** are each of the following responses by **Jack** in this situation?*

6. Report Mr Whitehall to the GMC
   a. A very appropriate thing to do
   b. Appropriate, but not ideal
   c. Inappropriate, but not awful
   d. A very inappropriate thing to do

7. Ask another medical student for help
   a. A very appropriate thing to do
   b. Appropriate, but not ideal
   c. Inappropriate, but not awful
   d. A very inappropriate thing to do

8. Talk to Mr Whitehall in private and raise his concerns
   a. A very appropriate thing to do
   b. Appropriate, but not ideal
   c. Inappropriate, but not awful
   d. A very inappropriate thing to do

9. Talk to the theatre manager about his concerns
   a. A very appropriate thing to do
   b. Appropriate, but not ideal
   c. Inappropriate, but not awful
   d. A very inappropriate thing to do

10. Confront Mr Whitehall in front of the theatre team
   a. A very appropriate thing to do
   b. Appropriate, but not ideal
   c. Inappropriate, but not awful
   d. A very inappropriate thing to do

11. Do nothing
    a. A very appropriate thing to do
    b. Appropriate, but not ideal
    c. Inappropriate, but not awful
    d. A very inappropriate thing to do

Question Set 3

Michael is a first-year medical student who is sitting his end of year exam. After the exam, lots of the medical students go to the pub. Jacob and Michael talk about the exam and Jacob mentions how he cheated in the exam by downloading a leaked question bank online. Michael knows that Jacob has violated their medical school's code of conduct but is unsure what to do.

*How **appropriate** are each of the following responses by **Michael** in this situation?*

12. Report Jacob to the Medical School
    a. A very appropriate thing to do
    b. Appropriate, but not ideal
    c. Inappropriate, but not awful
    d. A very inappropriate thing to do

13. Talk to Jacob and about his concerns and suggest he talks to the medical school
    a. A very appropriate thing to do
    b. Appropriate, but not ideal
    c. Inappropriate, but not awful
    d. A very inappropriate thing to do

14. Asks his advisor for advice
    a. A very appropriate thing to do
    b. Appropriate, but not ideal
    c. Inappropriate, but not awful
    d. A very inappropriate thing to do

15. Tweet about Jacob's cheating
    a. A very appropriate thing to do
    b. Appropriate, but not ideal
    c. Inappropriate, but not awful
    d. A very inappropriate thing to do

16. Ask another student for advice
    a. A very appropriate thing to do
    b. Appropriate, but not ideal
    c. Inappropriate, but not awful
    d. A very inappropriate thing to do

17. Do nothing
    a. A very appropriate thing to do
    b. Appropriate, but not ideal
    c. Inappropriate, but not awful
    d. A very inappropriate thing to do

Question Set 4

Susan is a junior doctor working an on-call weekend shift. She is called to a general medical ward by one of the nurses called Jeremy. Jeremy explains to Susan that he is worried for one of his patients, an elderly man called Bill. Susan assessed Bill early in the day and concluded his condition was stable and not serious, but Jeremy explained that Bill seems disorientated and is worried his condition is deteriorating. Susan is very busy and is unsure whether she should reassess Bill.

*How **appropriate** are each of the following responses by **Michael** in this situation?*

18. Reprimand Jeremy for wasting her time
    a. A very appropriate thing to do
    b. Appropriate, but not ideal
    c. Inappropriate, but not awful
    d. A very inappropriate thing to do

19. Don't assess Bill and tell Jeremy to call her if Bill's condition deteriorates
    a. A very appropriate thing to do
    b. Appropriate, but not ideal
    c. Inappropriate, but not awful
    d. A very inappropriate thing to do

20. Reassess Bill's condition
    a. A very appropriate thing to do
    b. Appropriate, but not ideal
    c. Inappropriate, but not awful
    d. A very inappropriate thing to do

21. Do nothing and walk away
    a. A very appropriate thing to do
    b. Appropriate, but not ideal
    c. Inappropriate, but not awful
    d. A very inappropriate thing to do

22. Report Jeremy to his supervisor for wasting her time
    a. A very appropriate thing to do
    b. Appropriate, but not ideal
    c. Inappropriate, but not awful
    d. A very inappropriate thing to do

23. Ask Bill some more questions to understand his concerns
    a. A very appropriate thing to do
    b. Appropriate, but not ideal
    c. Inappropriate, but not awful
    d. A very inappropriate thing to do

Question Set 5

Dr Lawton is a GP working in a London GP practice. One of his patients is a 22-year-old woman called Kimberly. Kimberly explains that she wants the contraceptive implant. However, Dr Lawton has a deeply held belief that contraception is morally wrong and so does not wish to perform the procedure to insert the implant.

How **appropriate** are each of the following responses by **Dr Lawton** in this situation?

24. Explain to Kimberly that she should not use contraception
    a. A very appropriate thing to do
    b. Appropriate, but not ideal
    c. Inappropriate, but not awful
    d. A very inappropriate thing to do

25. Refuse to perform the procedure
    a. A very appropriate thing to do
    b. Appropriate, but not ideal
    c. Inappropriate, but not awful
    d. A very inappropriate thing to do

26. Explain to Kimberley about his conscientious objection and refer her to another doctor
    a. A very appropriate thing to do
    b. Appropriate, but not ideal
    c. Inappropriate, but not awful
    d. A very inappropriate thing to do

27. Try to convince Kimberley not to use contraception
    a. A very appropriate thing to do
    b. Appropriate, but not ideal
    c. Inappropriate, but not awful
    d. A very inappropriate thing to do

Question Set 6

A group of nine third-year medical students are undertaking a group project which forms part of their grade. Their task is to create a presentation and every group member is required to contribute to the task. One of the group members, Chloe, has been consistently late to meetings and fails to complete her allocated work. Evie, the team leader, is becoming increasingly frustrated as Chloe's behaviour is impeding their process and she has noticed the rest of the group is becoming annoyed.

*How **appropriate** are each of the following responses by **Evie** in this situation?*

28. Complain about Chloe on social media
    a. A very appropriate thing to do
    b. Appropriate, but not ideal
    c. Inappropriate, but not awful
    d. A very inappropriate thing to do

29. Complain about Chloe to the rest of the group
    a. A very appropriate thing to do
    b. Appropriate, but not ideal
    c. Inappropriate, but not awful
    d. A very inappropriate thing to do

30. Report Chloe to their tutor
    a. A very appropriate thing to do
    b. Appropriate, but not ideal
    c. Inappropriate, but not awful
    d. A very inappropriate thing to do

31. Privately chat with Chloe and ask her why she is late to the meetings
    a. A very appropriate thing to do
    b. Appropriate, but not ideal
    c. Inappropriate, but not awful
    d. A very inappropriate thing to do

32. Speak to her advisor and ask for advice
    a. A very appropriate thing to do
    b. Appropriate, but not ideal
    c. Inappropriate, but not awful
    d. A very inappropriate thing to do

33. Wait and see if Evie's behaviour improves
    a. A very appropriate thing to do
    b. Appropriate, but not ideal
    c. Inappropriate, but not awful
    d. A very inappropriate thing to do

Question Set 7

Jane is a junior doctor working in a general surgery department. One of the patients on her ward is a 42-year-old man called Nick. A few weeks after Nick is discharged, Jane happens to meet him in a bar. He asks her if she wants to go on a date with him.

*How **important** to take into account are the following considerations for **Jane** when deciding how to respond to the situation?*

34. Jane was Nick's doctor
    a. Very important
    b. Important
    c. Of minor importance
    d. Not important at all

35. How Jane's decision may impact the public's trust in the medical profession
    a. Very important
    b. Important
    c. Of minor importance
    d. Not important at all

36. Nick is a man
    a. Very important
    b. Important
    c. Of minor importance
    d. Not important at all

37. Jane was not a key clinician in Nick's care
    a. Very important
    b. Important
    c. Of minor importance
    d. Not important at all

Question Set 8

John is a 42-year-old man who has been involved in a serious accident, and is rushed to A&E in an ambulance. On arrival, he is unconscious and therefore cannot communicate with the medical team. Due to the extensive nature of his injuries, he requires emergency surgery. However, the surgery is considered very high risk and John is unable to give consent. Dr Campbell believes the surgery is in John's best interests and that he will likely die without it.

*How **important** to take into account are the following considerations for **Dr Campbell** when deciding how to respond to the situation?*

38. John's right to make his own medical decisions
    a. Very important
    b. Important
    c. Of minor importance
    d. Not important at all

39. Whether John has an advanced directive
    a. Very important
    b. Important
    c. Of minor importance
    d. Not important at all

40. John's family's view on the surgery
    a. Very important
    b. Important
    c. Of minor importance
    d. Not important at all

41. John is 42 years old
    a. Very important
    b. Important
    c. Of minor importance
    d. Not important at all

42. Dr Campbell believes the surgery is in John's best interest
    a. Very important
    b. Important
    c. Of minor importance
    d. Not important at all

43. When John may regain capacity
    a. Very important
    b. Important
    c. Of minor importance
    d. Not important at all

Question Set 9

Dr Wickers is a new junior doctor working on a medical ward. It is her first job as a doctor, and she is very nervous about performing certain practical procedures. One of the senior nurses asks her to take a blood sample, a procedure Dr Wickers does not feel confident performing. Dr Wickers is unsure what to do.

*How **important** is it to take into account are the following considerations for __Dr Wickers__ when deciding how to respond to the situation?*

44. Dr Wicker's competence
    a. Very important
    b. Important
    c. Of minor importance
    d. Not important at all

45. The risks to the patient if she performs the procedure incorrectly
    a. Very important
    b. Important
    c. Of minor importance
    d. Not important at all

46. It was a nurse who requested it
    a. Very important
    b. Important
    c. Of minor importance
    d. Not important at all

47. Dr Wicker's professional development
    a. Very important
    b. Important
    c. Of minor importance
    d. Not important at all

48. Taking blood is an important skill for a doctor
    a. Very important
    b. Important
    c. Of minor importance
    d. Not important at all

Question Set 10

Holly is a junior doctor working in intensive care medicine and anaesthetics. She is on call for the intensive care unit. Two patients are admitted and require a specialised life support machine. However, only one machine is available. Holly must decide which patient should be given the machine.

*How **important** is it to take into account are the following considerations for **Holly** when deciding how to respond to the situation?*

49. The gender of the patients
    a. Very important
    b. Important
    c. Of minor importance
    d. Not important at all

50. The patient's age
    a. Very important
    b. Important
    c. Of minor importance
    d. Not important at all

51. The survival chance of the patients
    a. Very important
    b. Important
    c. Of minor importance
    d. Not important at all

52. Any legal responsibilities Holly has
    a. Very important
    b. Important
    c. Of minor importance
    d. Not important at all

53. The underlying disease in each patient
    a. Very important
    b. Important
    c. Of minor importance
    d. Not important at all

Question Set 11

Pete is a 26-year-old who has been diagnosed with a chronic illness. At their next follow up appointment, Pete informs Dr Arnott that he has stopped taking his medication as he believes that a combination of a vegan diet, essential oils and yoga will cure his illness. Dr Arnott is deeply concerned as he knows Pete will continue to deteriorate if he does not take the prescribed medication.

*How **important** is it to take into account are the following considerations for **<u>Dr Arnott</u>** when deciding how to respond to the situation?*

54. The side effects of the medications
    a. Very important
    b. Important
    c. Of minor importance
    d. Not important at all

55. Pete is male
    a. Very important
    b. Important
    c. Of minor importance
    d. Not important at all

56. The evidence behind Pete's alternative medicine
    a. Very important
    b. Important
    c. Of minor importance
    d. Not important at all

57. Pete's right to make his own decisions about his health
    a. Very important
    b. Important
    c. Of minor importance
    d. Not important at all

58. The consequence of Pete no taking his medication
    a. Very important
    b. Important
    c. Of minor importance
    d. Not important at all

Question Set 12

Rosie is a second-year medical student who lives with another medical student called Jacob. Jacob has noticed Rosie is becoming more distant and has become very socially isolated. Jacob is concerned it is starting to affect her studies as she is often late to medical school and is not completing the work.

*How **important** is it to take into account are the following considerations for **Jacob** when deciding how to respond to the situation?*

59. That Rosie may face consequences to her degree and future registration
    a. Very important
    b. Important
    c. Of minor importance
    d. Not important at all

60. Why Rosie is becoming more isolated
    a. Very important
    b. Important
    c. Of minor importance
    d. Not important at all

61. That Rosie's medical school performance is being affected
    a. Very important
    b. Important
    c. Of minor importance
    d. Not important at all

62. How it is affecting Rosie's clinical performance
    a. Very important
    b. Important
    c. Of minor importance
    d. Not important at all

Question Set 13

Joe is a 4th year medical student on her GP placement. The first patient in the clinic is a 19-year-old student called Alfie. The GP informs Alfie that he will have to stop driving until his condition has been treated. A few days later, Joe notices Mike driving a car through the city centre.

*How **important** is it to take into account are the following considerations for **Joe** when deciding how to respond to the situation?*

63. Joe is only a medical student
    a. Very important
    b. Important
    c. Of minor importance
    d. Not important at all

64. Alfie is 19 years old
    a. Very important
    b. Important
    c. Of minor importance
    d. Not important at all

65. Alfie's right to confidentiality
    a. Very important
    b. Important
    c. Of minor importance
    d. Not important at all

66. If Alfie continue driving, he could be a danger to the public
    a. Very important
    b. Important
    c. Of minor importance
    d. Not important at all

Question 67

Charlotte is a 3rd Year Medical Student shadowing a GP, Dr Fraser. Dr Fraser prescribes the patient some antibiotics. Charlotte has read the patient's notes and knows that he is severely allergic to this particular medication.

*Choose **both** the **one most appropriate action** and the **one least appropriate action** that **Charlotte** should take in response to this situation.*

*You will not receive any marks for this question unless you select **both** the most and least appropriate actions.*

Options:
    a. Ask the patient whether she is allergic to these antibiotics
    b. Gently interrupt Dr Fraser and remind her the patient is allergic to the antibiotics
    c. Do nothing

Question 68

Mike is a 1st Year Medical Student shadowing a cardiologist Dr Witty. The GP asks Mike to take an ABG (arterial blood gas). However, Mike has never performed an ABG before and does not believe he has the skill to carry it out.

*Choose **both** the **one most appropriate action** and the **one least appropriate action** that **Mike** should take in response to this situation.*

*You will not receive any marks for this question unless you select **both** the **most and least appropriate actions.***

Options:
    a. Ask Dr Witty for help and explain he has never performed an ABG before
    b. Do the procedure anyway
    c. Don't perform the procedure but don't tell anyone

Question 69

Dr Patterson is a GP trainee working in a large GP practice. The patient comes in with a suspected chest infection. Dr Patterson takes a medical history and decides it is appropriate to prescribe antibiotics. He decides to prescribe penicillin however, the patient says she is allergic to penicillin despite it not being recorded in her notes.

Choose **both** the **one most appropriate action** and the **one least appropriate action** that **<u>Dr Patterson</u>** *should take in response to this situation.*

You will not receive any marks for this question unless you select **both** *the* **most and least appropriate actions.**

Options:

    a. Report the incident via the appropriate reporting procedure

    b. Assume the patient is mistaken and take no further action

    c. Add the penicillin allergy into the patient's medical notes

Answers: Situational Judgement Mock

Question Set 1

Question 1: D

Very inappropriate – in some circumstances, disclosure of confidential information to the police is acceptable. This is governed by GMC guidance which states "Such a situation might arise, for example, if a disclosure would be likely to be necessary for the prevention, detection or prosecution of serious crime, especially crimes against the person. When victims of violence refuse police assistance, disclosure may still be justified if others remain at risk, for example from someone who is prepared to use weapons, or from domestic violence when children or others may be at risk." (GMC Confidentiality Guidelines, p34). The keyword is **'serious'**, taking drugs is not a serious criminal offence. Furthermore, you have to consider that by reporting patients for drug use (a very common occurrence), you are endangering the patient's trust in you and therefore restricting their access to healthcare. Therefore on balance, disclosure in this case **would not** be justified and this action would breach confidentiality. Therefore, this action would be **very inappropriate**.

Question 2: A

Very appropriate – this action would provide the patient with good medical care whilst not inappropriately disclosing medical information. Therefore, this action is **very appropriate**.

Question 3: D

Very inappropriate – in this case, disclosure would not be justified as drug use is not a serious crime. Therefore, by threatening to report the patient Dr Green would be lying to the patient which violates Good Medical Practice which states "Patients need good doctors. Good doctors… are honest and trustworthy, and act with integrity and within the law" (Good Medical Practice, p4). Therefore, this action is **very inappropriate**.

Question 4: D

Very inappropriate – in this case, disclosure would not be justified as drug use is not a serious crime. Therefore, by informing the patient's parents, Dr Green would be breaching confidentiality which violates Good Medical Practice which states "You must treat information about patients as confidential. This includes after a patient has died" (Good Medical Practice, p17). Therefore, this action is **very inappropriate**.

Question 5: C

Inappropriate but not awful – this action would not unnecessarily breach confidentiality which is consistent with GMC confidentiality guidelines. Therefore this action is **not** very inappropriate. However, this action would not address the patient's potential addiction and therefore is **not** appropriate. Therefore, this action is **inappropriate but not awful**.

Top Tip: There should be a presumption against breaking confidentiality, confidentiality should only be broken in very specific circumstances.

Question Set 2

Question 6: D

Very inappropriate – by taking this action Jack would unnecessarily escalate the situation without first talking to Mr Whitehall. Furthermore, this action would not tackle the immediate patient safety issue which violates Good Medical Practice which states "[you must] Take prompt action if you think that patient safety, dignity or comfort is being compromised" (Good Medical Practice, p11). Therefore, this action would be **very inappropriate**.

Question 7: B

Appropriate but not ideal – this action would allow Jack to seek advice from a colleague which is **appropriate**. This is outlined in "In providing clinical care you must: consult colleagues where appropriate" (Good Medical Practice, p8). However, this action is not very appropriate as Jack is involving another member of staff before talking to the surgeon and therefore is potentially spreading sensitive information about the surgeon. Therefore, this action would be **appropriate but not ideal**.

Question 8: A

Very appropriate – This action would allow Jack to protect patient safety and so he is abiding by the **key principle of protecting patients**. This principle is outlined in Good Medical Practice which states "[you must] Take prompt action if you think that patient safety, dignity or comfort is being compromised" (Good Medical Practice, p11). Jack is also being sensitive regarding the surgeon's drinking, as this action will allow him to ascertain whether the surgeon may require help which is in line with Good Medical Practice which states "You must treat colleagues fairly and with respect" (Good Medical Practice, p14). Therefore, this action would be **very appropriate**.

Question 9: B

Appropriate but not ideal – by taking this action, Jack would be protecting patient safety and so is consistent with Good Medical Practice which states "[you must] Take prompt action if you think that patient safety, dignity or comfort is being compromised" (Good Medical Practice, p11). However, Jack is involving another member of staff before talking to the surgeon and therefore is potentially spreading sensitive information about the surgeon. Remember, you should always try and address the issue with the person concerned before escalating your concerns. Therefore, this action would be **appropriate but not ideal**.

Question 10: D

Very inappropriate – by confronting the surgeon in front of other members of staff, Jack is being unnecessarily aggressive and disrespectful to Mr Whitehall. This violates Good Medical Practice which states "You must treat colleagues fairly and with respect" (Good Medical Practice, p14). Therefore, this action would be **very inappropriate**.

Question 11: D

Very inappropriate – if a surgeon was under the influence the alcohol, this could jeopardise patient safety. Jack's primary concern **must** be the patient's safety as outlined in Good Medical Practice which states "[you must] Take prompt action if you think that patient safety, dignity or comfort is being compromised" (Good Medical Practice, p11). Therefore, by doing nothing Jack would be knowingly jeopardising patient safety so, this action would be **very inappropriate**.

Top Tip: Remember, you should always try and address the issue with the person concerned before escalating your concerns.

Question Set 3

Question 12: B

Appropriate but not ideal – this action would allow Michael to raise his concerns about Jacob's cheating. As Jacob's cheating could jeopardise patient safety, this action is consistent with Good Medical Practice which states "[you must] Take prompt action if you think that patient safety, dignity or comfort is being compromised" (Good Medical Practice, p11). However, this action escalates his concerns without talking to Jacob first hence, this action is **appropriate** but **not** very appropriate. Therefore, this action is **appropriate but not ideal**.

Question 13: A

Very appropriate – this action allows Michael to raise his concerns (about cheating which could jeopardise patient safety) whilst still allowing Jacob to remedy his mistake before escalating his concerns. This complies with Good Medical Practice which states "[you must] Take prompt action if you think that patient safety, dignity or comfort is being compromised" (Good Medical Practice, p11) and "You must treat colleagues fairly and with respect" (Good Medical Practice, p14). Therefore, this action would be **very appropriate**.

Question 14: A

Very appropriate – asking for advice from a more senior colleague or a tutor regarding concerns around another student or healthcare professional will always be appropriate. This is outlined in GMC guidelines which state "If you're not sure whether you should raise a concern formally, you should ask your medical school or an experienced healthcare professional for advice. GMC guidance to doctors on raising concerns acknowledges issues like this, including, for example, if the person causing concern is part of the problem or the doctor doesn't have confidence that the concern will be addressed adequately based on previous experiences. You may therefore find this guidance helpful" (Achieving Good Medical Practice: Guidance for Medical Students, p22). Therefore, this action would be **very appropriate**.

Question 15: D

Very inappropriate – this action would not address the potential patient safety concerns caused by Jacob's cheating. Furthermore, this action would spread sensitive information about Jacob on a public forum which violates Good Medical Practice which states "You must treat colleagues fairly and with respect" (Good Medical Practice, p14). Therefore, this action would be **very inappropriate**.

Question 16: B

Appropriate but not ideal – asking another student for advice would help Michael to address the issue of Jacob's cheating and is consistent with Good Medical Practice which states "In providing clinical care you must: consult colleagues where appropriate" (Good Medical Practice, p8). However, by informing another student about the situation, Michael is potentially distributing sensitive information about Jacob and there are more suitable people to consult e.g. a tutor. Therefore, this action is **appropriate but not ideal**.

Question 17: D

Very inappropriate – by allowing a student to cheat on a medical exam, it may allow the graduation or progression of incompetent medical students which could jeopardise patient safety.

Therefore, Michael **must** act on his concerns as outlined in Good Medical Practice which states "[you must] Take prompt action if you think that patient safety, dignity or comfort is being compromised" (Good Medical Practice, p11). Therefore, this action is **very inappropriate**.

Top Tip: Patient safety must always be your primary consideration.

Question Set 4

Question 18: D

Very inappropriate – by reprimanding Jeremy for wasting her time, Susan is creating an environment where raising concerns is discouraged. This violates Good Medical Practice which states "You must promote and encourage a culture that allows all staff to raise concerns openly and safely" (Good Medical Practice, p11). Therefore, this action would be **very inappropriate**.

Question 19: C

Inappropriate but not awful – Susan has an obligation to work collaboratively with all her colleagues (including nurses) and to act on any concerns. Therefore, this action violates Good Medical Practice which states "You must work collaboratively with colleagues [colleagues include anyone a doctor works with, whether or not they are also doctors]" (Good Medical Practice, p14). Therefore, this action is **inappropriate**. However, this action is **not** very inappropriate because Susan puts a plan in place if Bill's condition gets worse and so Susan is protecting patient safety. Therefore, this action would be **inappropriate but not awful**.

Question 20: A

Very appropriate – this action would allow Susan to address Jeremy's concerns about Bill and ensure patient safety is being protected by reassessing Bill's condition. This is consistent with Good Medical Practice which states "You must work collaboratively with colleagues [colleagues include anyone a doctor works with, whether or not they are also doctors]" (Good Medical Practice, p14) and "[you must] Take prompt action if you think that patient safety, dignity or comfort is being compromised" (Good Medical Practice, p11). Therefore, this action would be **very appropriate**.

Question 21: D

Very inappropriate – this action would jeopardise patient safety as Susan is not addressing Jeremy concerns which violates Good Medical Practice which states "[you must] Take prompt action if you think that patient safety, dignity or comfort is being compromised" (Good Medical Practice, p11). Therefore, this action would be **very inappropriate**.

Question 22: D

Very inappropriate – by reporting Jeremy to his supervisor, Susan is creating an environment where raising concerns is discouraged. This violates Good Medical Practice which states "You must promote and encourage a culture that allows all staff to raise concerns openly and safely" (Good Medical Practice, p11). Therefore, this action would be **very inappropriate**.

Question 23: B

Appropriate but not ideal – this action would allow Susan to address Jeremy's concerns about Bill and so is **appropriate**. The reason this action is **not** very appropriate is because if a colleague is concerned about a patient, the ideal course of action would be to assess the patient as this would comply with Good Medical Practice which states "You must work collaboratively with colleagues [colleagues include anyone a doctor works with, whether or not they are also doctors]" (Good Medical Practice, p14). Therefore, this action is **appropriate but not ideal**.

Top Tip: Doctors have a responsibility to not only listen to their colleagues' concerns but also to promote a culture where concerns can be raised.

Question Set 5

Question 24: D

Inappropriate – doctors **must never** judge patients based on their own beliefs. If a doctor has a conscientious objection to a procedure, they must ensure the patient understands they are making no judgement on them. This is outlined in Good Medical Practice which states "You must explain to patients if you have a conscientious objection to a particular procedure. You must tell them about their right to see another doctor and make sure they have enough information to exercise that right. In providing this information you must not imply or express disapproval of the patient's lifestyle, choices or beliefs. If it is not practical for a patient to arrange to see another doctor, you must make sure that arrangements are made for another suitably qualified colleague to take over your role" (Good Medical Practice, p17). Therefore, by talking to Kimberly in a judgemental way, Dr Lawton's action would be **inappropriate**.

Question 25: D

Inappropriate – If a doctor has a conscientious objection to a procedure, they must ensure the patient understands they are making no judgement on them. This is outlined in Good Medical Practice which states "You must explain to patients if you have a conscientious objection to a particular procedure. You must tell them about their right to see another doctor and make sure they have enough information to exercise that right. In providing this information you must not imply or express disapproval of the patient's lifestyle, choices or beliefs.

If it is not practical for a patient to arrange to see another doctor, you must make sure that arrangements are made for another suitably qualified colleague to take over your role" (Good Medical Practice, p17). Therefore, by refusing to perform the procedure and not referring Kimberly to another doctor, Dr Lawton's action would be **inappropriate**.

Question 26: A

Appropriate – this action would allow Kimberly to get the procedure she requires and is also respectful of Kimberly's decision. This is consistent with Good Medical Practice which states "You must explain to patients if you have a conscientious objection to a particular procedure. You must tell them about their right to see another doctor and make sure they have enough information to exercise that right. In providing this information you must not imply or express disapproval of the patient's lifestyle, choices or beliefs. If it is not practical for a patient to arrange to see another doctor, you must make sure that arrangements are made for another suitably qualified colleague to take over your role" (Good Medical Practice, p17). Therefore, this action would be **appropriate**.

Question 27: D

Inappropriate – doctors **must never** judge patients based on their own beliefs. If a doctor has a conscientious objection to a procedure, they must ensure the patient understands they are making no judgement on them. This is outlined in Good Medical Practice which states "You must explain to patients if you have a conscientious objection to a particular procedure. You must tell them about their right to see another doctor and make sure they have enough information to exercise that right. In providing this information you must not imply or express disapproval of the patient's lifestyle, choices or beliefs. If it is not practical for a patient to arrange to see another doctor, you must make sure that arrangements are made for another suitably qualified colleague to take over your role" (Good Medical Practice, p17). Therefore, by talking to Kimberly in a judgemental way and not respecting her beliefs, Dr Lawton's action would be **inappropriate**.

Top Tip: If a doctor has a conscientious objection to a certain procedure, they must not be judgemental and they must offer the patient a consultation with another doctor who can perform the procedure.

Question Set 6

Question 28: D

Inappropriate – this action would be disrespectful to Chloe by complaining about her on social media. This violates Good Medical Practice which states "You must treat colleagues fairly and with respect" (Good Medical Practice, p14). Therefore, this action would be **inappropriate**.

Question 29: D

Inappropriate – this action would be disrespectful to Chloe by complaining about her to her peers. This violates Good Medical Practice which states "You must treat colleagues fairly and with respect" (Good Medical Practice, p14). Therefore, this action would be **inappropriate**.

Question 30: D

Inappropriate – by reporting Chloe to their tutor before trying to address the issue, Evie is unnecessarily escalating the situation. Remember, you should **always** try and address the issue before escalating it further. Therefore, this action would be **inappropriate**.

Question 31: A

Appropriate – this would be the ideal course of action as it allows Evie to address the issue of Chloe behaviour whilst being respectful to her. This is consistent with GMC guidelines which states "Persistent inappropriate attitude or behaviour [for a medical student includes] poor time management [and] non-attendance]" (Achieving Good Medical Practice: Guidance for Medical Students, p48) and "You must treat colleagues fairly and with respect" (Good Medical Practice, p14). Therefore, this action would be **appropriate**.

Question 32: A

Appropriate – it will always be appropriate to seek advice from an advisor if you have concerns about a colleague. This is outlined in GMC guidance which states "If you're not sure whether you should raise a concern formally, you should ask your medical school or an experienced healthcare professional for advice" (Achieving Good Medical Practice: Guidance for Medical Students, p22). Therefore, this action would be **appropriate**.

Question 33: D

Inappropriate – this action would not address the issue of Chloe's behaviour. This violates GMC guidance which states "It can be difficult to raise concerns about fellow students, who may be people you work with on projects or placements or your friends. But as a student choosing to join a regulated profession, it is your duty to put patients first and this includes patients you see on placements and those treated by your fellow students in the future." (Achieving Good Medical Practice: Guidance for Medical Students, p21). Therefore, this action would be inappropriate.

Top Tip: Questions about group work are very common in the SJT, so it is important to know how to answer them.

Question Set 7

Question 34: B

Important – a doctor **should not** enter a sexual or romantic relationship with a patient. This is outlined in Good Medical Practice which states "You must not use your professional position to pursue a sexual or improper emotional relationship with a patient or someone close to them" (Good Medical Practice, p18). Therefore, this consideration is **important**.

Question 35: B

Important – maintaining public trust is a key part of Good Medical Practice which states "You must make sure that your conduct justifies your patients' trust in you and the public's trust in the profession" (Good Medical Practice, p21). Therefore, this consideration is **important**.

Question 36: D

Not Important – Nick's gender is irrelevant to the situation as doctors must **never** discriminate against their patients for any reason, this principle is outlined in Good Medical Practice which states "You must not unfairly discriminate against patients or colleagues by allowing your personal views [This includes your views about a patient's or colleague's lifestyle, culture or their social or economic status, as well as the characteristics protected by legislation: age, disability, gender reassignment, race, marriage and civil partnership, pregnancy and maternity, religion or belief, sex and sexual orientation] to affect your professional relationships or the treatment you provide or arrange" (Good Medical Practice, p20). Therefore, this consideration is **not important**.

Question 37: D

Not Important – regardless of how involved Jane was involved in Nick's care, Jane was still in a position of trust as a result of her professional position and so it would be inappropriate to enter a sexual or romantic relationship with Nick. This is outlined in Good Medical Practice which states "You must not use your professional position to pursue a sexual or improper emotional relationship with a patient or someone close to them" (Good Medical Practice, p18). Therefore, this consideration is **not important**.

*Top Tip: Doctors **must not** enter into a sexual or romantic relationship with any of their patients.*

Question Set 8

Question 38: B

Important – the principle of autonomy is one of the four pillars of medical ethics. Autonomy is the right of a patient to control their own medical decisions. This principle is also outlined in Good Medical Practice which states "Respect patients' right to reach decisions with you about their treatment and care." (Good Medical Practice, p1). Therefore, this consideration is **important**.

Question 39: B

Important – checking for an advanced directive would allow Dr Campbell to determine whether Sarah has any specific wishes for her treatment and allow Dr Campbell to comply with GMC Consent Guidelines which state "If there is no evidence of a legally binding advance refusal of treatment, and no one has legal authority to make this decision for them, then you are responsible for deciding what would be of overall benefit to your patient." (Decision Making and Consent, p36). Therefore, this consideration is **important**.

Question 40: B

Important – considering what John's family believe would allow Dr Campbell to understand what John's wishes are. Therefore, this consideration is **important**.

Question 41: D

Not Important – John's age is irrelevant to the situation as doctors must not discriminate against patients based on any factors other than clinically relevant factors. This is outlined in Good Medical Practice which states "You must not unfairly discriminate against patients or colleagues by allowing your personal views [This includes your views about a patient's or colleague's lifestyle, culture or their social or economic status, as well as the characteristics protected by legislation: age, disability, gender reassignment, race, marriage and civil partnership, pregnancy and maternity, religion or belief, sex and sexual orientation] to affect your professional relationships or the treatment you provide or arrange" (Good Medical Practice, p20). Therefore, this consideration is **not important**.

Question 42: B

Important – Doctors must act in a patient's best interests. This is outlined in Good Medical Practice which states "They treat each patient as an individual. They do their best to make sure all patients receive good care and treatment that will support them to live as well as possible, whatever their illness or disability." (Good Medical Practice, p4). Therefore, this consideration is **important**.

Question 43: B

Important – If John may regain capacity in time to make a decision, then Dr Campbell must consider this as he has a responsibility to respect John's right to make his own decisions. This principle is also outlined in Good Medical Practice which states "[You should] respect patients' right to reach decisions with you about their treatment and care." (Good Medical Practice, p1). Therefore, this consideration is **important**.

Top Tip: If a patient does not have capacity, a doctor can give emergency treatment without consent if it is in their best interests.

Question Set 9

Question 44: A

Very Important – doctors **must** only perform procedures which they are competent to perform. This principle is outlined in Good Medical Practice which states "You must recognise and work within the limits of your competence" (Good Medical Practice, p7). Therefore, this consideration is **very important**.

Question 45: A

Very Important – patient safety **must** be your primary consideration and you **must** not do anything which endangers patient safety. This is outlined in Good Medical Practice which states "[you must] Take prompt action if you think that patient safety, dignity or comfort is being compromised" (Good Medical Practice, p11). Therefore, this consideration is **very important**.

Question 46: D

Not Important at all – the profession of the colleague requesting the procedure is irrelevant. Therefore, this factor **should not** be considered and so the consideration is **not important at all**.

Question 47: B

Important – doctors have a professional responsibility to keep their professional knowledge and skills up to date. This is outlined in Good Medical Practice which states "Patients need good doctors. Good doctors make the care of their patients their first concern: they are competent, keep their knowledge and skills up to date" (Good Medical Practice, p4). However, the reason this factor is **not** very important is because patient safety **must** be the primary consideration and Dr Wickers must not endanger it. Therefore, this consideration is **important**.

Question 48: B

Important – if Dr Wicker's is unable to perform a key practical procedure, she must take action to rectify this. This is outlined in Good Medical Practice which states "Patients need good doctors. Good doctors make the care of their patients their first concern: they are competent, keep their knowledge and skills up to date" (Good Medical Practice, p4). However, the reason this factor is **not** very important is because patient safety **must** be the primary consideration and Dr Wickers must not endanger it. Therefore, this consideration is **important**.

Top Tip: Doctors have a professional responsibility to maintain their professional skills and knowledge.

Question Set 10

Question 49: D

Not Important at All – the gender of the patients **must not** be considered as it is not clinically relevant and would likely be discriminatory. This violates Good Medical Practice which states "You must not unfairly discriminate against patients or colleagues by allowing your personal views [This includes your views about a patient's or colleague's lifestyle, culture or their social or economic status, as well as the characteristics protected by legislation: age, disability, gender reassignment, race, marriage and civil partnership, pregnancy and maternity, religion or belief, sex and sexual orientation] to affect your professional relationships or the treatment you provide or arrange" (Good Medical Practice, p20). Therefore, this factor **must not** be considered.

Question 50: B

Important – the principle of justice is one of the four pillars of medical ethics. Justice is the principle of ensuring doctor's actions are lawful, respect patient's rights and are fair. Part of this principle of fairness is ensuring that when resources are limited, they are distributed fairly. As the age of the patients may impact each patient's survival chance, this factor **should** be considered. The reason this factor is not very important is because their age is not the only factor which will affect the survival chance of the patients. Therefore, this factor **should** be considered.

Question 51: A

Very Important – the principle of justice is one of the four pillars of medical ethics. Justice is the principle of ensuring doctor's actions are lawful, respect patient's rights and are fair. Part of this principle of fairness is ensuring that when resources are limited, they are distributed fairly. Therefore, the survival chance of the patient's must be considered.

Question 52: A

Very Important – a key principle of medical ethics is that doctors must follow the law. This is outlined in Good Medical Practice which states "Patients need good doctors. Good doctors… act with integrity and within the law" (Good Medical Practice, p4). Therefore, this factor **must** be considered.

Question 53: B

Important – the principle of justice is one of the four pillars of medical ethics. Justice is the principle of ensuring doctor's actions are lawful, respect patient's rights and are fair. Part of this principle of fairness is ensuring that when resources are limited, they are distributed fairly. As the underlying disease may impact each patient's survival chance, this factor **should** be considered. The reason this factor is **not** very important is because their underlying disease is not the only factor which will affect the survival chance of each patient. Therefore, this factor **should** be considered.

Top Tip: Justice is one of the four pillars of medical practice. Justice is the principle of ensuring doctor's actions are lawful, respect patients' rights and are fair.

Question Set 11

Question 54: B

Important – Dr Arnott **must** take into account the benefits and risks (including side effects) of any medications. This principle is outlined in Good Medical Principle which states "You must work in partnership with patients, sharing with them the information they will need to make decisions about their care, including: their condition, its likely progression and the options for treatment, including associated risks and uncertainties" (Good Medical Practice, p16). However, the reason this factor is **not** very important is because in Dr Arnott's professional judgement, the medications are the most appropriate treatment option. Therefore, this consideration is **important**.

Question 55: D

Not Important at All – the gender of the patients **must not** be considered as it is not clinically relevant and would likely be discriminatory. This violates Good Medical Practice which states "You must not unfairly discriminate against patients or colleagues by allowing your personal views [This includes your views about a patient's or colleague's lifestyle, culture or their social or economic status, as well as the characteristics protected by legislation: age, disability, gender reassignment, race, marriage and civil partnership, pregnancy and maternity, religion or belief, sex and sexual orientation] to affect your professional relationships or the treatment you provide or arrange" (Good Medical Practice, p20). Therefore, this factor **must not** be considered.

Question 56: B

Important – Dr Arnott has a professional responsibility to use the best evidence to provide Pete with the best quality care. This principle is outlined in Good Medical Practice which states "In providing clinical care you must: provide effective treatments based on the best available evidence" (Good Medical Practice, p8). The reason this factor is **not** very important is because Dr Arnott knows alternative medicine is **not** the most appropriate treatment option. Therefore, this consideration is **important**.

Question 57: A

Very important – The principle of autonomy (the right to have control over your own treatment) is one of the four pillars of medical ethics. This principle is outlined in Good Medical Practice which states "You must work in partnership with patients, sharing with them the information they will need to make decisions about their care" (Good Medical Practice, p16). Therefore, Dr Arnott **must** consider Pete's right to autonomy, so this consideration is **very important**.

Question 58: A

Very Important – Dr Arnott's primary concern must be the best interest of the patient. This principle is contained in Good Medical Practice which states "In providing clinical care you must: provide effective treatments based on the best available evidence" (Good Medical Practice, p8). Therefore, if Dr Arnott is aware Pete is not receiving the most appropriate treatment, he **must** consider this factor. Therefore, this consideration is **very important**.

Top Tip: Whilst a doctor must provide the best clinical care to their patients, if a patient has capacity, they can make their own medical decision even if the doctor considers it inappropriate.

Question Set 12

Question 59: D

Not Important at all – patient safety and Rosie's wellbeing must be Jacob's primary considerations. Any other factors including his or Rosie's career must not be considered. Therefore, this consideration is **not important at all**.

Question 60: A

Very Important – the reason why Rosie is becoming more distant and isolated must be considered as it may be masking another problem e.g. bereavement. By understanding the problem, Jacob can understand any underlying reasons which would enable him to support Rosie or assist her to access the correct support.

This principle is outlined in GMC guidance which states "You must… support staff and fellow students, including those from other healthcare professions" (Achieving Good Medical Practice: Guidance for Medical Students, p30). Therefore, this consideration is **very important**.

Question 61: B

Important – Medical students have a professional responsibility to fully engage in the medical course. This principle is outlined in GMC guidance which states "You must engage fully with your medical course by attending educational activities, including lectures, seminars and placements, and by completing coursework" (Achieving Good Medical Practice: Guidance for Medical Students, p9). Therefore, if Rosie is not engaging in the course, this factor **should** be considered. The reason this factor is not very important is because patient safety is not directly at risk due to Rosie's lack of engagement. Therefore, this consideration is **important**.

Question 62: A

Very Important – if Rosie's performance in clinical settings is being affected, it may be jeopardising patient safety and therefore, Jacob must raise his concerns. This is outlined in GMC guidance which states "[you must] Take prompt action if you think that patient safety, dignity or comfort is being compromised" (Good Medical Practice, p11). Therefore, this consideration is **very important**.

Top Tip: If you have concerns about a fellow medical student, you must raise your concerns firstly with the person concerned and only escalate if necessary.

Question Set 13

Question 63: D

Not Important at all – As medical Students must follow the same ethical guidelines as doctors, it is irrelevant that Joe is a medical student. Therefore, this consideration is **not important at all**.

Question 64: D

Not Important at all – Alfie's age must not be considered as it is not clinically relevant and would likely be discriminatory. This violates Good Medical Practice which states "You must not unfairly discriminate against patients or colleagues by allowing your personal views [This includes your views about a patient's or colleague's lifestyle, culture or their social or economic status, as well as the characteristics protected by legislation: age, disability, gender reassignment, race, marriage and civil partnership, pregnancy and maternity, religion or belief, sex and sexual orientation] to affect your professional relationships or the treatment you provide or arrange" (Good Medical Practice, p20). Therefore, this factor is **not important at all**.

Question 65: A

Very Important – Confidentiality is a key principle of medical ethics, this is outlined in Good Medical Practice which states "You must treat information about patients as confidential. This includes after a patient has died." (Good Medical Practice, p17). The reason confidentiality is important is because it forms the basis of trust for the doctor-patient relationship. This is outlined in GMC guidelines which state "Trust is an essential part of the doctor-patient relationship and confidentiality is central to this. Patients may avoid seeking medical help, or may under-report symptoms, if they think their personal information will be disclosed by doctors without consent, or without the chance to have some control over the timing or amount of information shared." (GMC Confidentiality Guidelines, p10). Therefore, this factor is **very important.**

Question 66: A

Very Important – Doctors have an obligation to act if they believe public safety is at risk. This exception to confidentiality is outlined in the GMC Confidentiality Guidance which states "There are also important uses of patient information for purposes other than direct care… Other uses are not directly related to the provision of healthcare but serve wider public interests, such as disclosures for public protection reasons" (GMC Confidentiality Guidelines, p10). Therefore, this consideration is **very important**.

Top Tip: Confidentiality must be maintained unless specific exceptions are met for example, if someone else's safety is at risk.

Question 67

Most Appropriate – Gently interrupt Dr Fraser and remind her the patient is allergic to the antibiotics

Least Appropriate – Do nothing

Option 2 is the most appropriate option. This option protects patient safety by stopping Dr Fraser from prescribing the wrong medicine. This is consistent with Good Medical Practice which states "[you must] Take prompt action if you think that patient safety, dignity or comfort is being compromised" (Good Medical Practice, p11). Furthermore, by gently reminding Dr Fraser about the patient's allergy, Charlotte is showing respect for Dr Fraser which is consistent with Good Medical Practice which states "You must treat colleagues fairly and with respect" (Good Medical Practice, p14). Therefore, option 2 is the **most appropriate** option.

Option 1 is neither the most nor least appropriate option. This option would protect patient safety by reminding Dr Fraser of the patient's allergy which is consistent with Good Medical Practice which states "[you must] Take prompt action if you think that patient safety, dignity or comfort is being compromised" (Good Medical Practice, p11). However, as this action is not directly addressing the issue with Dr Fraser, it is **not** the most appropriate option. Therefore. option 1 is **neither** the most **nor** least appropriate option.

Option 3 is the least appropriate option. By doing nothing, Charlotte is knowingly allowing patient safety to be jeopardised. This violates Good Medical Practice which states "[you must] Take prompt action if you think that patient safety, dignity or comfort is being compromised" (Good Medical Practice, p11). Therefore, option 3 is the least appropriate option.

Top Tip: Remember, your first course of action should always be to address any patient safety concerns directly with the clinicians responsible.

Question 68

Most Appropriate – Ask Dr Witty for help and explain he has never performed an ABG before

Least Appropriate – Do the procedure anyway

Option C is the most appropriate option. This option protects patient safety by ensuring he is competent to perform the procedures. This is in line is with the GMC guidance which states *"As a medical student, this applies to you in relation to the time you'll spend with patients on a clinical placement. It also means you should only treat patients or give medical advice when you are under the supervision of a registered healthcare practitioner"* (Achieving Good Medical Practice: Guidance for Medical Students, p11). Furthermore, patient safety must be the top priority which is in line with Good Medical Practice which states *"[you must] Take prompt action if you think that patient safety, dignity or comfort is being compromised"* (Good Medical Practice, p11). Therefore, by taking this action, Mike is protecting patient safety and ensuring he is acting within his competency.

Option A is the least appropriate option. If Mike performs the procedure without being competent, he could cause harm to the patient. This violates Good Medical Practice which states *"[you must] Take prompt action if you think that patient safety, dignity or comfort is being compromised"* (Good Medical Practice, p11).

Option B is neither the most nor least appropriate option. Whilst this option would protect patient safety in the short term, it would endanger it in the long term as it would stop the patient from getting a key test. Therefore, this option violates Good Medical Practice which states *"[you must] Take prompt action if you think that patient safety, dignity or comfort is being compromised"* (Good Medical Practice, p11).

Top Tip: You must never perform a procedure that you are not competent to perform or if you might endanger patient safety.

Question 69

Most Appropriate – Report the incident via the appropriate reporting procedure

Least Appropriate – Assume the patient is mistaken and take no further action

Option C is the least appropriate action. By assuming the patient is mistaken instead of recording her penicillin action, Dr Patterson is jeopardising patient safety which violates Good Medical Practice which states *"[you must] Take prompt action if you think that patient safety, dignity or comfort is being compromised"* (Good Medical Practice, p11). Therefore, this action is the least appropriate option.

Option B is the most appropriate action as it addresses the patient safety issue and ensures that the mistakes which led to it can be rectified by reporting the incident. This is outlined in Good Medical Practice which states *"To help keep patients safe you must: contribute to adverse event recognition"* (Good Medical Practice, p10). Therefore, this action is the most appropriate.

Option A is neither the most nor least appropriate option. Whilst option 1 protects patient safety, it does not help to prevent the incident from occurring again and therefore does not comply with Good Medical Practice which states *"To help keep patients safe you must: contribute to adverse event recognition"* (Good Medical Practice, p10). Therefore, option 1 is neither the most nor the least appropriate option.

Top Tip: Remember, whilst it is important to protect patient safety by taking immediate action, you must also take action to prevent similar mistakes in the future.

UCAT Mock 1

Verbal Reasoning Mock 1

Question Set 1

Naomi Osaka's withdrawal from the French Open, after the tennis player was threatened with suspension for refusing to attend press conferences for the sake of her mental health, is the most recent example of the war playing out between celebrities and the establishment, through which the public justify their own grievances.

These incidents may seem like confected media culture war events – flaring up just as quickly as they die down, and fuelled by the cheap kindling of social media, then doused by our low attention spans. But there is something more substantive about them in that they define, or give shape to, a much more significant clash between two value systems.

In one corner, there are those who ask or demand that their personal experiences and identity be respected, that they are treated better, that first and foremost, they are believed. In the opposing corner stand those who chafe against this new world in which people's feelings are indulged at the expense of established institutions, processes and practices – be it press conferences, university curriculums or royal protocol.

Osaka personifies two contested issues: race and mental health. Equal rights between races and the validity of mental health issues are universally accepted principles. There is no shortage of high-profile figures willing to talk about their own mental health struggles.

But still we argue over the most basic ways of showing support for these causes, such as taking the knee, or about whether we believe people's mental health claims. What is becoming clear is that there is broad consensus that racism is bad and that we need to care about mental health, but very little appetite for actually doing anything to make the world fairer or more accommodating.

Source:
https://www.theguardian.com/commentisfree/2021/jun/07/naomi-osaka-value-systems-racism-mental-health-celebrity

1. What would the author most likely agree with?
    a. Naomi Osaka has depression
    b. Mental health should be the top priority in sport
    c. More should be done to protect people's mental health
    d. Journalists should be excluded from talking to athletes

2. What cannot be inferred from the passage?
    a. Press conferences can be damaging to athletes mental health
    b. There have been opposing views regarding the royal protocol
    c. The public solve their own problems by getting involved in celebrity fights
    d. Celebrities often do not want to talk to the press

3. What would the author most likely agree with regards to media?
    a. The Media culture war described in the passage will flare up and die down quickly
    b. Most people spend too much time on social media
    c. There are many famous people willing to talk about their mental health
    d. Media can help advance athlete's careers

4. What does the word appetite mean in the context of the passage?
    a. To be hungry
    b. To be interested
    c. To believe
    d. To care

Question Set 2

The US Food and Drug Administration (FDA) approval yesterday, May 21st 2021, of the first new drug for Alzheimer's disease in eighteen years was welcomed by some people looking for hope against an intractable condition. But, for many researchers, it came as a surprise — and a disappointment.

Aducanumab — developed by biotechnology company Biogen in Cambridge, Massachusetts — is the first approved drug that attempts to treat a possible cause of the neurodegenerative disease, rather than just the symptoms. But the approval has sparked a contentious debate over whether the drug is effective. Many experts, including an independent panel of neurologists and biostatisticians, advised the FDA that clinical-trial data did not conclusively demonstrate that aducanumab could slow cognitive decline.

The FDA instead relied on an alternative measure of activity, which sets a dangerous precedent, some researchers warn.

Current Alzheimer's drugs address only disease symptoms, for instance by delaying memory loss by a few months. Aducanumab clears out clumps of a protein in the brain called amyloid-β, which some researchers think is the root cause of Alzheimer's.
This theory is known as the amyloid hypothesis. The FDA approved the drug on the basis of its ability to reduce the levels of these plaques in the brain.

Amended from Nature: https://www.nature.com/articles/d41586-021-01546-2

5. What can be said to be true about the drug Aducanumab?
   a. It will cure Alzheimer's
   b. It clears proteins associated with the Alzheimer's
   c. It addresses symptoms of Alzheimer's
   d. It is the first Alzheimer's drug

6. Why are some researchers sceptical of Aducanumab?
   a. They don't believe the drugs target is the definitive cause of Alzheimer's
   b. They think the data of the clinical trial was tampered with
   c. They think symptoms are more important and should be targeted
   d. They don't trust the FDA

7. When was the last drug, before the current new one, discovered?
   a. 2002
   b. 2003
   c. 2004
   d. 2005

8. What had all previous Alzheimer's drugs targeted?
   a. Tau bodies
   b. Amyloid- beta plaques
   c. Neuronal pathways
   d. Symptoms of Alzheimer's

Question Set 3

When the sequencing of the human genome was announced two decades ago by the Human Genome Project and biotech firm Celera Genomics, the sequence was not truly complete. About 15% was missing: technological limitations left researchers unable to work out how certain stretches of DNA fitted together, especially those where there were many repeating letters (or base pairs). Scientists solved some of the puzzle over time, but the most recent human genome, which geneticists have used as a reference since 2013, still lacks 8% of the full sequence.

Now, researchers in the Telomere-to-Telomere (T2T) Consortium, an international collaboration that comprises around 30 institutions, have filled in those gaps. In a 27 May preprint1 entitled 'The complete sequence of a human genome', genomics researcher Karen Miga at the University of California, Santa Cruz, and her colleagues report that they've sequenced the remainder, in the process discovering about 115 new genes that code for proteins, for a total of 19,969.

"It's exciting to have some resolution to the problem areas," says Kim Pruitt, a bioinformatician at the US National Center for Biotechnology Information in Bethesda, Maryland, who calls the result a "significant milestone".

The newly sequenced genome — dubbed T2T-CHM13 — adds nearly 200 million base pairs to the 2013 version of the human genome sequence. This time, instead of taking DNA from a living person, the researchers used a cell line derived from what's known as a complete hydatidiform mole, a type of tissue that forms in humans when a sperm inseminates an egg with no nucleus. The resulting cell contains chromosomes only from the father, so the researchers don't have to distinguish between two sets of chromosomes from different people.

Source: https://www.nature.com/articles/d41586-021-01506-w

9. What can be inferred from the passage?
    a. The entire human genome was sequenced in 2013
    b. The US National Center for Biotechnology is in Washington D.C.
    c. The entire genome has 200 million base pairs
    d. A hydatidiform mole was used to discover the missing bases

10. What organisation managed to fill in the missing gaps of the genome?
    a. Celera Genomics
    b. Human genome sequencing organisation
    c. Telomere-to-Telomere (T2T) Consortium
    d. University of California

11. What is a hydatidiform mole?
    a. A cell without a nucleus
    b. A tissue formed when an eggs is inseminated that does not have a nucleus
    c. A type of DNA replication molecule
    d. A sequence of base pairs

12. What percentage of the human genome was missing after the very first sequencing?
    a. 15%
    b. 8%
    c. 10%
    d. 12%

Question Set 4

Booooo! Has become their ritual, England's footballers took the knee this weekend. And as has become their ritual, a section of the England fans, newly permitted to congregate at stadiums post-pandemic, took the opportunity to barrack those for whom taking the knee has become a statement, a gesture of belonging, solidarity and a token of faith.

If you ask those who take the knee why they do so, I am sure the reasons will differ. Some are black players who want to challenge the perception that their status as sporting superstars protects them from the realities of being black in Britain, in a white-dominated country, in a white-dominated sport. They have always felt it; taking the knee allows them to articulate it.

Some are young black sportsmen who want to show that whatever their own exalted fortunes, their existence within the bubble of elite sport does not blind them to the realities of what life is like for those outside that bubble, who can't walk safely, who can't get jobs, who don't have futures, who have police officers ram their knees on to their necks.

Some are not black but bond day in and day out with those black men and want to support them. Some may just have become part of the ritual and see no harm in it.

Source:
https://www.theguardian.com/commentisfree/2021/jun/09/boo-take-the-knee-fans-boris-johnson-england-footballers

13. What can be said about England's football fans?
    a. They are racist
    b. There are different opinions between fans
    c. Some of them take the knee with the players
    d. They were all very excited to be back in the stadium

14. What cannot be inferred from the passage?
    a. Some fans are not happy about the players taking the knee
    b. The football clubs fully support their players
    c. Players want to raise awareness of racism they and others face
    d. Football is largely white dominated in the UK

15. What would the author agree with are the reasons young black players take the knee?
    a. To show solidarity with others that have not been as fortunate as them to play professional football
    b. To show that they are not blind to the realities faced by black people out
    c. To allow them to be part of a movement
    d. To combat the police

16. What can be inferred from the passage?
    a. There are black and non-black players taking the knee
    b. Football is generally quite diverse
    c. Players lose money for taking the knee
    d. Many football fans believe football should not include politics

Question Set 5

China's mass detention of Uyghur Muslims – the largest of a religio-ethnic group since the second world war – is not the inevitable or predictable outcome of Chinese communist policies towards ethnic minorities. I've spent the past 20 years studying ethnicity in China and, when viewing the present situation in Xinjiang through the prism of history, one thing becomes clear: this is not what was "supposed" to happen.

In the early 1950s the Chinese Communist party (CCP) was holding on to revolutionary victory by its fingernails. The postwar economy was in shambles, and the outbreak of the Korean war brought a nuclear hegemon to its doorstep, in the form of the United States. Not the moment most regimes would choose to enlarge their to-do lists. The CCP did, however, committing to officially recognising more minority peoples than any other Chinese regime in history. While Chiang Kai-shek's nationalists had begrudgingly accepted the official existence of five groups in the 1930s and 40s, the Communists recognised 55 in all (plus the Han majority), many with populations under 10,000.

A remarkable amount of time and capital was dedicated to the celebration and bolstering of these groups. Perhaps the largest social survey in human history sent thousands of researchers into minority communities, filling libraries with their reports. Linguists created writing systems for minorities who did not already have them. The scale of the People's Republic of China's investment in groups it designated as "minorities" has been staggering.

Source:
https://www.theguardian.com/commentisfree/2021/jun/10/china-celebrating-diversity-suppressing-xinjiang-communist-party

17. The state of China has always detested Uyghur Muslims
    a. True
    b. False
    c. Can't Tell

18. The Korean war was in the 1950s
    a. True
    b. False
    c. Can't Tell

19. The largest social survey in human history was conducted in China, involving minority groups.
    a. True
    b. False
    c. Can't Tell

20. Many minority groups in China did not yet have writing systems when the social survey was conducted.
    a. True
    b. False
    c. Can't Tell

Question Set 6

Anyone who thought the world had four oceans will now have to think again, after the National Geographic Society announced it would recognise a new Southern Ocean in Antarctica, bringing the global total to five.

The National Geographic, a non-profit scientific and educational organisation whose mapping standards are referenced by many atlases and cartographers, said the Southern Ocean consists of the waters surrounding Antarctica, out to 60-degrees south latitude.

National Geographic Society geographer Alex Tait said scientists have long known that the waters surrounding Antarctica form a "distinct ecological region defined, by ocean currents and temperatures".

Tait told the Washington Post that the span of water is yet to be officially recognized as an ocean by the relevant international body: "But we thought it was important at this point to officially recognize it."

"People look to us for geographic fact: How many continents, how many countries, how many oceans? Up until now, we've said four oceans," Tait said, referring to the Arctic, Atlantic, Indian and Pacific.

The US Board of Geographic Names, a federal body created in 1890 to establish and maintain "uniform geographic name usage" through the federal government, already recognizes the Southern ocean as occupying the same territory, but this is the first time the National Geographic has done so.

Source:
https://www.theguardian.com/environment/2021/jun/10/new-ocean-global-total-five-national-geographic

21. How many oceans are officially recognised by relevant international bodies?
   a. 3
   b. 4
   c. 5
   d. 6

22. What is the function of the US Board of Geographic Names?
   a. To ensure every geographic structure has a name
   b. To unify geographic names used across the US
   c. To unify names used for geographic structures across the world
   d. To make Geography a more popular subject to study

23. How far has National Geographic determined does the Southern ocean reach from Antarctica?
   a. 60-degrees south latitude
   b. 90-degrees south latitude
   c. 40- degrees south latitude
   d. 50- degrees south latitude

24. According to the article, what kind of organisation is The National Geographic?
   a. A non- profit scientific organisation
   b. A non- profit scientific and educational magazine
   c. A non-profit scientific and educational organisation
   d. A for profit educational organisation

Question Set 7

Of all the prevailing ideas for how black holes emerge, none could account for the existence of an impossibly large type of black hole detected in 2019 – but now we may know how it could have formed.

In May 2019, researchers at the Laser Interferometer Gravitational-Wave Observatory (LIGO) in the US and its Italian counterpart Virgo measured ripples in space-time called gravitational waves and determined that their signal was the result of two black holes merging.

Stellar-mass black holes like these arise when a star becomes too large to support its own weight and explodes in a supernova, its inner layers collapsing in on themselves.

However, this process was thought to only produce black holes up to about 65 times the mass of the sun because the winds that blow away the outer layers of the star during the supernova remove so much mass that it limits the size of the resulting black hole.

The larger of the two black holes detected by LIGO and Virgo had a mass 85 times that of the sun, so seems to be larger than previously thought possible.

Jorick Vink at the Armagh Observatory & Planetarium in Northern Ireland and his colleagues performed simulations of stars that may have formed billions of years ago and found that they could be the progenitors of larger black holes.

Source:

https://www.newscientist.com/article/2280062-impossibly-huge-black-holes-may-have-come-from-weird-ancient-stars/#ixzz6xOFsNrUU

25. How do stellar- mass black holes arise?
    a. When many black holes merge
    b. They arise from a supernova
    c. From a star that has become too big
    d. When gravity pulls at a black hole

26. According to the passage, what are undulations through space and time called?
    a. Gravitational waves
    b. Space ripples
    c. Gravity undulation
    d. Gravitational radiation

27. What was previously thought to be the limit mass of Stellar-mass black holes in comparison to the sun?
    a. Fifty-five times the sun
    b. Sixty-five times the su
    c. Eighty-five times the sun
    d. One hundred times the sun

28. What was special about the black hole detected in 2019?
    a. It was older than any previous black hole detected
    b. It was so large no previous theory could explain its existence
    c. It had appeared suddenly
    d. It was the largest in the universe

Question Set 8

"QUANTUM supremacy" is a phrase that has been in the news a lot lately. Several labs worldwide have already claimed to have reached this milestone, at which computers exploiting the wondrous features of the quantum world solve a problem faster than a conventional classical computer feasibly could. Although we aren't quite there yet, a general-purpose "universal" quantum computer seems closer than ever – a revolutionary development for how we communicate and encrypt data, for virtual reality, artificial intelligence and much more.

These prospects excite me as a theoretical physicist too, but my colleagues and I are captivated by an even bigger picture. The quantum theory of computation originated as a way to deepen our understanding of quantum theory, our fundamental theory of physical reality. By applying the principles we have learned more broadly, we think we are beginning to see the outline of a radical new way to construct laws of nature.

It means abandoning the idea of physics as the science of what's actually happening, and embracing it as the science of what might or might not happen. This "science of can and can't" could help us tackle some of the big questions that conventional physics has tried and failed to get to grips with, from delivering an exact, unifying theory of thermodynamics and information to getting round conceptual barriers that stop us merging quantum theory with general relativity, Einstein's theory of gravity. It might go even further and help us to understand how intelligent thought works, and kick-start a technological revolution that would make quantum supremacy look modest by comparison.

Source:
https://www.newscientist.com/article/mg25033300-300-quantum-computers-are-revealing-an-unexpected-new-theory-of-reality/#ixzz6xOQKC4L3

29. Physics has been a science dealing with what is actually happening up until now.
    a. True
    b. False
    c. Can't Tell

30. Quantum theory has reconstructed the laws of nature.
    a. True
    b. False
    c. Can't Tell

31. Thermodynamics is the hardest area of physics
    a. True
    b. False
    c. Can't Tell

32. Computers exploring the quantum are now faster at solving problems than conventional classic computers.
    a. True
    b. False
    c. Can't Tell

Question Set 9

A radio telescope in Canada has detected 535 fast radio bursts, quadrupling the known tally of these brief, highly energetic phenomena in one go. The long-awaited results show that these enigmatic events come in two distinct types — most bursts are one-off events, with a minority repeating periodically and lasting at least ten times longer on average.

The findings strongly suggest that fast radio bursts could be the result of at least two distinct astrophysical phenomena. "I think this really just nails it that there is a difference," says study co-author Kiyoshi Masui, an astrophysicist at the Massachusetts Institute of Technology in Cambridge.

The overnight jump in the available data has put the radio astronomy community into a tizzy. "I woke up this morning and all my Slack channels were full of people talking about the papers," says Laura Spitler, an astrophysicist at the Max Planck Institute for Radio Astronomy in Bonn, Germany, who co-discovered the first repeating burst2 in 2016 using the now-collapsed Arecibo telescope in Puerto Rico.

The Canadian Hydrogen Intensity Mapping Experiment (CHIME) collected the events in its first year of operation, between 2018 and 2019. The team announced its results during a virtual meeting of the American Astronomical Society on 9 June 2021, and posted four preprints on the online repository arXiv.

Source: https://www.nature.com/articles/d41586-021-01560-4

33. What was roughly the amount of radio bursts recorded, before the recent radio burst discovery?
    a. 535 bursts
    b. 400 bursts
    c. 135 bursts
    d. 45 bursts

34. Why was the discovery of the new radio burst such big news?
   a. Because it vastly changed the amount of information available on radio bursts
   b. Because it led to many new theories
   c. Because the lead scientists who discovered it were Canadian
   d. Because it completely changed existing knowledge

35. Using what device are radio bursts recorded?
   a. Using a mapping device
   b. Using a telescope
   c. Using a repository device
   d. Using an X-ray

36. What can be said to be true about the fast radio burst according to the passage?
   a. They are all about the same length
   b. Not much is known about them
   c. There seem to be two distinct types
   d. There may be many more than two types

Question Set 10

The name Berlin appears for the first time in recorded history in 1244, seven years after that of its sister town, Kölln, with which it later merged. Both were founded near the beginning of the 13th century. In 1987 both East and West Berlin celebrated the city's 750th anniversary. Whatever the date of foundation, it is certain that the two towns were established for geographic and mercantile reasons, as they commanded a natural east-west trade route over the Spree River.

In 1411 the mark of Brandenburg came under the governorship of the Nürnberg feudal baron Frederick VI. This began Berlin's association with the Hohenzollerns, who from the end of the 15th century as electoral princes of Brandenburg established Berlin-Kölln as their capital and permanent residence.

The Thirty Years' War of 1618–48 laid a heavy financial burden on the city, and the population was reduced from 12,000 to 7,500. When Frederick William the Great Elector assumed power in 1640, he embarked on a building program, which included fortifications that enabled him to expel Swedish invaders. His rule also marked the beginning of the development of canals, which by 1669 provided a direct link between Breslau (now Wrocław, Pol.) in the east and Hamburg and the open sea in the west. His successor, Frederick III, crowned Prussian king (as Frederick I) in 1701 in Königsberg (now Kaliningrad, Russia), made Berlin the royal residence city. In 1709 the framework of Greater Berlin was laid when Berlin-Kölln and the newer towns of Friedrichswerder, Dorotheenstadt, and Friedrichstadt were put under a single magistrate. The population grew from 12,000 in 1670 to 61,000 in 1712, including 6,000 French Huguenot refugees.

37. Why was Berlin founded?
   a. Due to its good access to clean water
   b. Due to having access to good business opportunities
   c. Due to its natural resources
   d. Due to invaders pushing people in the country inwards

38. Which ruler developed the canals between Hamburg and the sea?
   a. Fredrick I
   b. Frederick III
   c. Fredrick William
   d. Fredrick William III

39. When did Berlin's association with the Hollenzollerns begin?
   a. 1244
   b. 1411
   c. 1618
   d. 1709

40. Where would Königsberg be located today?
   a. Germay
   b. France
   c. Russia
   d. Poland

Question Set 11

Almost half of the litter found in the world's oceans is plastic made by takeaway food and drinks, new research has shown.

In the first comprehensive study of its kind, researchers from 15 institutions in 10 countries analysed 12m data points from 36 global data sets on litter pollution, discovering that plastic accounts for 80 per cent of human-made products dumped in the world's seas.

Although they analysed 112 different litter categories, 75 per cent of the ocean's waste came from just 10 plastic products. And half of all the objects comprised only four items: single-use bags, food containers, wrappers and bottles, each in about equal proportion.

Given these findings, Andres Cozar, the study's coordinator who works at Spain's University of Cadiz, said governments need to do more to tackle the heart of the problem.

While well-intentioned, policies aimed at cutting the manufacture of plastic stirrers, straws and cotton buds – responsible for a tiny fraction of the overall pollution – do not solve the key issues, he explained.

"Here we show that restrictions on the use of plastic items, such as straws, cotton buds and drink stirrers, while sound, do not yet address the core problem," Mr Cózar warned.

The researchers believe that authorities should ban avoidable plastic products used for take-aways, and levy a deposit on those deemed essential.

More easily degradable materials should also be used in the manufacturing process where possible, the authors added.

Source:

https://www.independent.co.uk/climate-change/news/oceans-plastic-pollution-takeaways-b18 64109.html

41. If 100 pieces of plastic were pulled from the ocean, roughly how many of these would be bottles?
    a. 13 bottles
    b. 20 bottles
    c. 50 bottles
    d. 100 bottles

42. What would the researchers mentioned in the passage most likely agree with?
    a. Plastic straws, drink stirrers and cotton buds are a big problem for ocean pollution
    b. There should be a deposit paid for essential plastic products
    c. There have been several studies such as this one, all with similar findings
    d. There are not yet enough sustainable alternatives

43. What is the main component of the trash found in the ocean?
    a. Plastic from straws
    b. Plastic bags
    c. Plastic bottles
    d. Plastic from takeaways

44. What cannot be inferred from the passage?
    a. Plastic straws only make up a tiny proportion of the ocean plastic
    b. Plastic is the main item humans dispose of in the oceans
    c. Plastic in the oceans provides a big threat to marine life
    d. If the ten most common plastic products were no longer dumped in the ocean this would make a huge difference

Answers: Verbal Reasoning Mock 1

Question Set 1

Question 1: C

Statement A: Keyword: illness
Although the passage states that Noami Osaka was removed due to her mental health there is no support for her having depression. Even if she has a mental illness we do not know it is depression.

Statement B: Keyword: priority
Although, the author supports mental health having a higher priority in society and sport there is no statement that says it should be the top priority. This is too extreme of a statement.

Statement C: Keyword: protect
In the last paragraph the author says very little is being done to combat racism and poor mental health. The passage would therefore support that the author believes more should be done.

Statement D: Keyword: journalists
The passage is about Naomi Osaka not wanting to talk to journalists during the French Open. There is nothing to indicate that the author thinks none of the athletes should talk to journalists.

Top Tip: For author opinion questions always make sure to read the first and the last sentence fully.

Question 2: D

Statement A: This can be inferred from the passage, as Naomi Osaka, who is an athlete, does not want to talk to the journalists due to her mental health.

Statement B: In the third paragraph it says, 'In the opposing corner stand those who chafe against this new world in which people's feelings are indulged at the expense of established institutions, processes and practices – be it press conferences, university curriculums or royal protocol.' Therefore, the royal protocol is mentioned as another example where there have been opposing views.

Statement C: The last sentence of the first paragraph states 'the war playing out between celebrities and the establishment, through which the public justify their own grievances'. The statement is therefore supported by the passage as problem is a synonym for grievance.

Statement D: There is no mention of other celebrities in the passage or how they might feel about the press. The statement is therefore not supported by the passage.

Top Tip: Look out for extreme language when examining statements.

Question 3: C

Statement A: Although the author states that 'These incidents may seem like confected media culture war events – flaring up just as quickly as they die down', the same paragraph later states that 'there is something more substantive about them in that they define, or give shape to, a much more significant clash between two value systems.' It therefore seems that the author would not agree that this situation will simply flare up and die down.

Statement B: This is not talked about or mentioned in the passage.

Statement C: This is supported by the third paragraph where the author states 'There is no shortage of high-profile figures willing to talk about their own mental health struggles'.

Statement D: This is not discussed in the passage and therefore not supported by it.

Question 4: B

The word appetite is used in the last sentence 'but very little appetite for actually doing anything to make the world fairer or more accommodating'. In this context it is synonymous with being interested.

Question Set 2

Question 5: B

B is the only option supported by the passage. It is mentioned in the last paragraph that 'Aducanumab clears out clumps of a protein in the brain called amyloid-β'. The other three statements are not supported by the passage.

Question 6: A

In the last paragraph it says 'Aducanumab clears out clumps of a protein in the brain called amyloid-β, which some researchers think is the root cause of Alzheimer's'. This implies that many researchers do not believe this to be the root cause. Amyloid beta plaques are the target but not the definitive cause and therefore statement A is correct.

Question 7: B

The first sentence of the passage states that the announcement of the new drug happened on May 21st 2021. The next sentence states that this was 'the first new drug for Alzheimer's disease in eighteen years'. 2021-18 = 2003.

Question 8: D

This is stated in the first sentence of the last paragraph where it says, 'Current Alzheimer's drugs address only disease symptoms'.

Question Set 3

Question 9: D

Statement A: In the first paragraph it says that 15% of the genome was still missing in the 2013 version, therefore not making it possible to infer this from the passage.

Statement B: In the third paragraph it says the US National Center for Biotechnology Information is in Bethesda, Maryland, not in Washington D.C.

Statement C: Keyword: 200. 200 million can be found in the last paragraph where it says, 'The newly sequenced genome — dubbed T2T-CHM13 — adds nearly 200 million base pairs to the 2013 version of the human genome sequence'. This statement is therefore false, as 200 million new bases were discovered but the entire genome is much larger.

Statement D: Keyword: hydatidiform mole. The last paragraph states 'the researchers used a cell line derived from what's known as a complete hydatidiform mole'. Therefore this statement can be inferred from the passage.

Question 10: C

The second paragraph states 'researchers in the Telomere-to-Telomere (T2T) Consortium, an international collaboration that comprises around 30 institutions, have filled in those gaps'.

Question 11: B

The last paragraph states 'hydatidiform mole, a type of tissue that forms in humans when a sperm inseminates an egg with no nucleus'. Therefore statement B is the correct answer.

Question 12: A

In the first paragraph 15% is stated as the percentage that was missing when the genome was first sequenced

Question Set 4

Question 13: B

Statement A: Saying they are all racist is using extreme language and is not supported by the passage.

Statement B: The first paragraph implies there are different opinions between fans, by referring to a 'a section of the England fans'. It implies that not all England fans are booing at the players for taking the knee but some are.

Statement C: This is not mentioned nor supported by the passage

Statement D: The first paragraph states that the players were 'newly permitted to congregate at stadiums post-pandemic', but nothing is mentioned about them being excited or not.

Question 14: B

Statement B is not mentioned in the passage and can therefore not be inferred.

Question 15: B

Although none of these answer options are completely false B best represents the opinion of the author presented in paragraph three when they talk about young black sportsmen.

Question 16: A

Statement A: The last paragraph mentions non- black players also taking the knee; therefore option A is correct.

Statement B: The second paragraph described Britain and football as being a 'white-dominated country, in a white-dominated sport'. Therefore, this statement cannot be inferred from the passage.

Statement C: There is no mention of players losing money.

Statement D: There is no mention that football should not include politics or that many fans believe this.

Question Set 5

Question 17: B

The first paragraph states that this 'is not the inevitable or predictable outcome of Chinese communist policies towards ethnic minorities. This statement is therefore false.

Question 18: A

The second paragraph states 'In the early 1950s the Chinese Communist party (CCP) was holding on to revolutionary victory (...) and the outbreak of the Korean war brought a nuclear hegemon to its doorstep'. This implies that the Korean war started in the early 1950s.

Question 19: C

The passage states '**Perhaps** the largest social survey in human history'. Therefore, from the passage alone we cannot know for sure if it was the largest.

Question 20: C

The third paragraph states 'Linguists created writing systems for minorities who did not already have them'. From this we cannot know if it was many, most or only a few minority groups that did not yet have writing systems.

Question Set 6

Question 21: B

Although the National Geographic Society now recognizes there are five, the relevant international bodies are said not to have recognized the Southern Ocean yet (paragraph 4).

Question 22: B

In the last paragraph it says it was established to 'maintain "uniform geographic name usage" through the federal government', implying the US.

Question 23: A

In the second paragraph it is stated that 'the Southern Ocean consists of the waters surrounding Antarctica, out to 60-degrees south latitude'.

Top Tip: Numbers are easy keywords to spot.

Question 24: C

The second paragraph states 'The National Geographic, a non-profit scientific and educational organisation'. Therefore, option C is correct.

Question Set 7

Question 25: C

The third paragraph states 'Stellar-mass black holes like these arise when a star becomes too large to support its own weight and explodes in a supernova, its inner layers collapsing in on themselves'. Therefore, option C is correct.

Question 26: A

In the second paragraph it states 'measured ripples in space-time called gravitational waves'. Undulation is a synonym for ripples.

Question 27: B

The fourth paragraph states: 'this process was thought to only produce black holes up to about 65 times the mass of the sun'.

Question 28: B

Only B is supported by the passage. In the first paragraph it states: 'Of all the prevailing ideas for how black holes emerge, none could account for the existence of an impossibly large type of black hole detected in 2019'. Although, this black hole is the largest to have been discovered by humans so far we do not know it to be the largest in the universe.

Common Trap: Watch out for inferences that over exaggerate from the information you have been given in the passage.

Question Set 8

Question 29: A

In the first sentence of the third paragraph, it says we would have to abandon the 'idea of physics as the science of what's actually happening'. This implies this is what physics currently is.

Question 30: B

The second paragraph states 'The quantum theory of computation originated as a way to deepen our understanding of quantum theory (...). By applying the principles we have learned more broadly, we think we are beginning to see the outline of a radical new way to construct laws of nature'. This means the laws of nature have not been reconstructed yet.

Question 31: C

The passage says that there is not a unifying theory of thermodynamics yet, but it does not say whether or not it is the hardest.

Question 32: B

The first paragraph states that we are not far from this happening, but that it has not happened yet.

Question Set 9

Question 33: C

The first paragraph states that the 535 radio bursts detected quadrupled the previous known tally. A quarter of 535 is about 135.

Question 34: A

The third paragraph states 'The overnight jump in the available data has put the radio astronomy community into a tizzy'. It has therefore greatly increased the amount of information available.

Question 35: B

The first sentence states 'A radio telescope in Canada has detected 535 fast radio bursts. Therefore, option B is correct.

Question 36: D

Statement A: The first passage states that some are shorter while others can be ten times as long. This is therefore not correct.

Statement B: The passage is about the data available on the radio bursts increasing. It is therefore not correct to say not much is known about them.

Statement C: The first passage states 'The long-awaited results show that these enigmatic events come in two distinct types'.

Statement D: This is not mentioned in the passage.

Question Set 10

Question 37: B

The first paragraph states 'it is certain that the two towns were established for geographic and mercantile reasons, as they commanded a natural east-west trade route over the Spree River'. Therefore option B is correct.

Question 38: C

The third paragraph states that Fredrick William who assumed power in 1640, began developing the canals.

Question 39: B

The second paragraph states 'In 1411 the mark of Brandenburg came under the governorship of the Nürnberg feudal baron Frederick VI. This began Berlin's association with the Hohenzollerns'. Therefore 1411 is the correct answer.

Question 40: C

The third paragraph states 'in Königsberg (now Kaliningrad, Russia)'.

Question Set 11

Question 41: A

The third paragraph states 'half of all the objects comprised only four items: single-use bags, food containers, wrappers and bottles, each in about equal proportion.' Since the question states that 100 pieces of plastic were pulled from the ocean, 50 of these would be either single-use bags, food containers, wrappers, or bottles. As each of the four items are present in equal proportion there would be 50/4 bottles and therefore about 13.

Question 42: B

Statement A: Although these are a problem they are said to be said to be 'responsible for a tiny fraction of the overall pollution'.

Statement B: This is stated in the seventh paragraph where it says 'and levy a deposit on those deemed essential'.

Statement C: The second paragraph states that this study is 'the first comprehensive study of its kind'. Therefore, it seems there have not been many studies like it before.

Statement D: The passage does not mention this or discuss this topic at all. Although one can presume the researchers would agree with this it is not supported by the passage.

Question 43: D

The first sentence of the passage states 'Almost half of the litter found in the world's oceans is plastic made by takeaway food and drinks, new research has shown'.

Question 44: C

Statement A: This is stated in the fifth paragraph where it says 'While well-intentioned, policies aimed at cutting the manufacture of plastic stirrers, straws and cotton buds - responsible for a tiny fraction of the overall pollution'.

Statement B: The second paragraph states that 'plastic accounts for 80 per cent of human-made products dumped in the world's seas.' Therefore, this statement can be inferred from the passage.

Statement C: Although from outside knowledge we know this to be true, the passage does not mention marine life and therefore this statement cannot be inferred from the passage.

Statement D: This statement can be inferred, as the third paragraph states that '75 per cent of the ocean's waste came from just 10 plastic products.' Therefore, if dumping of these 10 plastic products into the oceans was stopped there would be a 75% reduction in plastic disposed of in the ocean.

Decision Making Mock 1

Question 1

Four siblings are helping their mother cook a meal together in the kitchen. Joel, Derek, Alex and Mary must complete the one task which they dislike doing: either setting the table, cutting onions, washing the plates or peeling the carrots.

When asked to do their task, each sibling has a different reaction. One huffs, one complains, one smirks, and one leaves.

Joel smirked at his chore.
Derek hates cutting onions and Alex hates setting the table.
The sibling that huffs likes cutting onions.
The sibling that dislikes peeling the carrots is the one that leaves.
The sibling that doesn't like cutting onions always complains.

Which of the following must be true?
    a. Joel does not like washing up
    b. Derek leaves
    c. Alex complains
    d. Mary likes peeling carrots.

Question 2

Four brothers wanted to go travelling but they had different destinations in mind. Vernon, Sam, Jack and Aaron, each wanted to go somewhere different; Madrid, Berlin, Edinburgh and Dublin. Each brother also wanted to travel in different ways; one brother wanted to fly, one wanted to drive, one wanted to sail, and another wanted to go by train.

Vernon wanted to sail.
Sam wants to go to Paris and Jack wants to go to Madrid.
The brother who wants to fly does not want to go to Dublin.
The brother who wants to drive wants to go to Edinburgh.

Which of the following must be true?
    a. Aaron wants to fly
    b. Jack wants to travel by train
    c. Vernon wants to go to Dublin
    d. Sam wants to drive

Question 3

A girl has a small pack of mixed seeds that she wants to plant which contain 16 chilli seeds, 10 Strawberry seeds and 8 Pumpkin.

Will she increase the chance of picking a strawberry seed if she removes three of each seed variety from her pack?
   a. No, the chance of selecting a strawberry seed remains the same when an equal number of each seed variety is removed
   b. No, the chance of selecting a strawberry seed decreases when an equal number of each seed variety is removed
   c. Yes, the likelihood of selecting a strawberry seed increases when there are fewer chilli seeds and pumpkin seeds
   d. Yes, the likelihood of picking a particular seed variety increases when the total number of seeds decrease

Question 4

Lu has an odd number of pencils. This the average number of pencils that both Charlie and Harry have. Molly has 8 pencils and Amit has half as many pencils as Molly. Charlie has more pencils than Amit but fewer pencils than Molly. Harry has 2 more pencils than Charlie.

Which of the following must be true?
   a. Harry and Molly have the same number of pencils
   b. Amit and Charlie have a total of 11 pencils
   c. Charlie and Molly have the same number of pencils
   d. Amit and Harry have total of 13 pencils

Question 5

The NHS should pay for everyone to be taught CPR at schools because it will ultimately help save lives.

Regarding the above statement, which of the following is the strongest argument?
   a. Yes, because there are many people who require first aid in the UK each year
   b. Yes, because other countries do it already
   c. No, first aid should be just for medical professionals who have been trained in providing medical care.
   d. No, because it will be expensive to teach CPR, and more lives could be saved by providing more ambulances instead.

Question 6

Should children be encouraged to keep pets to gain a sense of responsibility and how to look after other?

Regarding the above statement, which of the following is the strongest argument?
  a. Yes, scientists have proven that owning a pet reduces anxiety
  b. Yes, pets require regular grooming and therefore there is a duty of care when owning a pet
  c. No, children could put pets in danger
  d. No, many children are not well behaved enough to look after animals.

Question 7

Should schools increase the daily intake of fruit and vegetables by subsidising school meals?

Regarding the above statement, which of the following is the strongest argument?
  a. Yes, it will encourage greater production of fruit and vegetables from farmers and so be helpful to the economy
  b. Yes, fruit and vegetables are essential to maintain a healthy lifestyle
  c. No, they are expensive to buy
  d. No, schools regularly provide free meals already to many, instead the government should subsidise fruit and vegetables.

Question 8

A code is made up of four letters: A, B,C and D. The following conditions apply to the code:
→ *D is in third place*
→ *If A is in first place, then B is in the third place*
→ *If B is next to the second place, then A is in the fourth place*

Which of the following must be true?
  a. Only three combinations fulfil all the criteria
  b. All possible answers have the same letter in fourth place
  c. The letter B cannot be in second place
  d. Two of the possible combinations have A in second place

Question 9

Should GPs charge patients a fee for missed appointments?

Regarding the above statement, which of the following is the strongest argument?
   a.   Yes, GPs can use the extra funding to cover the budget cut by the government
   b.   Yes, patients will be encouraged to attend or cancel in advance
   c.   No, people could miss appointments due to unforeseen situations
   d.   No, it will always be unethical to ask an absent patient to pay for an appointment and could prove challenging.

Question 10

Should drivers be forced to retake their driving test at regular intervals?

Regarding the above statement, which of the following is the strongest argument?
   a.   Yes, having up to date knowledge of road rules is important
   b.   Yes, the fees which are collected from repeated tests could be used to fund new roads
   c.   No, most people would just pretend to drive well during the test and the continue being reckless when not in test conditions
   d.   No, even though a lot of people forget the details of the highway code, they still drive safely, even when they have passed the test many years beforehand

Question 11

Ryan is having a conversation with his coworker and says the following:
→ *When I'm on holiday, I Jet ski*
→ *When I am not on holiday, I don't go on a diet*
→ *I am currently on a diet*
→ *When I am happy, I jet ski and when I am not happy I do not.*

Select Yes if the conclusion follows and NO if it does not
   a.   Ryan is not on holiday
   b.   Ryan is not happy
   c.   When Ryan is on holiday, he goes on a diet
   d.   If Ryan is not happy, he is not on holiday
   e.   If Ryan does not jet ski then he is not happy.

Question 12

Eight world class chess players enter a meeting and sit around a round table. They get talking and realise that when you add up the total number of medals won by any two chess players sitting opposite each other, it always gives a total of 13. The following conversation ensues:

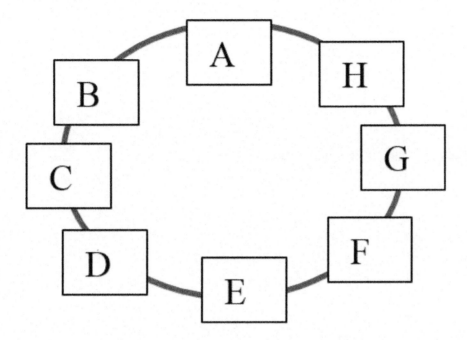

A: 'I have won three fewer medals than F'
B: 'I know for a fact that G and E have 17 medals altogether'
C: 'I know for a fact that A and D have won 17 medals altogether'
D: 'I have won two more than F'

How many medals has G won?

    a. 6
    b. 7
    c. 9
    d. 10

Question 13

All of Harry's books are horrors. Some of Daisy's books are non-fiction, but none of her books are novels. Book A is either Harry's or Daisy's

Which of the following is true?
a. Book A is a novel
b. Book A is not non-fiction
c. Book A is Daisy's
d. If book A is not Harry's, it is not a novel

Question 14

8 friends are competing in the 100m sprint at their school's sports day.

→ *Mary wins the race*
→ *Hamesh finished behind Kavita*
→ *Rosie was close behind Mary*
→ *Bilraj and Cathy did not beat Ander, but they win against Timothy*
→ *Kavita finished just behind Timothy*

Which position did Timothy finish in?
a. 3rd
b. 4th
c. 5th
d. 6th

Question 15

Kiki has only two friends to whom she gives food. JJ gives sweets to Kiki who returns the favour. Everyone in their neighbourhood gives food to El.

Answer YES if the conclusion follows and NO if it does not.
a. If someone is given food by Kiki, then they must be JJ or El.
b. Everyone gets food from JJ.
c. If someone receives food from Nick, then they must be El.
d. El gives sweets to everyone in the neighbourhood.
e. El has food, he must have gotten it from Kiki

Question 16

There are five siblings in a room: Bea, Holly, Jim, Emma and Mick. Emma is older than Bea and Mick is twice the age of Emma. Jim is older than two of his siblings.

Which of the following must be true?
a. Holly is the eldest
b. Mick is the eldest
c. Mick is the youngest
d. Mick is older than Jim

Question 17

All the people in the student accommodation except for Mason like to drink tea. More than one person in the accommodation like milkshakes.

Answer YES if the conclusion follows and NO if it does not.
a. Mason likes milkshakes
b. If someone in the accommodation does not like milkshakes they must like tea
c. If someone does not like to drink tea it must be Mason
d. If only two people like milkshakes one has to be Mason
e. Someone in the accommodation likes both tea and milkshakes.

Question 18

Should the legal voting age be lowered to 17 to overcome the issue of bad voter turn-out?

Select the strongest argument from the statements below.
a. Yes, If under 18s could vote, their issues would be considered in the court of law
b. Yes, it will mean more people will be eligible to vote
c. No, 17 year olds are not mature enough to be able to make valid political decisions
d. No, Increasing the number of people who can vote won't necessarily increase turn-out on election day.

Question 19

There are 54 people in the cinema who are either adults or children. There are 6 more males than females. 24 of the 32 adults are male.

How many male children are there in the cinema?
  a. 6
  b. 8
  c. 10
  d. 12

Question 20

A teacher makes a seating plan for her class. June sits in the first seat and April sits as far away from her as possible. Joey sits in an odd numbered seat. Suma is sat next to William who is adjacent to Joey does not sit opposite to April and has people sitting on both sides. Ross is not neighbours with Joey.

5	6	7	8
1	2	3	4

Which of the following must not be true?
  a. Ross is opposite June
  b. June is opposite Joey
  c. Joey is opposite William
  d. Suma is sat in seat number 6.

Question 21

Should we focus more on rehabilitating offenders rather than punishing them for the crimes they commit?

Select the strongest argument from the statements below.
- a. Yes, crimes could be committed by people that had poor living circumstances
- b. Yes, rehabilitating some will lead to a reduction in crime in the future.
- c. No, A crime is still a crime regardless of the cause
- d. No, It will not provide justice to the victims of the crime.

Question 22

In a shop there are 40 people. 24 are looking for onions and 18 are looking for cabbages. 8 are looking for something else entirely.

How many have both?
- a. 10
- b. 12
- c. 14
- d. 16

Question 23

60% of children play football. 50% play cricket. 30% play rugby.

Answer Yes if the conclusion follows and No if it does not.
- a. At most 10% play football and cricket
- b. At least 20% of kids play neither cricket nor rugby
- c. Some play all three
- d. At most 10% do not play football or rugby
- e. 50% of children must only play cricket

Question 24

Jess goes to the cinema with her younger brother and two older sisters, Molly and Holly. One of them buys a hot dog, one buys nachos, one buys a pack of sweets and one buys nothing.
→ *The eldest picks something savoury*
→ *Jess does not get nachos*
→ *Youngest has savoury too*
→ *The one who picks no snack is a girl.*

Who picked the bag of sweets?
   a.   Jess
   b.   Holly
   c.   Molly
   d.   Their Brother

Question 25

If Jos eats a kebab, he drinks a pint of water. When he drinks hot chocolate, he doesn't feel hungry. When he eats breakfast, he has a dessert the same day. He always has a latte when he eats a kebab for dinner.

Place 'Yes' if the conclusion does follow. Place 'No' if the conclusion does not follow.
   a.   If he feels hungry, he must have had dessert
   b.   If he finishes his dinner without drinking latte afterwards, he must not have had a kebab
   c.   When he has burgers, he has a latte
   d.   He will have cocktails when he has desserts

Question 26

If A is lighter than B and C, and if D is heavier than B, which of the following must be true?
   a.   D is lighter than A
   b.   D is lighter than B
   c.   D could be lighter than C
   d.   D is heavier than c

Question 27

All hungry people are mean. No food lover is rude. Some food lovers are hungry.

Which of the following contradicts the above passage?
   a.   Some food lovers are mean
   b.   Some mean people are rude
   c.   All mean people are rude
   d.   Some hungry people are also food lovers.

Question 28

Alice did a survey within a group of 15 people attending a specialist autoimmune clinic to find out which condition they have.

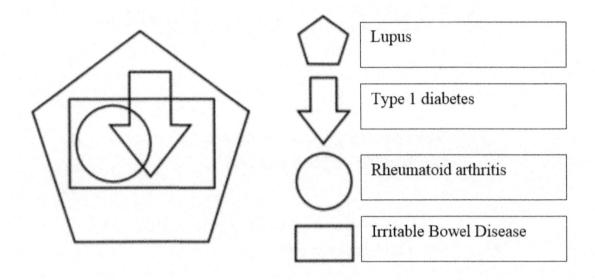

Based on the above, which statement is true about all the individuals who have type 1 diabetes?
- a. They also have lupus
- b. They also have Irritable Bowel Disease
- c. They have only one autoimmune condition
- d. They have at least three other autoimmune conditions

Question 29

A wall has 5 shelves built into it. Eileen puts either one cup or two cups on each of the five shelves.

If the total number of cups on the wall is eight, on how many shelves did Eileen put two cups?
- a. 1
- b. 2
- c. 3
- d. 4

1:1 UCAT TUTORING

 Delivered by UCAT experts, who scored in the top 10% of the exam

 A personalised 1:1 approach, tailored to your unique needs

 Proven success, with Medic Mind students achieving an average score of 2810 (top 10% nationally)

Book your FREE consultation now

Visit the link or scan the QR code below for more information:
www.medicmind.co.uk/ucat-tutoring

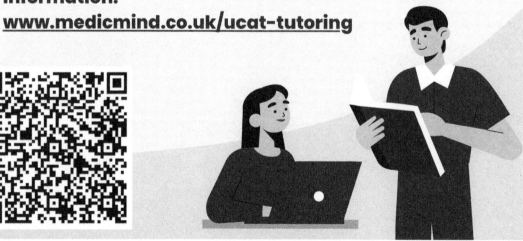

UCAT ONLINE COURSE

 100+ tutorials, designed by our UCAT experts, to guide you through every section of the exam

 Access to our UCAT Question Bank, with 8,000+ practice questions to use in your revision

 Invites to regular UCAT webinars, live classes and interactive sessions

Buy Now!

Visit the link or scan the QR code below for more information:
https://www.medicmind.co.uk/ucat-online-course/

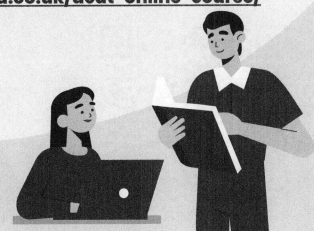

1:1 MEDICINE INTERVIEW TUTORING

 Delivered by Medicine Interview experts, who scored in the top 10% of the exam

 A personalised 1:1 approach, tailored to your unique needs

 Proven success, with Medic Mind students acing their Medicine Interview.

Book your FREE consultation now

Visit the link or scan the QR code below for more information:
www.medicmind.co.uk/interview-tutoring/

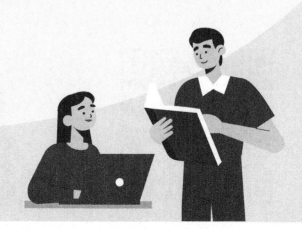

MEDICINE INTERVIEW ONLINE COURSE

 100+ tutorials, and 200+ MMI stations , designed by our Medicine interview experts

 Learn how to answer questions on motivation for Medicine, personal skills, work experience, hot topics, and more

 A range of packages available, including a live day of teaching and 1:1 tutoring

Buy Now!

Visit the link or scan the QR code below for more information:
www.medicmind.co.uk/interview-online-course/

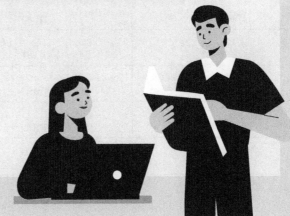

Answers: Decision Making Mock 1

Question 1: A

For this question it is helpful to make a table on your whiteboard. And start by filling in the information you already know, for example, we know that the sibling that leaves is the one that dislikes peeling carrots and that Joel smirks at his task. We know that they are all doing something they dislike and so the second statement that says the sibling that huffs likes cutting onions tells us that they are not the ones cutting onions. This means that Alex is setting the table. The one that dislikes cutting onions is the one that complains and this must be Derek. We also know that Alex must be setting the table as that is what she hates. Alex must be the one that huffs as the other three responses are accounted for.

We now know that the answer must be A as that is the only task left to fill.

Names	Task	Response
Joel		Smirks
	Peeling carrots	Leaves
Derek	Cutting onions	Complains
Alex	Setting the table	Huffs

Question 2: C

Make a table and start with the clearest information like we do in our lesson on ordered logical puzzles.

The text in red is the easy info we are given. We know that Aaron must want to drive to Edinburgh because all the other brothers have at least one box filled in the table

Names	Task	Response
Vernon	Dublin	Sail
Sam	Paris	
Jack	Madrid	
Aaron	London	Drive

We can fill in the information from here and see that Vernon must want to go to Dublin.

Question 3: B

To work this out we need to know the original probability of her picking a strawberry seed from the bag. Total number of seeds= 34.

Strawberry seeds= 10/34= 0.29

If three seeds of each variety are removed, the chance of picking a strawberry seed is reduced because:

Total number of seeds is now 25

Strawberry seeds: 7/25= 0.28

Question 4: A

We know that the average number of pencils that Charlie and Harry have is an odd number from the first sentence. Charlie is mentioned most in this scenario so let's focus on him first- Charlie must have more than 4 but fewer than 8 toys as we know he has more than Amit but fewer than Molly. The last sentence then tells us that Harry has 2 more than Charlie. Remember that the average of Charlie and Harry's pencils is an odd number. This means that the only number between 4 and 8 that Charlie can have is 6 and so harry must have 8 pencils.

6+8=14. 14/2= 7. This makes the answer A as we are told that Molly has 8 pencils and we worked out that so does Harry.

Question 5: D

Top Tip: Read through each statement carefully to see if they refer to all the key topics in the questions and select the strongest argument based on this. The main topics of focus in this question are cost and lifesaving.

A does not deal with the cost aspect of the statement and also does not explain why the NHS should be the ones paying. **B** is weak as it does not answer either. **C** is incorrect as it fails to address the issue of saving more lives as it just focuses on medical professionals. **D** is the strongest argument because it addresses the cost aspect and also argues that more lives could be saved in a different way.

Question 6: B

The fact that pets require regular duties of care means that children would be exposed to more responsibility, satisfying both themes of the statement.

The other options do not mention looking after others and nor does it suggest anything to do with gaining more responsibility.

Question 7: D

The main themes here are schools as a provider of the fruit and veg, consumption and subsidising.

A. The point here is not to necessarily increase but to subsidise costs to encourage consumption.

B. This lightly touches on the theme of consumption as the more important they are for your survival, the more likely you are to consume them however, this point does not cover whether subsidies would be a useful tool in increasing consumptions.

C. This could potentially touch on the idea against subsidising fruit and vegetables but there is not much given to make this a strong argument.

D is the strongest argument here and it provides a counter argument by suggesting that schools already have other costs to handle and provides and alternative solution.

Question 8: A

Start with what we know to be true, the fact that D is in third place. Looking at the second point, this means that A cannot be in first place as this would put B in third which we know cannot be true. This gives us the following possible combinations:

1. _ _ D A
2. _ A D _

If B is in first place, then it is next to second place (third bullet point) and A should be in fourth- therefore leaving the possible combination of BCDA. B could be in second place as we are not told that it cannot be. There is no condition that means anything should happen to other letters if B is in second. Therefore, leaving us with the possible combination of CBDA.

Top Tip: You can cancel out C as the correct answer here as nothing proves to us that B cannot be in second place- so if you have to guess due to lack of time then you have narrowed the possible right answers down which increases your chance of guessing the right answer!

If we look at one of the 2 combinations that we worked out above, _A D _: If B is in first place then it means B is next to second and so A must be last, which contradicts the fact that it actually is in second place. Therefore B cannot be in first place and has to be in last place, leaving CADB as our last possible combination.

Question 9: B

The reason for charging is to discourage people from missing appointments at all or cancel in advance so the space could be left free for someone else.

Option A misses the point that charging for missed appointments is to prevent patients from missing appointments and not implemented to substitute for government budget cuts. The point of using the money for other things is not a topic that is being discussed in the stem.

Option C offers a reasonable point but that does not mean that charging cannot be put in place. As option B shows, patients could still call and cancel.

Option D, though this is also reasonable, just because something is unfair and challenging does not mean it cannot be put in place.

Question 10: D

This is the strongest answer as it is a direct argument against the stem as it suggests that regular testing is unnecessary, and drivers can be safe regardless. This is why it is stronger than option A as it builds on it. The scope of A is too narrow and assumes that people lose their knowledge of rules as they get older which is speculative as it could be argued that with practice you actually remember rules better.

Question 11

A. **No** - When not on holiday, he does not go on a diet. Since he is currently on a diet then it means he must be on holiday

B. **No** - since we know he is on holiday, then it means he jet skis. We know that when he is happy he jet skis and so he must be happy.

C. **No** - We know that he is not on a holiday, he is not on a diet. But we don't know when the condition is that he is on holiday.

D. **Yes** - if he is not happy then he will not jet ski. We know that on holiday he jet skis too. So this means that when he is not jet skiing then he isn't on holiday.

E. **Yes** - when happy, he jet skis and so when he does not jet ski he is not happy.

Question 12: D

Lets start by working out who we know most information about. We know most about A, D and F. A won 3 less than F and D won 2 more than F and when we add the totals of A and d we get 17. from this information we can conclude the following:

A > F > D

D has 5 more medals than A.

A = 6 medals

D= 11 medals

F= 9 medals

A is sat opposite E and so E must have 7 medals. This is important to work out as we are told that E and G have a total of 17 medals too. This means that G must have 10 medals.

Common Trap: you might be tempted to start by working out what number of medals C has as they are sat opposite G but we have zero information about C so it is best to avoid this.

Question 13: D

The stated fact here is that all of Harry's books are Horrors. Daisy has non-fiction books and does not have any novels. If the book is not hers it is Harry's.

Option A is incorrect as if the book is Harry's, it is not a novel, it is a horror.

Option B is incorrect- if it is not non-fiction then it is a horror. But the book could be Daisy's which would mean it could be non-fiction.

Question 14: D

The stated fact here is that Mary wins the race. We also know that Rosie comes second. We need to now focus on what we know about Tim- since he did not finish first and the options given to us suggest that he did not finish last either we need to figure out how many people finished before him. Ander beat Bilraj and Cathy and Bilraj and Cathy beat Tim.

However, Timothy beats Mary and Hamesh. This therefore places Timothy sixth.

Question 15

A. **Yes** - We know that everyone gives food to El and that Kiki gives food to JJ and someone else.

B. **No** - We cannot conclude that he gives food to anyone other than Kiki.

C. **No** - the question implies that El is the only person that gets food from Nick which is not necessarily the case.

D. **No** - she gets food but we do not know about giving.

E. **No** - El gets food from everyone in their neighbourhood so it might not necessarily from Kiki. 'must' is use of extreme language.

Question 16: D

Since there are 5 children in this family and Jim is older than two of his siblings then he must be third oldest. We know that Emma is older than at least Ben and younger than Mick- making Emma the fourth or second oldest. Meaning Mick is either eldest or second eldest. We cannot exactly pinpoint if she is oldest and so cannot select B.

Question 17

A. **No** - we don't have any information to conclude that he likes milkshakes

B. **No** - we do not know if they prefer drinking something else like coffee

C. **Yes** - everyone there likes tea except from Mason

D. **No** - he could like coffee or something else

E. **Yes** - more than one person likes milkshake and only Mason does not like tea, so at least one person must like both.

Question 18: D

All other options do not address the theme of voter turn out.

Question 19: A

If 24 of the 32 are adult males then 8 of the 32 Adults are females. So 22 of the 54 must be children.

There are 6 more males than females. We can write this into an equation:

24 MA (male adults) + MC (male children) = 8 FA +FC +6

Knowing that 22 are children, we can work out the answer to be 6

Question 20: D

We know that June is in seat 1. And so April has to be in number 8. William must be in 7 as he is adjacent to April. And so Suma must be in seat 6 as she is next to William.

Question 21: B

Deals with the outcome of rehabilitation whilst the others only offer opinions.

Question 22: A

An equation can be written, assume X is the number who are looking for both cabbages and onions.

(24-x) +x + (18-x)=32 (as 8 are removed)

24+18-x=32

24+18=32+x

42-32=x

10=x

Question 23

A. **No** - it is possible that all who play football also play cricket

B. **Yes** - the minimum percentage of kids who play neither cricket nor rugby is 20%

C. **Yes** - we know that at least 20% of kids do not play cricket or rugby. The use of the words 'some' suggests that some can play all three

D. **No** - If all those who play rugby also play football, then 30% of students play both, 30% play football and not rugby ad 40% of students play neither.

E. **No** - just because 50% play cricket we cannot assume that ONLY 50% play cricket.

Question 24: D

Jess must be the youngest girl. She therefore has bought a savoury snack and so can be excluded. We are told that she does not like nachos so it is unlikely that she got this and so must have gotten a hot dog. One of the girls has picked no snack which leaves the brother with the bag of sweets.

Question 25

A. **No** – we know he does not feel hungry when he has hot chocolate but not about the effect of dessert on his hunger.

B. **Yes** – we know he has latte after he has kebab for dinner. So he must not have had kebab for dinner if he has not had a black coffee

C. **No** – we cannot make this assumption

D. **No** – not enough information to make this assumption.

Question 26: C

We know that A is lighter than B and we know B is lighter than D:

A>B >D.

We know that C is heavier than A but we don't know where it fits in relation to B and D.

Question 27: C

We know that some food lovers are hungry and that all hungry people are mean. We can conclude that some food lovers are mean. We can also conclude that some food lovers are mean but not rude. Therefore, it is not true that all mean people are rude.

Question 28: A

This is because the shape representing type 1 diabetes is the arrow and is within the large pentagon that represents lupus.

Question 29: C

This is because she must put one cup on each of the five shelves, leaving three cups. She does not place three cups on any of the shelves as said in the stem, so there must be three racks that hold two cups.

TOP TIP: Use your whiteboard to draw out 5 shelves if you struggle to visualise things in your mind.

Quantitative Reasoning Mock 1

Question 1

The table below shows the temperatures in 8 different countries. Temperatures are given in either Fahrenheit (°F) or Celsius (°C).

Country	Temperature
Egypt	35.1 °C
Ghana	84.0 °F
Cuba	75.7 °F
Australia	53.0 °F
Taiwan	26.0 °C
Peru	19.0 °C
Netherlands	63.2 °F
Uzbekistan	33.0 °C

Temperature in °C multiplied by 1.8, then add 32 = Temperature in °F

How much higher is the temperature in Ghana than the temperature in Peru?
  a. 16.8 °F
  b. 17.8 °F
  c. 18.3 °F
  d. 19.4 °F
  e. 20.1 °F

Question 2

The table below shows the temperatures in 8 different countries. Temperatures are given in either Fahrenheit (°F) or Celsius (°C).

Country	Temperature
Egypt	35.1 °C
Ghana	84.0 °F
Cuba	75.7 °F
Australia	53.0 °F
Taiwan	26.0 °C
Peru	19.0 °C
Netherlands	63.2 °F
Uzbekistan	33.0 °C

Temperature in °C multiplied by 1.8, then add 32 = Temperature in °F

What is the temperature in Cuba in °C?
  a. 21.1 °C
  b. 22.6 °C
  c. 22.9 °C
  d. 23.1 °C
  e. 24.8 °C

Question 3

The table below shows the temperatures in 8 different countries. Temperatures are given in either Fahrenheit (°F) or Celsius (°C).

Country	Temperature
Egypt	35.1 °C
Ghana	84.0 °F
Cuba	75.7 °F
Australia	53.0 °F
Taiwan	26.0 °C
Peru	19.0 °C
Netherlands	63.2 °F
Uzbekistan	33.0 °C

Temperature in °C multiplied by 1.8, then add 32 = Temperature in °F

The temperature in Josh's village is halfway between that in Egypt, and that in Taiwan. What is his village's temperature in °F?

a. 78.8 °F
b. 87.0 °F
c. 95.2 °F
d. 102.1 °F
e. 106.7 °F

Question 4

The table below shows the temperatures in 8 different countries. Temperatures are given in either Fahrenheit (°F) or Celsius (°C).

Country	Temperature
Egypt	35.1 °C
Ghana	84.0 °F
Cuba	75.7 °F
Australia	53.0 °F
Taiwan	26.0 °C
Peru	19.0 °C
Netherlands	63.2 °F
Uzbekistan	33.0 °C

Temperature in °C multiplied by 1.8, then add 32 = Temperature in °F

The temperature in Amir's city is exactly half the temperature in Uzbekistan. What is the temperature in Amir's city in °F?

    a. 42.6 °F
    b. 43.9 °F
    c. 44.1 °F
    d. 45.7 °F
    e. 46.3 °F

Question 5

A sustainable haberdashery sources all of its supplies from ethical businesses. It purchases its four most popular types of material, in boxes of either 6 metres or 8 metres each, and sells the material in rolls of 5 or 8 m.

	Buys		Sells	
MATERIAL	Metres per roll	Price per metre	Price per 8 metres of material	Price per 5 metres of material
White cotton	8	$4.00	$38.00	$24.00
Green silk	8	$24.50	$220.00	$150.00
Blue denim	6	$2.90	$26.00	$18.65
Lilac rayon	6	$1.95	$18.00	$12.99

Profit = Selling price – Buying price

Kimberley visits the haberdashery one day. How much more will be spent per metre, if she buys 8 metres of white cotton instead of 8 metres of lilac rayon?

    a. 11.1 %
    b. 12.3 %
    c. 13.1 %
    d. 14.2 %
    e. 15.6 %

Question 6

A sustainable haberdashery sources all of its supplies from ethical businesses. It purchases its four most popular types of material, in boxes of either 6 metres or 8 metres each, and sells the material in rolls of 5 or 8 m.

	Buys		Sells	
MATERIAL	Metres per roll	Price per metre	Price per 8 metres of material	Price per 5 metres of material
White cotton	8	$4.00	$38.00	$24.00
Green silk	8	$24.50	$220.00	$150.00
Blue denim	6	$2.90	$26.00	$18.65
Lilac rayon	6	$1.95	$18.00	$12.99

Profit = Selling price – Buying price

A trader buys 20 8-metre rolls of green silk, and sells them at a price which is 35% higher per metre, than the haberdashery sold them as. How much is the trader selling each roll at?

    a. $256.00
    b. $279.00
    c. $297.00
    d. $298.00
    e. $299.70

Question 7

A sustainable haberdashery sources all of its supplies from ethical businesses. It purchases its four most popular types of material, in boxes of either 6 metres or 8 metres each, and sells the material in rolls of 5 or 8 m.

	Buys		Sells	
MATERIAL	Metres per roll	Price per metre	Price per 8 metres of material	Price per 5 metres of material
White cotton	8	$4.00	$38.00	$24.00
Green silk	8	$24.50	$220.00	$150.00
Blue denim	6	$2.90	$26.00	$18.65
Lilac rayon	6	$1.95	$18.00	$12.99

Profit = Selling price – Buying price

How much more does the haberdashery charge for an 8-metre roll of lilac rayon, than they pay for a 6-metre roll of the same material?

- a. 53.8%
- b. 54.8%
- c. 55.9%
- d. 56.2%
- e. 61.1%

Question 8

A sustainable haberdashery sources all of its supplies from ethical businesses. It purchases its four most popular types of material, in boxes of either 6 metres or 8 metres each, and sells the material in rolls of 5 or 8 m.

	Buys		**Sells**	
MATERIAL	**Metres per roll**	**Price per metre**	**Price per 8 metres of material**	**Price per 5 metres of material**
White cotton	8	$4.00	$38.00	$24.00
Green silk	8	$24.50	$220.00	$150.00
Blue denim	6	$2.90	$26.00	$18.65
Lilac rayon	6	$1.95	$18.00	$12.99

Profit = Selling price – Buying price

A buyer wants to purchase a 5-metre roll for their upcoming sewing project. What is the second-cheapest option?
   a. White cotton
   b. Green silk
   c. Blue denim
   d. Lilac rayon
   e. Can't tell

Question 9

Jude is drafting a map of his school grounds. On his map, the Anderson tennis courts, occupy an area of 864 m2 in total. There are three rectangular tennis courts in total, which require special permission from the PE department to play on.

What is the scale of Jude's map, if each tennis court measures 15 cm by 160 cm on it?
   a. 1 to 4
   b. 1 to 12
   c. 1 to 200
   d. 1 to 1200
   e. 1 to 12000

Question 10

Whilst attending a national conference on medical leadership, Ron notices that the ratio of conference volunteers to organisers is 4 to 1, and there are 2 female speakers for every 10 conference volunteers. Meanwhile, the ratio of male to female speakers is 2 to 5.

If there are 30 conference organisers, how many more women than men are speaking at the leadership conference?
   a. 2
   b. 8
   c. 12
   d. 20
   e. 30

Question 11

A group of friends have started a local music festival every year, to increase awareness of the benefits of classical music.

The festival hosted five orchestral concerts in its first year.

There were two orchestral and two choral concerts in the second year of the festival. On average, the number of people who attended all four concerts was exactly 30% greater than the average number in the first year, which was 50 in the first year.

How many people attended all of the concerts in the festival's second year?
   a. 50
   b. 65
   c. 210
   d. 260
   e. 285

Question 12

Margot sends a carrier pigeon to her aunt, which flies a total distance of 50.5 miles in 94 minutes.

What is the speed of the carrier pigeon in miles per hour (mph)?
   a. 8.4 mph
   b. 13.3 mph
   c. 32.3 mph
   d. 61.8 mph
   e. 94.0 mph

Question 13

The number of people with a type I diabetes diagnosis in City Z is exactly one quarter of that in City X. However, the number of people diagnosed with type I diabetes in City X is 46% more than in City Y.

If there are 1600 people who have been diagnosed with type I diabetes in City Z, how many more people have a type I diabetes diagnosis in City Y, compared to City X?
   a. 2944
   b. 2964
   c. 3120
   d. 8642
   e. 9344

Question 14

In Sanne's county, there are 1900 people who are double-jointed. However, the double-jointed population in Vasili's county is one third of that in Corinne's county, whilst the double-jointed population in Sanne's county is 40% of that in Vasili's county.

How many people are double-jointed in Corinne's county?
   a. 4750
   b. 9625
   c. 14250
   d. 16950
   e. 17460

Question 15

Whilst out for a walk, Jock and Carol notice that apple trees are being planted on a plot of land measuring 48 m by 52 m. On their map, the footpath next to the plot, is 12 cm long, but measures 76.8 m in real life.

What is the area of this plot on the map?
   a. 58.62 cm²
   b. 59.84 cm²
   c. 60.94 cm²
   d. 61.83 cm²
   e. 63.94 cm²

Question 16

Priya and Olly take the train to Dumfries for their four-week hospital placement. On Saturday afternoon, their train journey home takes 110 minutes.

Their journey to Dumfries took three and a half hours.

How much longer was their train journey to Dumfries, compared to their journey back?
- a. 84%
- b. 88%
- c. 91%
- d. 96%
- e. 102%

Question 17

On a day trip to the zoo, Mila notices that the ratio of penguins to giraffes is 5 to 3. Meanwhile, the ratio of giraffes to pandas is 12 to 1.

If there are 4 pandas at the zoo, how many penguins are there?
- a. 80
- b. 84
- c. 90
- d. 91
- e. 96

Question 18

The number of sparrowhawks in Abundin is 40% of that of Limeton. The number of sparrowhawks in Feiser is 70% of the number of sparrowhawks in Limeton.

If there are 620 sparrowhawks in Abundin, how many are there in Feiser?
- a. 620
- b. 730
- c. 810
- d. 980
- e. 1085

Question 19

On Saturday morning, Matt runs around a running track with a perimeter of 600 metres.

What is his speed in kilometres per second (km/s), if he runs 6 laps around the track in twelve and a half minutes?
   a.   0.0036 km/s
   b.   0.0048 km/s
   c.   0.048 km/s
   d.   0.086 km/s
   e.   4.8 km/s

Question 20

The table below shows the number of live births and fertility rates in Country P over the period 2012-2020.

Country P, 2012-2020

Year	Number of live births	Fertility rate
2012	451,842	1.8
2013	464,726	1.9
2014	452,948	2.3
2015		2.4
2016	456,534	2.2
2017	488,628	2.3
2018	469,992	
2019	414,966	2.4
2020	409,592	2.6

The fertility rate is calculated as the number of live births per 1,000 women of childbearing age.

In 2018, there were 187,752,488 women of childbearing age living in Country P.

What was the fertility rate for Country P in 2018?
   a. 0.25
   b. 2.5
   c. 2.7
   d. 2.8
   e. 2.9

Question 21

The table below shows the number of live births and fertility rates in Country P over the period 2012-2020.

Country P, 2012-2020

Year	Number of live births	Fertility rate
2012	451,842	1.8
2013	464,726	1.9
2014	452,948	2.3
2015		2.4
2016	456,534	2.2
2017	488,628	2.3
2018	469,992	
2019	414,966	2.4
2020	409,592	2.6

The fertility rate is calculated as the number of live births per 1,000 women of childbearing age.

In 2018, there were 187,752,488 women of childbearing age living in Country P.

On average, approximately how many live births were there per year in the period 2016-2020?
   a. 429,50018
   b. 432,90042
   c. 439,200174
   d. 457,80036
   e. 447,90042

Question 22

The table below shows the number of live births and fertility rates in Country P over the period 2012-2020.

Country P, 2012-2020

Year	Number of live births	Fertility rate
2012	451,842	1.8
2013	464,726	1.9
2014	452,948	2.3
2015		2.4
2016	456,534	2.2
2017	488,628	2.3
2018	469,992	
2019	414,966	2.4
2020	409,592	2.6

The fertility rate is calculated as the number of live births per 1,000 women of childbearing age.

In 2018, there were 187,752,488 women of childbearing age living in Country P.

Overall, what was the percentage increase in the fertility rate of Country P between 2012 and 2020?
   a. 41%
   b. 42%
   c. 44%
   d. 48%
   e. 51%

Question 23

The table below shows the number of live births and fertility rates in Country P over the period 2012-2020.

Country P, 2012-2020

Year	Number of live births	Fertility rate
2012	451,842	1.8
2013	464,726	1.9
2014	452,948	2.3
2015		2.4
2016	456,534	2.2
2017	488,628	2.3
2018	469,992	
2019	414,966	2.4
2020	409,592	2.6

The fertility rate is calculated as the number of live births per 1,000 women of childbearing age.

In 2018, there were 187,752,488 women of childbearing age living in Country P.

If the number of women of childbearing age in Country P decreased by 3.4% between 2015 and 2018, approximately how many live births were there in 2015?
   a. 466,466500
   b. 478,500466
   c. 481,500462
   d. 485,800786
   e. 489,900964

Question 24

A research organisation is reviewing the governmental expenditures of a country in the past twenty years. The government spent $300 million and $525 million respectively on general public services and environmental protection, for the period 2012-2013. In this same period, government spending totalled $950 million. The governmental expenditure on foreign aid and welfare funding comprised less than one-fifth of the expenditure on general public services. The rest of the total budget was spent on health and social services.

Approximately, what was the government's spending on health and social services in the period 2012-2013?
  a. $42 million
  b. $48 million
  c. $52 million
  d. $65 million
  e. $75 million

Question 25

The table below shows the number of people who have passed their driving tests in a sixth-form, across both year groups attending the sixth-form.

Driving test status	Year 12		Year 13	
	Boys	Girls	Boys	Girls
Passed	34	20	42	35
Not passed	31	45	27	32

What is the ratio of boys to girls in this sixth-form?
  a. 65 : 62
  b. 66 : 67
  c. 66 : 78
  d. 67 : 66
  e. 134 : 131

Question 26

The table below shows the number of people who have passed their driving tests in a sixth-form, across both year groups attending the sixth-form.

Driving test status	Year 12		Year 13	
	Boys	Girls	Boys	Girls
Passed	34	20	42	35
Not passed	31	45	27	32

Of all the Year 12 students, what percentage had not passed their driving test?
- a. 58.9%
- b. 59.2%
- c. 60.1%
- d. 61.4%
- e. 62.9%

Question 27

The table below shows the number of people who have passed their driving tests in a sixth-form, across both year groups attending the sixth-form.

Driving test status	Year 12		Year 13	
	Boys	Girls	Boys	Girls
Passed	34	20	42	35
Not passed	31	45	27	32

The new intake for Year 12 at another school totals 300. This sixth-form is representative of the new Year 12 intake. Based on the data shown, how many people in the new Year 12 cohort have passed their driving test?
- a. 125
- b. 54
- c. 77
- d. 153
- e. 108

Question 28

The table below shows the number of people who have passed their driving tests in a sixth-form, across both year groups attending the sixth-form.

Driving test status	Year 12		Year 13	
	Boys	Girls	Boys	Girls
Passed	34	20	42	35
Not passed	31	45	27	32

Half of the boys in Year 13 who have passed their driving tests have green eyes, and one-fifth of the girls in Year 13 and a quarter of the girls in Year 12 who have passed are green-eyed. The Year 12 boys who have passed their tests are not green-eyed. Of those who have passed, which is the closest estimate of the proportion of students who also have green eyes?

    a. 22.2%
    b. 24.1%
    c. 25.2%
    d. 26.2%
    e. 27.5%

Question 29

The estate agent Muller-Franck owns four properties in a district: A, B, C, and D. The table below shows the average annual expenses for their upkeep: allowable expenses include spending on maintenance and fixtures, whilst capital expenses include spending on furnishings and interior decorations. The graph shows their annual rental income over the last three years.

Both the graph and the table give their figures in pounds.

Property	Allowable expenses	Capital expenses
A	1450	590
B	910	462
C	9983	2489
D	1840	754

Rental income				
Year	A	B	C	D
2018	14840	10320	20742	16550
2019	14620	12480	20480	16520
2020	14680	12598	21020	16840

Profit = Rental income – total annual expenses

What was the total combined profit from properties A, B, and C in 2019?
- a. £12478
- b. £13592
- c. £14486
- d. £15884
- e. £16842

Question 30

The estate agent Muller-Franck owns four properties in a district: A, B, C, and D. The table below shows the average annual expenses for their upkeep: allowable expenses include spending on maintenance and fixtures, whilst capital expenses include spending on furnishings and interior decorations. The graph shows their annual rental income over the last three years.

Both the graph and the table give their figures in pounds.

Property	Allowable expenses	Capital expenses
A	1450	590
B	910	462
C	9983	2489
D	1840	754

Rental income				
Year	A	B	C	D
2018	14840	10320	20742	16550
2019	14620	12480	20480	16520
2020	14680	12598	21020	16840

Profit = Rental income – total annual expenses

How did Property D's profits change from 2019 to 2020?
- a. Increase by 1.3%
- b. Increase by 2.3%
- c. Decrease by 2.4%
- d. Decrease by 2.5%
- e. Can't tell

Question 31

The estate agent Muller-Franck owns four properties in a district: A, B, C, and D. The table below shows the average annual expenses for their upkeep: allowable expenses include spending on maintenance and fixtures, whilst capital expenses include spending on furnishings and interior decorations. The graph shows their annual rental income over the last three years.

Both the graph and the table give their figures in pounds.

Property	Allowable expenses	Capital expenses
A	1450	590
B	910	462
C	9983	2489
D	1840	754

Rental income				
Year	A	B	C	D
2018	14840	10320	20742	16550
2019	14620	12480	20480	16520
2020	14680	12598	21020	16840

Profit = Rental income – total annual expenses

Which of Muller-Franck's properties made the most profit in 2018?
  a. Property A
  b. Property B
  c. Property C
  d. Property D
  e. Can't tell

Question 32

The estate agent Muller-Franck owns four properties in a district: A, B, C, and D. The table below shows the average annual expenses for their upkeep: allowable expenses include spending on maintenance and fixtures, whilst capital expenses include spending on furnishings and interior decorations. The graph shows their annual rental income over the last three years.

Both the graph and the table give their figures in pounds.

Property	Allowable expenses	Capital expenses
A	1450	590
B	910	462
C	9983	2489
D	1840	754

Rental income				
Year	A	B	C	D
2018	14840	10320	20742	16550
2019	14620	12480	20480	16520
2020	14680	12598	21020	16840

Profit = Rental income – total annual expenses

By what percentage did the rental income from property C increase from 2018 to 2020?
   a. 0.013%
   b. 0.15%
   c. 1.3%
   d. 1.5%
   e. 13%

Question 33

The table below shows the flight prices for the different destinations which an airline flies to, from one airport. The off-peak discount is applied to the summer rate at the pricing shown, but only for spring, autumn, and winter travel. All flights are one-way, whilst flights to and from Porto are stopped in winter.

Destination	Summer rate	Off-peak discount
Dublin	£12.10	20%
Rome	£9.80	6%
Marseille	£24.00	35%
Porto	£10.68	10%
Ibiza	£58.40	28% 42.05

Adam, Mark, and Lea are planning to go on a holiday in September. How much would each person save if they bought a return ticket to Porto, instead of Ibiza?

    a. £50.96
    b. £51.59
    c. £52.66
    d. £53.82
    e. £54.66

Question 34

The table below shows the flight prices for the different destinations which an airline flies to, from one airport. The off-peak discount is applied to the summer rate at the pricing shown, but only for spring, autumn, and winter travel. All flights are one-way, whilst flights to and from Porto are stopped in winter.

Destination	Summer rate	Off-peak discount
Dublin	£12.10	20%
Rome	£9.80	6%
Marseille	£24.00	35%
Porto	£10.68	10%
Ibiza	£58.40	28% 42.05

Which destination is the most expensive to fly to in April?
   a. Dublin
   b. Marseille
   c. Ibiza
   d. Rome
   e. Porto

Question 35

The table below shows the flight prices for the different destinations which an airline flies to, from one airport. The off-peak discount is applied to the summer rate at the pricing shown, but only for spring, autumn, and winter travel. All flights are one-way, whilst flights to and from Porto are stopped in winter.

Destination	Summer rate	Off-peak discount
Dublin	£12.10	20%
Rome	£9.80	6%
Marseille	£24.00	35%
Porto	£10.68	10%
Ibiza	£58.40	28% 42.05

A couple are considering a holiday to Rome. How much would they save if they flew on this airline in December instead of July?

 a. £2.53
 b. £2.68
 c. £3.92
 d. £3.98
 e. £4.01

Question 36

The table below shows the flight prices for the different destinations which an airline flies to, from one airport. The off-peak discount is applied to the summer rate at the pricing shown, but only for spring, autumn, and winter travel. All flights are one-way, whilst flights to and from Porto are stopped in winter.

Destination	Summer rate	Off-peak discount
Dublin	£12.10	20%
Rome	£9.80	6%
Marseille	£24.00	35%
Porto	£10.68	10%
Ibiza	£58.40	28% 42.05

Last summer, Ellen bought a return ticket to Ibiza for June. How much would she have saved if she bought two return tickets to Rome in the same month?

- a. 193.6%
- b. 194.2%
- c. 196.5%
- d. 197.9%
- e. 198.9%

Answers: Quantitative Reasoning Mock 1

Question 1: B

1. Work out the temperature in Peru in °F:
(19 x 1.8) + 32 = 66.2 °F

2. Work out the difference between the temperatures:
84 – 66.2 = 17.8 °F

Top Tip: do not hurry to the calculator. Make sure you have a clear target in mind, before you make any calculations. Use the whiteboard to quickly note down your calculations if helpful.

Question 2: D

Convert the temperature from °F to °C:

(Temperature in °C x 1.8) + 32 = 75.7

Temperature in °C x 1.8   ≈ 41.5

Temperature in °C   = 23.0555(...)

Top Tip: do not hurry to the calculator without a clear target calculation in mind. Use the whiteboard to quickly note down your calculations if helpful.

Question 3: B

1. Convert the temperatures in Egypt and Taiwan to °F:
For Taiwan: (26 x 1.8) + 32 = 78.8
For Egypt: (35.1 x 1.8) + 32 = 95.18

2. Work out the difference between these temperatures:
95.18 – 78.8 = 16.38

3. Work out the midpoint (temperature in Josh's village):
(16.38/2) + 78.8 = 86.99 °F

Common Trap: UCAT question options may be numbers which are part of calculating the actual answer, to trip test-takers up.

Question 4: D

1. Convert the temperature in Uzbekistan to °F:
(33 x 1.8) + 32 = 91.4

2. Work out half of this temperature:
91.4/ 2 = 45.7

Top Tip: convert earlier on to the units in the answer options – this will make your final calculations quicker and less confusing.

Question 5: A

1. Work out how much is spent per metre when buying 8 metres of cotton:
38 / 8 = $4.75 per metre

2. Work out how much is spent per metre when buying 8 metres of rayon:
18 / 8 = $2.25 per metre

3. Work out the difference between the two prices:
4.75 – 2.25 = $2.50

4. Hence, work out the percentage difference:
2.50 / 2.25 = 1.111(...)

2.25 x 111.11(...)% = 2.50 – indicating an increase of 11.1 %.

Top Tip: make good use of the whiteboard. It is there for you to jot down multiple figures, to come back to them at different times during your calculations.

Question 6: C

1. Work out how much the haberdashery charged per metre, on the 8-metre silk rolls:
220 / 8 = $27.50 per metre

2. Work out how much the trader is charging per metre, on them:
$27.5 x 1.35 = $37.125

3. Work out how much the trader is charging per roll:
37.125 x 8 = $297

Top Tip: the UCAT answer options can be very similar. Reading the answers carefully is crucial to not missing easy marks.

Question 7: A

1. Work out how much the haberdashery pays for a 6 m roll:
$1.95 x 6 = $11.70

2. Work out the percentage difference between the haberdashery's buying and selling prices:
(18 – 11.7) / 11.7 x 100 = 53.846(...)%

Top Tip: do not hurry to the calculator. Make sure you have a clear target in mind, before you make any calculations. Use the whiteboard to quickly note down your calculations if helpful.

Question 8: C

Eyeball the prices for the 5-metre rolls the haberdashery is selling:
Blue denim is priced most cheaply at $18.65 per 5-metre roll, next to lilac rayon at $12.99 per roll – so this is the correct option.

Timing Tip: Be prepared to eyeball and estimate without calculating, to save time and potential marks.

Question 9: D

1. Work out the area of each tennis court on the map (in metres):
0.15 x 1.6 = 0.24 m2

2. Work out the area of each tennis court in real life:
864 / 3 = 288 m2

3. Work out how many times bigger the real-life area is than that on the map:
288 / 0.24 = 1200

4. Hence, set up the ratio/map scale:
0.24 : 288 = 1 : 1200

Top Tip: make good use of the whiteboard. It is there for you to jot down multiple figures, to come back to them at different times during your calculations.

Top Tip: do not hurry to the calculator. Make sure you have a clear target in mind, before you make any calculations. Use the whiteboard to quickly note down your calculations if helpful.

Question 10: C

1. Using the ratio given, work out the number of volunteers:
4 : 1 = volunteers : 30
Volunteers = 4 x 30 = 120

2. Using the ratio given, work out the number of female speakers:
Female speakers : volunteers = 2 : 10 = speakers : 120
Female speakers = (120 / 10) x 2 = 20

3. Work out the number of male speakers:
Male speakers : female speakers = 2 : 5 = male : 20
Male speakers = (20 / 5) x 2 = 8

4. Work out the difference between the two speaker numbers:
20 – 8 = 12

Timing Tip: practise basic mental maths. This will give you more time to tackle other questions in the QR section.

Question 11: D

1. Work out the average audience size in the first year:
250 / 5 = 50

2. Work out the average size in the second year:
50 x 1.3 = 65

3. Work out the total number of concert attendees in the second year:
65 x 4 = 260

Common Trap: UCAT question options may be numbers which are part of calculating the actual answer, to trip test-takers up.

Question 12: C

1. Work out the number for scaling down 94 minutes to 1 hour:
94 x (scale factor) = 60 minutes
Scale factor = 94 / 60 = 1.56

2. Work out how many miles the carrier pigeon would fly in 1 hour:
50.5 / 1.56 = 32.3 miles per hour

Common Trap: UCAT question options may be numbers which are part of calculating the actual answer, to trip test-takers up.

Question 13: A

1. Work out the number of people diagnosed with diabetes in City X:

A = 1600 x 4 = 6400

2. Work out the number in City Y:

B = 6400 x 1.46 = 9344

3. Work out the difference between Cities X and Y:

9344 – 6400 = 2944

Top Tip: the UCAT answer options can be very similar. Reading the answers carefully is crucial to not missing easy marks.

Question 14: C

1. Work out the double-jointed population in Vasili's county:

1900 = 0.4 x V

X = 1900 / 0.4 = 4750

2. Work out the population in Corinne's county:

4750 = Y / 3

Y = 4750 x 3 = 14250

Top Tip: do not hurry to the calculator. Make sure you have a clear target in mind, before you make any calculations. Use the whiteboard to quickly note down your calculations if helpful.

Question 15: C

1. Work out the map scale:

12 cm : 76.8 m = 12 cm : 7680 cm = 1 cm : (7680 / 12) cm

= 1 : 640

2. Work out the dimensions of the plot on the map:

With a scale of 1: 640, the plot of land has a length of (5200 / 640 =) 8.125 cm, and a width of (4800 / 640 =) 7.5 cm.

3. Work out the area of the plot on the map:

8.125 x 7.5 cm = 60.9375 cm^2

Top Tip: make good use of the whiteboard. It is there for you to jot down multiple figures, to come back to them at different times during your calculations.

Question 16: C

1. Convert three and a half hours to minutes:
3.5 x 60 = 210 minutes

2. Work out the difference between both times:
210 – 110 = 100 minutes

3. Work out the percentage increase, from 110 minutes to three and a half hours:
(210 – 110) / 110 = 100 / 110 = 0.90909(…), or 91%.

Timing Tip: practise basic conversions, such as those from minutes to seconds and vice versa. This will save you crucial time for other calculations.

Question 17: A

1. Using the ratio given, work out how many giraffes there are:
Giraffes: pandas = 12 : 1 = giraffes : 4
4 x 12 = 48

2. Hence, work out how many penguins there are:
Penguins: giraffes = 5 : 3 = penguins : 48
Penguins = (48 / 3) x 5 = 80

Top Tip: familiarise yourself with carrying out accurate conversions quickly, to boost your score and save time.

Question 18: E

1. Work out the sparrowhawk number in Limeton:
620/0.4 = 1550

2. Work out the sparrowhawk number in Feiser:
1550 x 0.7 = 1085

Top Tip: do not hurry to the calculator. Make sure you have a clear target in mind, before you make any calculations. Use the whiteboard to quickly note down your calculations if helpful.

Question 19: B

1. Work out the total distance Matt ran:
600 x 6 = 3600 m

2. Convert to seconds:
(12.5 x 60) = 750 seconds

3. Work out how many metres per second Matt ran:
3600 m in 750 seconds – 3600 / 750 is the speed = 4.80 metres per second

4. Convert to kilometres per second:
4.8 / 1000 = 0.0048 km per second

Top Tip: practise basic mental maths (like 600 x 6 for step 1 here) – this will save your time to tackle other questions in the QR section.

Question 20: B

1. Set up the ratio for live births: women of childbearing age:
= 469,992 : 187,752,488

2. Hence work out the number of live births per 1000 women:
To scale the total number of women of childbearing age down to 1000, we need to divide the total number by x.
187,752,488 / 1000 = x = 187,752.488
469,992 / 187,752.488 = 2.503(...) = 2.5

Top Tip: do not hurry to the calculator. Make sure you have a clear target in mind, before you make any calculations. Use the whiteboard to quickly note down your calculations if helpful.

Question 21: E

1. Work out the total number of live births over this time period:
456,534 + 488,628 + 469,992 + 414,966 + 409,592 = 2,239,712

2. Divide by the number of years in this time period:
2,239,712 / 5 = 447,942.4

Question 22: C

1. Work out the difference between the fertility rates in 2012 and 2020:
2.6 – 1.8 = 0.8

2. Divide by the 2012 fertility rate to work out the percentage increase:
(0.8 / 1.8) x 100 = 44%

Timing Tip: practise basic mental maths. This will give you more time to tackle other questions in the QR section.

Question 23: A

1. Work out the number of women of childbearing age in 2015:
2015 population x (1-0.034) = 187,752,488
2015 population = 187,752,488 / 0.966 = 194,360,753.6(...) or 194,360,754 approx.

2. Work out the number of live births in 2015:
Fertility rate in 2015 = 2.4 per 1000
 1. x (194,360,754 / 1000) = 466,465.8(...) or 466,466

Top Tip: the UCAT answer options can be very similar. Reading the answers carefully is crucial to not missing easy marks.

Question 24: D

1. Work out how much the government spent on foreign aid and welfare funding:
300 / 5 = 60 (million dollars)

2. Work out how much the government spent on all services except health and social services:
300 + 525 + 60 = 885 (million dollars)

3. Work out how much the government spent on health and social services:
Total spending = 950 – 885 = 65 (million dollars)

Top Tip: make good use of the whiteboard. It is there for you to jot down multiple figures, to come back to them at different times during your calculations.

Question 25: D

1. Work out the total number of girls:
20 + 45 + 35 + 31 = 132

2. Work out the total number of boys:
34 + 31 + 42 + 27 = 134

3. Set up the ratio:
Boys : girls = 134 : 132, which can be simplified down to 67 : 66

Top Tip: the UCAT answer options can be very similar. Reading the answers carefully is crucial to not missing easy marks.

Question 26: A

1. Work out the total number of students who had not passed:
31 + 45 = 76

2. Work out the total number of students in Year 12:
34 + 20 + 31 + 45 = 130

3. Work out the percentage of students who had not passed:
(76 / 130) x 100 = 58.46(...) = 58.9%

Top Tip: do not hurry to the calculator. Make sure you have a clear target in mind, before you make any calculations. Use the whiteboard to quickly note down your calculations if helpful.

Question 27: A

1. Work out how many people in Year 12 have passed (in this sixth-form):
34 + 20 = 54

2. Work out the percentage of Year 12s who have passed:
(54 / 130) x 100 = 41.53(...)%

3. Work out how many Year 12s in the new intake have passed:
41.53 % of 300 = 0.4153 x 300 = 124.59, which rounds to 125

Timing Tip: practise basic mental maths. This will give you more time to tackle other questions in the QR section.

Question 28: C

1. Work out how many green-eyed Year 13 boys have passed their tests:
42 / 2 = 21

2. Work out how many green-eyed Year 12/13 girls have passed their tests:
35 / 5 = 7
20 / 4 = 5

3. Work out the proportion of students who have passed, who are green-eyed:
Total number who have passed = (34 + 20+ 42 + 35) = 131
Total number who have passed and are green-eyed = (7 + 5 + 21) = 33
(33/131) x 100 = 25.2%

Top Tip: the UCAT answer options can be very similar. Reading the answers carefully is crucial to not missing easy marks.

Question 29: D

1. Work out the total 2019 rental income:
14620 + 12480 + 20480 = 47580

2. Work out the total 2019 spending on these properties:
1450 + 590 + 910 + 462 + 9983 + 2489 = 15884

3. Hence, work out the profit:
47580 – 15884 = 31696

Top Tip: do not hurry to the calculator. Make sure you have a clear target in mind, before you make any calculations. Use the whiteboard to quickly note down your calculations if helpful.

Question 30: B

1. Work out the profit in 2019:
16520 – (1840 + 754) = 13926

2. Work out the profit in 2020:
16840 – (1840 + 754) = 14246

3. Hence, work out the percentage increase from 2019 to 2020:
((14246 – 13926) / 13926) x 100 = 2.3% (to 1 decimal place)

Top Tip: the UCAT answer options can be very similar. Reading the answers carefully is crucial to not missing easy marks.

Question 31: D

1. Eyeball and/or estimate the total spending for each property:
Approximately £2000 is spent on Property A; £1300-1400 on B; £10-11000 on C; and £2500 on D.
Property A had the lowest annual expenses in 2020, and Property C had the most.

2. Eyeball and/or estimate the profit for each property:
Property A has made approximately (£14000 – £2000=) £12000.
Property B has made less profit than A, as its total 2020 income was approximately £12,000.
Property C has made less profit than A (approximately £21000 – £10000 or £11000, which is less than £12000).
Property D has roughly the same annual expenses as A, but has generated a much higher income. Therefore, Property D is clearly the most profitable.

Timing Tip: Be prepared to eyeball and estimate without calculating, to save time and potential marks.

Question 32: C

1. Calculate the difference between the 2018 and 2020 rental incomes:
21020 – 20742 = 278

2. Hence, work out the percentage difference:
(278 / 20742) x 100 = 1.3%

Common Trap: UCAT question options may be numbers which are part of calculating the actual answer, to trip test-takers up.

Question 33: A

1. Work out the price of 1 return journey to Porto (with the off-peak discount):
0.9 x 10.68 x 2 = 19.224

2. Work out the price of 1 return journey to Ibiza:
0.78 x 58.4 x 2 = 91.104

3. Work out the difference in cost:
91.104 – 19.224 = 52.656

Top Tip: do not hurry to the calculator. Make sure you have a clear target in mind, before you make any calculations. Use the whiteboard to quickly note down your calculations if helpful.

Question 34: C

1. Eyeball and eliminate the cheapest options:
Even with the off-peak discount, we can tell that Dublin (A), Rome (D), and Porto (E) will cost less than the other destinations, as their original summer rates are substantially cheaper.

2. Eyeball and compare Marseille and Ibiza:
A 28% discount on £58.40 is a smaller discount (and more expensive rate) than a 35% discount on £24.00. This 28% discount is for Ibiza, making it the correct answer.

Timing Tip: getting used to eyeballing without using the calculator, will enable you to save valuable time for other questions in the QR section.

Question 35: A

1. Work out the return fare to Rome in July:
$9.8 \times 2 \times 2 = £39.20$

2. Work out the return fare to Rome in December:
$9.8 \times 0.94 \times 2 \times 2 = £36.848$

3. Work out the difference in cost:
$£39.20 - £36.848 = £2.532$

Top Tip: make good use of the whiteboard. It is there for you to jot down multiple figures, to come back to them at different times during your calculations.

Question 36: D

1. Work out how much the return ticket to Ibiza cost:
$58.4 \times 2 = £116.80$

2. Work out how much the two return tickets to Rome would have cost:
$9.8 \times 2 \times 2 = £39.20$

3. Work out the percentage difference between these two choices:
$(116.80 - 39.20) / 39.20 \times 100 = 197.9(...)\%$

Top Tip: do not hurry to the calculator. Make sure you have a clear target in mind, before you make any calculations. Use the whiteboard to quickly note down your calculations if it helps.

Abstract Reasoning Mock 1

Questions 1-5

SET A

SET B

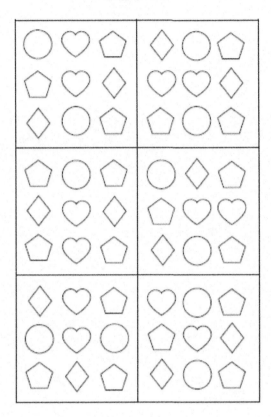
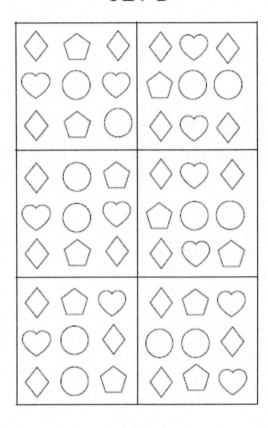

Question 1:

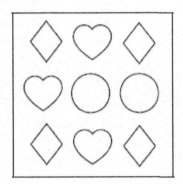

a. Set A
b. Set B
c. Neither

Question 2

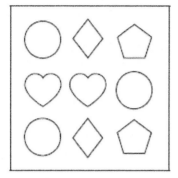

    a. Set A
    b. Set B
    c. Neither

Question 3

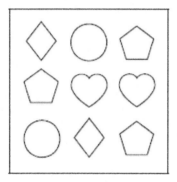

    a. Set A
    b. Set B
    c. Neither

Question 4

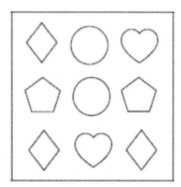

    a. Set A
    b. Set B
    c. Neither

Question 5

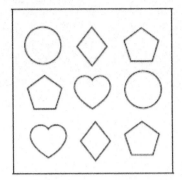

    a.   Set A
    b.   Set B
    c.   Neither

Questions 6-10

SET A

SET B

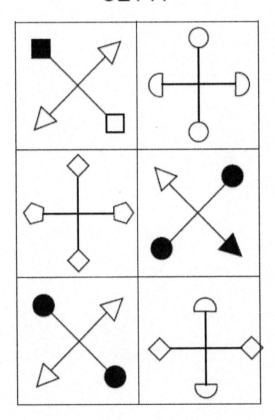
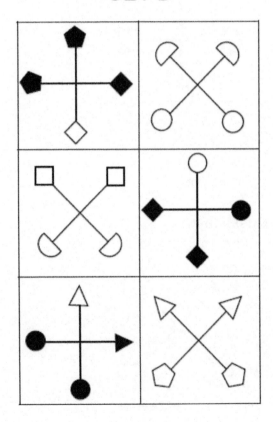

Question 6

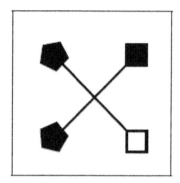

a.   Set A
b.   Set B
c.   Neither

Question 7

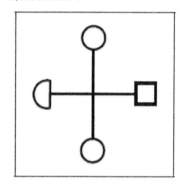

a.   Set A
b.   Set B
c.   Neither

Question 8

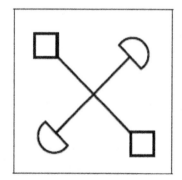

a.   Set A
b.   Set B
c.   Neither

Question 9

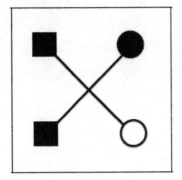

a. Set A
b. Set B
c. Neither

Question 10

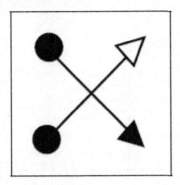

a. Set A
b. Set B
c. Neither

Questions 11-15

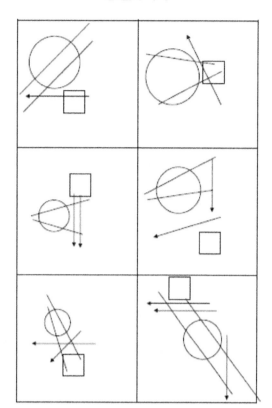

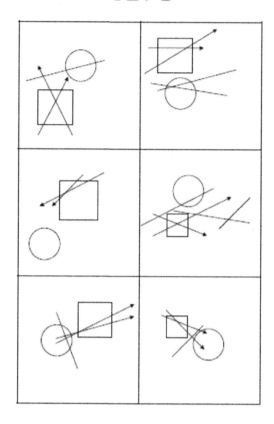

Question 11

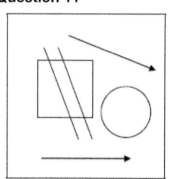

a. Set A
b. Set B
c. Neither

Question 12

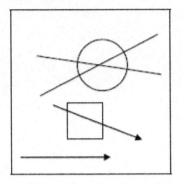

    a. Set A
    b. Set B
    c. Neither

Question 13

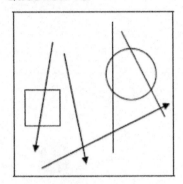

    a. Set A
    b. Set B
    c. Neither

Question 14

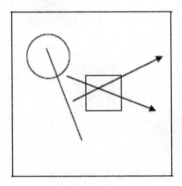

    a. Set A
    b. Set B
    c. Neither

Question 15

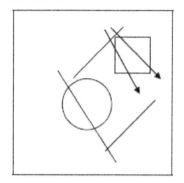

   a. Set A
   b. Set B
   c. Neither

Questions 16-20

SET A

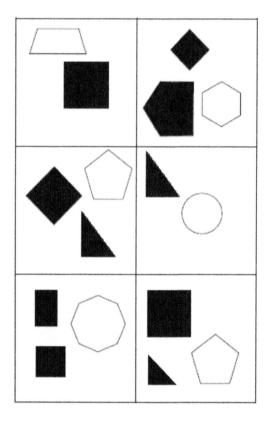

SET B

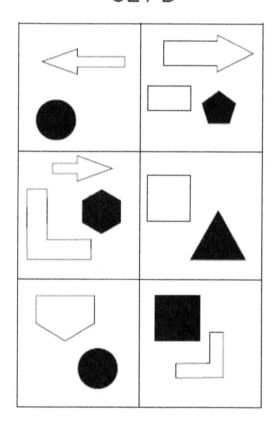

Question 16

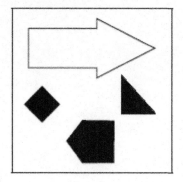

a. Set A
b. Set B
c. Neither

Question 17

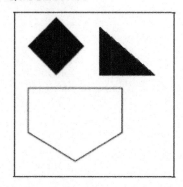

a. Set A
b. Set B
c. Neither

Question 18

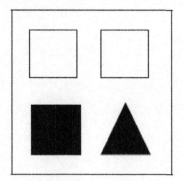

a. Set A
b. Set B
c. Neither

Question 19

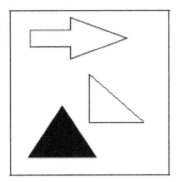

a. Set A
b. Set B
c. Neither

Question 20

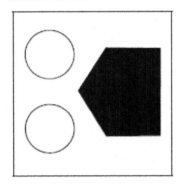

a. Set A
b. Set B
c. Neither

Questions 21-25

SET A   SET B

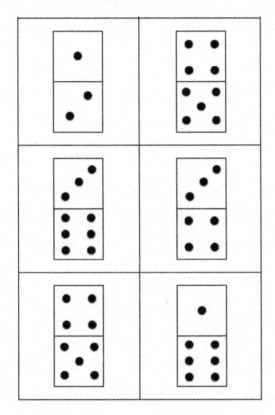 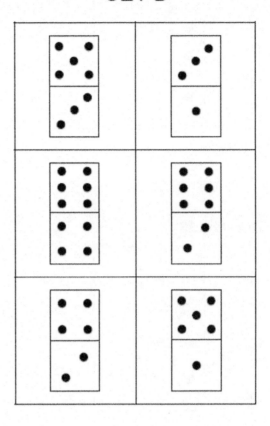

Question 21

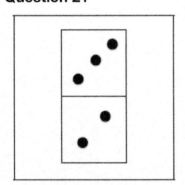

    a. Set A
    b. Set B
    c. Neither

Question 22

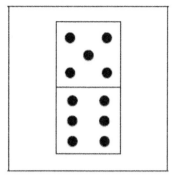

   a. Set A
   b. Set B
   c. Neither

Question 23

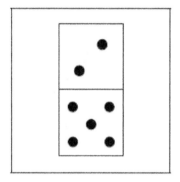

   a. Set A
   b. Set B
   c. Neither

Question 24

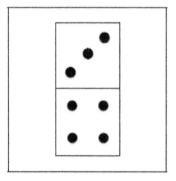

   a. Set A
   b. Set B
   c. Neither

Question 25

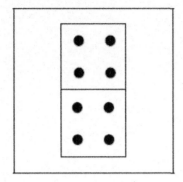

a. Set A
b. Set B
c. Neither

Questions 26-30

SET A

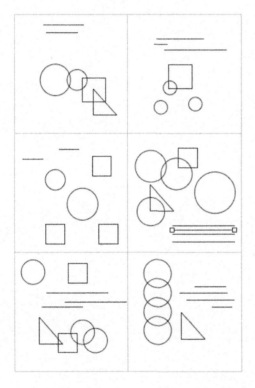

SET B

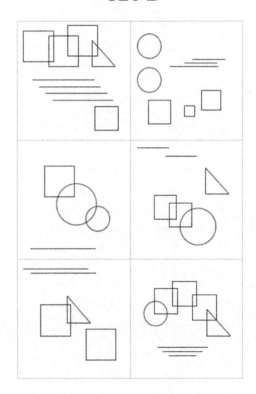

Question 26

Which of the following test shapes belongs in Set A?

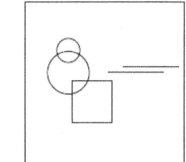

a.

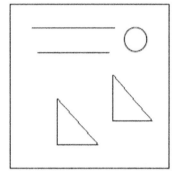

b.

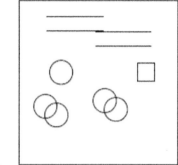

c.

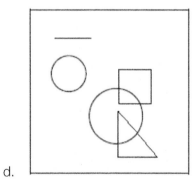

d.

Question 27

Which of the following test shapes belongs in Set A?

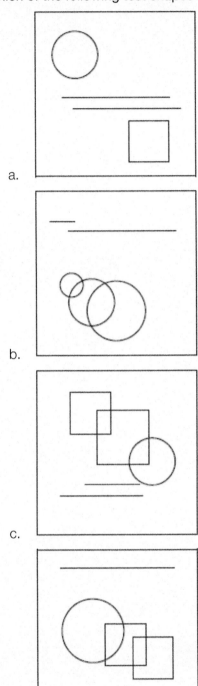

a.

b.

c.

d.

Question 28

Which of the following test shapes belongs in Set B?

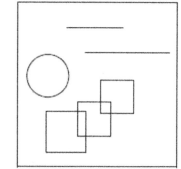

a.

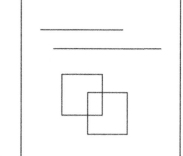

b.

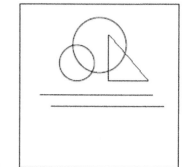

c.

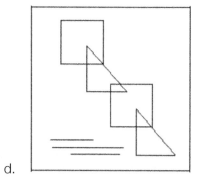

d.

Question 29

Which of the following test shapes belongs in Set A?

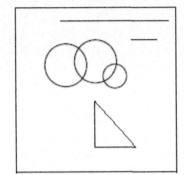

a.

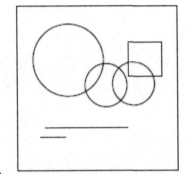

b.

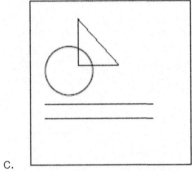

c.

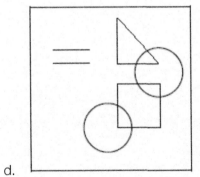

d.

Question 30

Which of the following test shapes belongs in Set B?

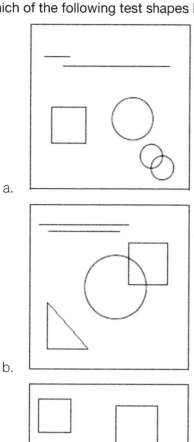

a.

b.

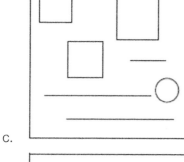

c.

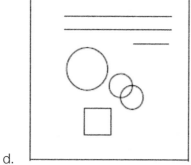

d.

Questions 31-35

SET A

N S	Y E
J G	K W
S I	U L

SET B

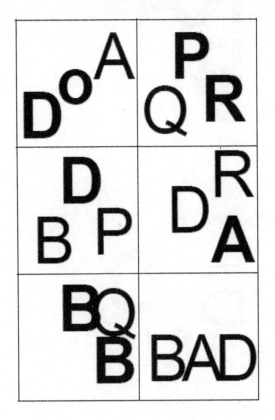

Question 31

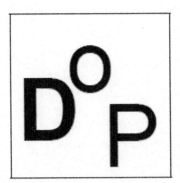

a. Set A
b. Set B
c. Neither

Question 32

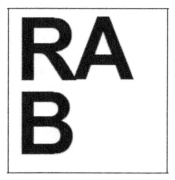

a. Set A
b. Set B
c. Neither

Question 33

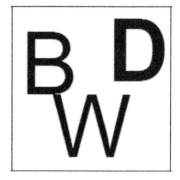

a. Set A
b. Set B
c. Neither

Question 34

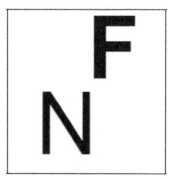

a. Set A
b. Set B
c. Neither

Question 35

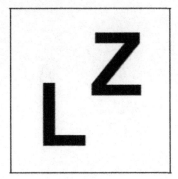

a.   Set A
b.   Set B
c.   Neither

Question 36

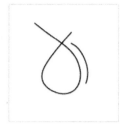 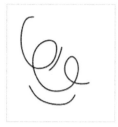 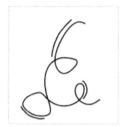 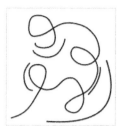

Which figure completes the series?

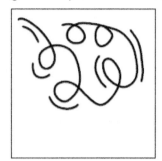

a.

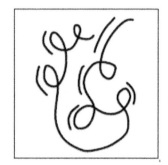

b.

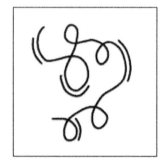

c.

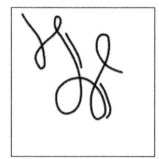

d.

Question 37

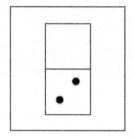 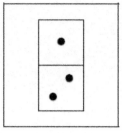 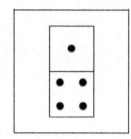 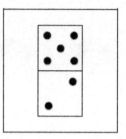

Which figure completes the series?

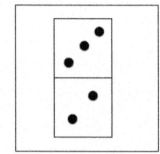

a.

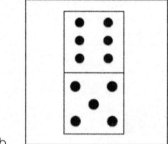

b.

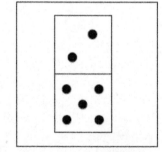

c.

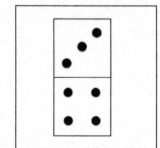

d.

Question 38

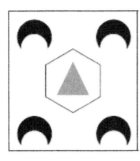

is to

as

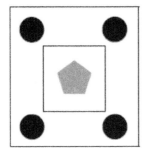

is to

Which of the following completes the statement?

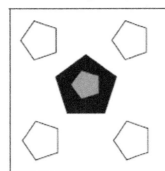

a.

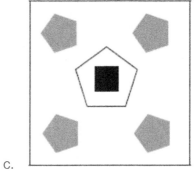

c.

b.

d.

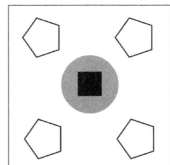

Question 39

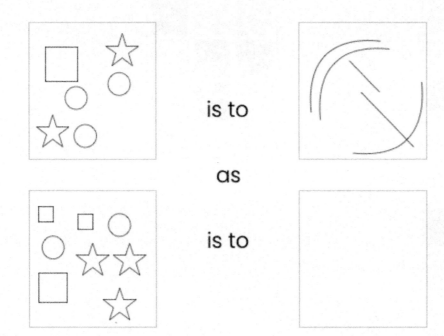

Which of the following completes the statement?

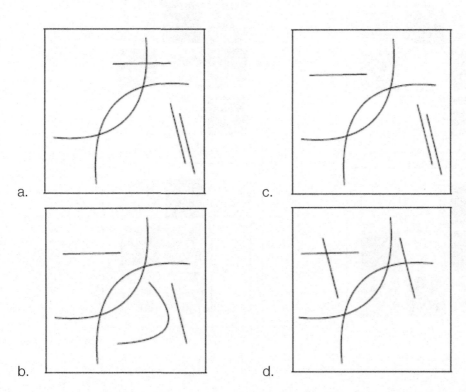

a.

b.

c.

d.

Question 40

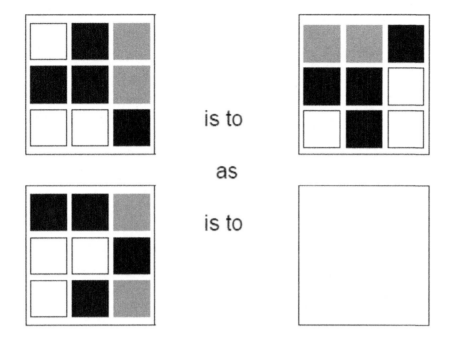

Which of the following completes the statement?

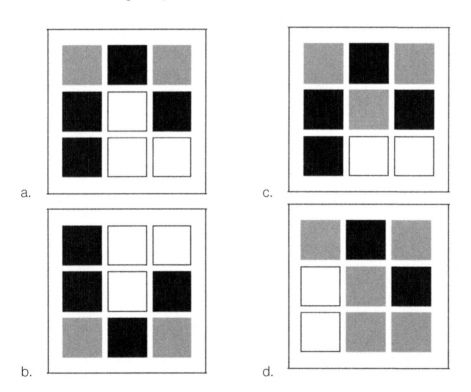

Question 41-45

SET A

SET B

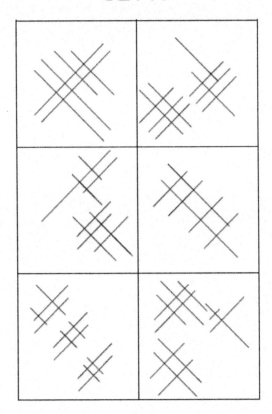 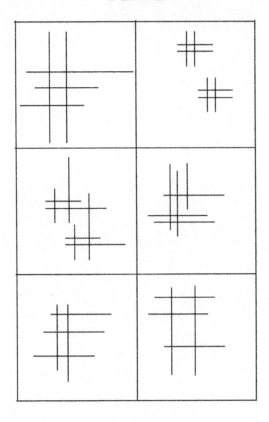

Question 41

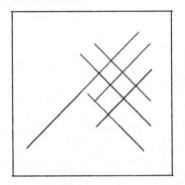

a. Set A
b. Set B
c. Neither

Question 42

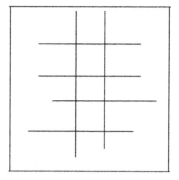

a. Set A
b. Set B
c. Neither

Question 43

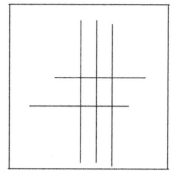

a. Set A
b. Set B
c. Neither

Question 44

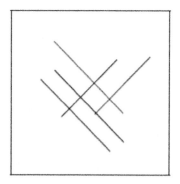

a. Set A
b. Set B
c. Neither

Question 45

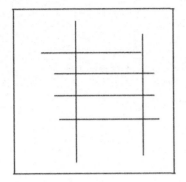

    a. Set A
    b. Set B
    c. Neither

Questions 46-50

Set A

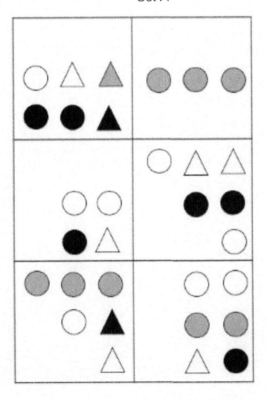

Set B

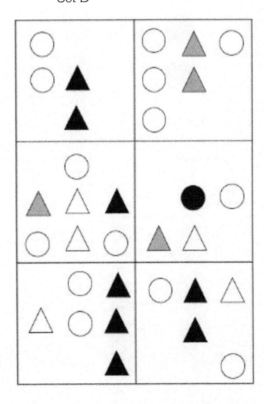

Question 46

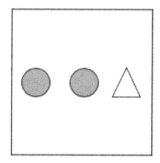

    a. Set A
    b. Set B
    c. Neither

Question 47

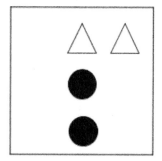

    a. Set A
    b. Set B
    c. Neither

Question 48

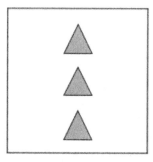

    a. Set A
    b. Set B
    c. Neither

Question 49

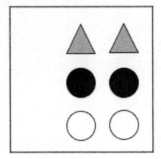

 a. Set A
 b. Set B
 c. Neither

Question 50

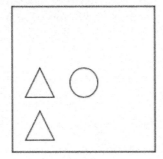

 a. Set A
 b. Set B
 c. Neither

Answers: Abstract Reasoning Mock 1

Questions 1-5

Question 1: C

Set A: In Set A, there are always pentagons in the right corners, and each box contains a pair of adjacent hearts but no other adjacent pairs.

Set B: In Set B, there are always diamonds in the left corners, and each box contains a pair of adjacent circles but no other adjacent pairs.

Neither: Although the box has diamonds in the left corners and a pair of adjacent circles, meaning that the box would fit Set B, there are also adjacent hearts present, so the test shape fits in neither set.

Top Tip: If you see lots of similar shapes in all boxes, the pattern is likely to do with the Position of shapes relative to each other.

Question 2: A

Set A: In Set A, there are always pentagons in the right corners, and each box contains a pair of adjacent hearts but no other adjacent pairs.

Set B: In Set B, there are always diamonds in the left corners, and each box contains a pair of adjacent circles but no other adjacent pairs.

There are pentagons in the right corners and two adjacent hearts, so this test shape fits Set A.

Question 3: A

Set A: In Set A, there are always pentagons in the right corners, and each box contains a pair of adjacent hearts but no other adjacent pairs.

Set B: In Set B, there are always diamonds in the left corners, and each box contains a pair of adjacent circles but no other adjacent pairs.

There are pentagons in the right corners and two adjacent hearts, so this test shape fits Set A.

Question 4: B

Set A: In Set A, there are always pentagons in the right corners, and each box contains a pair of adjacent hearts but no other adjacent pairs.

Set B: In Set B, there are always diamonds in the left corners, and each box contains a pair of adjacent circles but no other adjacent pairs.

There are diamonds in the left corners and two adjacent circles, so it fits Set B.

Question 5: A

Set A: In Set A, there are always pentagons in the right corners, and each box contains a pair of adjacent hearts but no other adjacent pairs.

Set B: In Set B, there are always diamonds in the left corners, and each box contains a pair of adjacent circles but no other adjacent pairs.

There are pentagons in the right corners and two adjacent hearts, so this test shape fits Set A.

Questions 6-10

Question 6: C

Set A: In Set A, there are two opposite pairs of shapes in a '+' shape. If any of the shapes are shaded, then an 'x' shape is formed.

Set B: In Set B, there are two opposite pairs of shapes in an 'x' shape. If three of the shapes are shaded, then a '+' shape is formed.

All the shapes are paired in A however this is is not a pair therefore it is C.

Top Tip: If you see lots of similar shapes in all boxes, the pattern is likely to do with the Position of shapes relative to each other. It also worth checking if the colour of shapes seems to be important, or if it could be a distractor.

Question 7: C

Set A: In Set A, there are two opposite pairs of shapes in a '+' shape. If any of the shapes are shaded, then an 'x' shape is formed.

Set B: In Set B, there are two opposite pairs of shapes in an 'x' shape. If three of the shapes are shaded, then a '+' shape is formed.

Neither: There aren't two pairs of shapes.

Question 8: C

Set A: In Set A, there are two opposite pairs of shapes in a '+' shape. If any of the shapes are shaded, then an 'x' shape is formed.

Set B: In Set B, there are two opposite pairs of shapes in an 'x' shape. If three of the shapes are shaded, then a '+' shape is formed.

Question 9: C

Set A: In Set A, there are two opposite pairs of shapes in a '+' shape. If any of the shapes are shaded, then an 'x' shape is formed.

Set B: In Set B, there are two opposite pairs of shapes in an 'x' shape. If three of the shapes are shaded, then a '+' shape is formed.

Question 10: C

Set A: In Set A, there are two opposite pairs of shapes in a '+' shape. If any of the shapes are shaded, then an 'x' shape is formed.

Set B: In Set B, there are two opposite pairs of shapes in an 'x' shape. If three of the shapes are shaded, then a '+' shape is formed.

Questions 11-15

Question 11: C

Set A: In Set A, there is always a square and a circle present. Two lines will always transect the circle but will never cross each other. The arrows are distractors.

Set B: In Set B, there is always a circle and a square present. Two arrows will always transect the square and will also always intersect each other. The straight lines are distractors.

Neither: Two straight lines, rather than arrows, transect the square, and they do not intersect each other.

Top Tip: If you see arrows, always consider the direction they point, or the shape they point at. If you see overlapping shapes, count the NUMBER of intersections, regions or segments.

Question 12: C

Set A: In Set A, there is always a square and a circle present. Two lines will always transect the circle but will never cross each other. The arrows are distractors.

Set B: In Set B, there is always a circle and a square present. Two arrows will always transect the square and will also always intersect each other. The straight lines are distractors.

Neither: Although two straight lines transect the circle, they intersect each other, so the test shape cannot fit Set A.

Question 13: A

Set A: In Set A, there is always a square and a circle present. Two lines will always transect the circle but will never cross each other. The arrows are distractors.

Set B: In Set B, there is always a circle and a square present. Two arrows will always transect the square and will also always intersect each other. The straight lines are distractors.

Question 14: B

Set A: In Set A, there is always a square and a circle present. Two lines will always transect the circle but will never cross each other. The arrows are distractors.

Set B: In Set B, there is always a circle and a square present. Two arrows will always transect the square and will also always intersect each other. The straight lines are distractors.

Question 15: C

Set A: In Set A, there is always a square and a circle present. Two lines will always transect the circle but will never cross each other. The arrows are distractors.

Set B: In Set B, there is always a circle and a square present. Two arrows will always transect the square and will also always intersect each other. The straight lines are distractors.

The arrows in the square are not intersecting each other so it should be C.

Questions 16-20

Question 16: A

Set A: In Set A, the number of right angles within the black shapes are equal to the number of sides on the white shapes.

Set B: In Set B, the number of right angles within the white shapes are equal to the number of sides on the black shapes, plus 1.

Top Tip: When you see very few shapes, look at Number as a pattern, e.g number of sides, right angles, etc.

Question 17: A

Set A: In Set A, the number of right angles within the black shapes are equal to the number of sides on the white shapes.

Set B: In Set B, the number of right angles within the white shapes are equal to the number of sides on the black shapes, plus 1.

Question 18: B

Set A: In Set A, the number of right angles within the black shapes are equal to the number of sides on the white shapes.

Set B: In Set B, the number of right angles within the white shapes are equal to the number of sides on the black shapes, plus 1.

Question 19: C

Set A: In Set A, the number of right angles within the black shapes are equal to the number of sides on the white shapes.

Set B: In Set B, the number of right angles within the white shapes are equal to the number of sides on the black shapes, plus 1.

Neither: In order to fit Set B, there should be 4 right angles within the white shapes, but there are only 4.

Question 20: A

Set A: In Set A, the number of right angles within the black shapes are equal to the number of sides on the white shapes.

Set B: In Set B, the number of right angles within the white shapes are equal to the number of sides on the black shapes, plus 1.

Questions 21-25

Question 21: C

Set A: In Set A, there is always an odd total number of dots, and there are more dots on the bottom half of the domino.

Set B: In Set B, there is always an even total number of dots, and there are more dots on the top half of the domino.

Neither: Odd total number of dots but cannot fit Set A as there are more dots on the top half of the domino.

Question 22: A

Set A: In Set A, there is always an odd total number of dots, and there are more dots on the bottom half of the domino.

Set B: In Set B, there is always an even total number of dots, and there are more dots on the top half of the domino.

Question 23: A

Set A: In Set A, there is always an odd total number of dots, and there are more dots on the bottom half of the domino.

Set B: In Set B, there is always an even total number of dots, and there are more dots on the top half of the domino.

Question 24: A

Set A: In Set A, there is always an odd total number of dots, and there are more dots on the bottom half of the domino.

Set B: In Set B, there is always an even total number of dots, and there are more dots on the top half of the domino.

Question 25: C

Set A: In Set A, there is always an odd total number of dots, and there are more dots on the bottom half of the domino.

Set B: In Set B, there is always an even total number of dots, and there are more dots on the top half of the domino.

Neither: Even total number of dots but cannot fit Set B as there are equal numbers of dots on each half of the domino.

Questions 26-30

Question 26: A

In Set A, the number of lines corresponds to the number of circles in the box. In Set B, the number of lines corresponds to the number of squares in the box. The intersections are distractors.

Top Tip: If you see lots of similar shapes in all boxes, the pattern is likely to do with the Position or Number of shapes relative to each other. Be wary of distractor shapes which aim to waste your time!

Question 27: D

In Set A, the number of lines corresponds to the number of circles in the box. In Set B, the number of lines corresponds to the number of squares in the box. The intersections are distractors.

Question 28: B

In Set A, the number of lines corresponds to the number of circles in the box. In Set B, the number of lines corresponds to the number of squares in the box. The intersections are distractors.

Question 29: D

In Set A, the number of lines corresponds to the number of circles in the box. In Set B, the number of lines corresponds to the number of squares in the box. The intersections are distractors.

Question 30: C

In Set A, the number of lines corresponds to the number of circles in the box. In Set B, the number of lines corresponds to the number of squares in the box. The intersections are distractors.

There are 3 lines in the box, and three squares. None of the other boxes have equal numbers of both squares and lines.

Questions 31-35

Question 31: B

Set A: In Set A, there are two letters per box, and none of the letters have enclosed spaces.

Set B: In Set B, there are three letters per box, and each of the letters have at least one enclosed space. Colour is irrelevant to both sets.

Top Tip: when you see shapes with letters, focus on those with and without enclosed spaces, or those with and without curved lines.

Question 32: B

Set A: In Set A, there are two letters per box, and none of the letters have enclosed spaces.

Set B: In Set B, there are three letters per box, and each of the letters have at least one enclosed space. Colour is irrelevant to both sets.

Question 33: C

Set A: In Set A, there are two letters per box, and none of the letters have enclosed spaces.

Set B: In Set B, there are three letters per box, and each of the letters have at least one enclosed space. Colour is irrelevant to both sets.

Neither: Contains three letters but has both letters with enclosed spaces and letter without.

Question 34: A

Set A: In Set A, there are two letters per box, and none of the letters have enclosed spaces.

Set B: In Set B, there are three letters per box, and each of the letters have at least one enclosed space. Colour is irrelevant to both sets.

Question 35: A

Set A: In Set A, there are two letters per box, and none of the letters have enclosed spaces.

Set B: In Set B, there are three letters per box, and each of the letters have at least one enclosed space. Colour is irrelevant to both sets.

Question 36: A

With each box in the series, the number of enclose spaces per box, and the number of lines, increase by one.

Top Tip: Focus closely on adjacent boxes – there is no use comparing box 1 to box 4. If you see unusual shapes, such as the crescent moon or curved arrows, then consider that it could be a curved shape pattern.

Question 37: B

Each domino adds to the next consecutive prime number (in ascending order from 2).

Top Tip: Focus closely on adjacent boxes – there is no use comparing box 1 to box 4.

Question 38: D

The inner grey shape becomes the 4 white shapes in the outer corners, and it rotates 90 degrees anticlockwise. The black corner shapes become the inner grey. The white shape becomes the inner black shape.

Question 39: C

Number of squares = number of intersections, number of circles = number of curved lines, number of stars = number of straight lines

Top Tip: When there are very few shapes, then it may be worth your while counting and considering number.

Question 40: A

Whole box rotates 90 degrees anticlockwise.

Top Tip: Remember, if you see lots of similar shapes in all boxes, the pattern is likely to do with the Position of shapes relative to each other.

Question 41-45

Question 41: A

Set A: Set A only has diagonal lines and has 3 enclosed spaces.

Set B: Set B only has vertical or horizontal lines and has 2 enclosed spaces.

Top Tip: If you see overlapping shapes, count the NUMBER of intersections, regions or segments.

Question 42: C

Set A: Set A only has diagonal lines and has 3 enclosed spaces.

Set B: Set B only has vertical or horizontal lines and has 2 enclosed spaces.

Neither: has three enclosed spaces so cannot fit Set B.

Question 43: B

Set A: Set A only has diagonal lines and has 3 enclosed spaces.

Set B: Set B only has vertical or horizontal lines and has 2 enclosed spaces.

Question 44: C

Set A: Set A only has diagonal lines and has 3 enclosed spaces.

Set B: Set B only has vertical or horizontal lines and has 2 enclosed spaces.

Neither: only has one enclosed space so cannot fit Set A.

Question 45: C

Set A: Set A only has diagonal lines and has 3 enclosed spaces.

Set B: Set B only has vertical or horizontal lines and has 2 enclosed spaces.

Neither: has three enclosed spaces so cannot fit Set B.

Questions 46-50

Question 46: A

Set A: Circles of the same shading are always horizontally adjacent.

Set B: Triangles of the same shading are always vertically adjacent.

There are two grey circles and they are both horizontally adjacent.

Question 47: C

Set A: Circles of the same shading are always horizontally adjacent.

Set B: Triangles of the same shading are always vertically adjacent.

There are two circles which have the same shading but are vertically aligned. The two triangles are horizontally aligned, so this cannot belong to set A nor set B.

Question 48: B

Set A: Circles of the same shading are always horizontally adjacent.

Set B: Triangles of the same shading are always vertically adjacent.

There are three triangles with identical shading which are all vertically aligned.

Question 49: A

Set A: Circles of the same shading are always horizontally adjacent.

Set B: Triangles of the same shading are always vertically adjacent.

All the circles of the same shading are horizontally aligned, so this belongs to set A.

Question 50: B

Set A: Circles of the same shading are always horizontally adjacent.

Set B: Triangles of the same shading are always vertically adjacent.

There are two triangles with the same shading which are vertically aligned, so this belongs to set B.

Top Tip: The only colours used in the UCAT exam will be black, white and grey. Grey does not appear frequently, so if it does, look for a colour pattern.

Situational Judgement Mock 1

Question Set 1

Alice is a doctor working in a busy Emergency Department. A man who has consumed large amounts of alcohol, and possibly other substances, begins to run around A&E, shouting at staff that he wants to be seen now. He is verbally abusive to staff and other patients.

*How **appropriate** are each of the following responses by **Alice** in this situation?*

1. Calmly talking to the drunk patient, telling him that he will be seen soon and that he needs to wait in the waiting area.
    a. A very appropriate thing to do
    b. Appropriate, but not ideal
    c. Inappropriate, but not awful
    d. A very inappropriate thing to do

2. Call security immediately
    a. A very appropriate thing to do
    b. Appropriate, but not ideal
    c. Inappropriate, but not awful
    d. A very inappropriate thing to do

3. Asking the patient to leave the hospital as he is acting inappropriately
    a. A very appropriate thing to do
    b. Appropriate, but not ideal
    c. Inappropriate, but not awful
    d. A very inappropriate thing to do

4. Ignoring the patient entirely.
    a. A very appropriate thing to do
    b. Appropriate, but not ideal
    c. Inappropriate, but not awful
    d. A very inappropriate thing to do

Question Set 2

Holly is a junior doctor in the hospital. She is starting the morning ward round when she notices her colleague Marcus, is not washing his hands between patients. This is the first time she has noticed Marcus failing to comply with hand hygiene measures.

*How **appropriate** are each of the following responses by **Holly** in this situation?*

5. Remind Marcus that he needs to wash his hand between patients
    a. A very appropriate thing to do
    b. Appropriate, but not ideal
    c. Inappropriate, but not awful
    d. A very inappropriate thing to do

6. Tell a senior member of staff of what she has seen
    a. A very appropriate thing to do
    b. Appropriate, but not ideal
    c. Inappropriate, but not awful
    d. A very inappropriate thing to do

7. Wait for the ward round to end before approaching Marcus
    a. A very appropriate thing to do
    b. Appropriate, but not ideal
    c. Inappropriate, but not awful
    d. A very inappropriate thing to do

8. Call infection control straight away to tell them what she has witnessed.
    a. A very appropriate thing to do
    b. Appropriate, but not ideal
    c. Inappropriate, but not awful
    d. A very inappropriate thing to do

Question Set 3

Three medical students are on a placement at the local general practice. One of the students, Harry makes sexist jokes towards another student, Molly. The third student, Jack, feels uncomfortable when Harry makes these comments as he knows it upsets his good friend Molly.

*How **appropriate** are each of the following responses by **Jack** in this situation?*

9. Apologise to Molly for Harry's attitude
    a. A very appropriate thing to do
    b. Appropriate, but not ideal
    c. Inappropriate, but not awful
    d. A very inappropriate thing to do

10. Speak to Harry and tell him his comments are inappropriate
    a. A very appropriate thing to do
    b. Appropriate, but not ideal
    c. Inappropriate, but not awful
    d. A very inappropriate thing to do

11. Tell the doctor they are shadowing of Harry's bullying
    a. A very appropriate thing to do
    b. Appropriate, but not ideal
    c. Inappropriate, but not awful
    d. A very inappropriate thing to do

12. Jack is not directly involved so should not get involved
    a. A very appropriate thing to do
    b. Appropriate, but not ideal
    c. Inappropriate, but not awful
    d. A very inappropriate thing to do

Question Set 4

Lucy is a medical student at her university hospital. A patient, Mr Brown, needs bloods taken and Lucy is tasked with this. She goes to gain consent from Mr Brown and it quickly becomes obvious that he is behaving aggressively and threatens to harm Lucy if she comes near him.

*How **appropriate** are each of the following responses by **Lucy** in this situation?*

13. Ask him to calm down and explain why it is important that she takes a blood sample from him
    a. A very appropriate thing to do
    b. Appropriate, but not ideal
    c. Inappropriate, but not awful
    d. A very inappropriate thing to do

14. Tell him to leave the hospital as he is being rude and aggressive
    a. A very appropriate thing to do
    b. Appropriate, but not ideal
    c. Inappropriate, but not awful
    d. A very inappropriate thing to do

15. Refuse to take blood from him
    a. A very appropriate thing to do
    b. Appropriate, but not ideal
    c. Inappropriate, but not awful
    d. A very inappropriate thing to do

16. Ask another medical student to take blood from him instead
    a. A very appropriate thing to do
    b. Appropriate, but not ideal
    c. Inappropriate, but not awful
    d. A very inappropriate thing to do

Question Set 5

A medical student, Joshua, is told by a patient, that a doctor swears loudly on the ward which makes him feel so uncomfortable that he does not want to stay in hospital. Joshua tells a nurse on the ward and she tells him that she has not ever witnessed this behaviour by the doctor. The nurse suggests that the patient might just dislike being in hospital. Joshua is unsure what to do because the doctor is also an examiner at his university.

*How **important** to take into account are the following considerations for **Joshua** when deciding how to respond to the situation?*

17. The doctor is an examiner at his university and could potentially be marking his work.
    a. Very important
    b. Important
    c. Of minor importance
    d. Not important at all

18. A patient has told him directly that he feels uncomfortable and does not want to be in hospital as a result
    a. Very important
    b. Important
    c. Of minor importance
    d. Not important at all

19. Other patients could have the same feelings as the doctor swears loudly on the ward
    a. Very important
    b. Important
    c. Of minor importance
    d. Not important at all

20. The nurse has never witnessed this behaviour from the doctor in question
    a. Very important
    b. Important
    c. Of minor importance
    d. Not important at all

Question Set 6

Sal, a medical student, is on a placement in his university hospital. A fellow medical student, Gemma, who is on a different ward calls Sal and asks him to access the file of a patient currently in the emergency department. Gemma explains that the patient is a friend of hers and she would like to know how he is getting along.

*How **appropriate** are each of the following responses by **Sal** in this situation?*

21. Tell Gemma that unfortunately he cannot give out patient information
    a. A very appropriate thing to do
    b. Appropriate, but not ideal
    c. Inappropriate, but not awful
    d. A very inappropriate thing to do

22. Tell Gemma that she should just visit her friend herself and see how he is doing
    a. A very appropriate thing to do
    b. Appropriate, but not ideal
    c. Inappropriate, but not awful
    d. A very inappropriate thing to do

23. Tell her to stay on the phone while he finds her friends file
    a. A very appropriate thing to do
    b. Appropriate, but not ideal
    c. Inappropriate, but not awful
    d. A very inappropriate thing to do

24. Tell Gemma to speak to the doctor involved in her friend's care directly as they are likely to have more information.
    a. A very appropriate thing to do
    b. Appropriate, but not ideal
    c. Inappropriate, but not awful
    d. A very inappropriate thing to do

Question Set 7

Alice is a final-year medical student currently on placement at a local general practice. Whilst on placement she is allowed to see patients by herself before seeking senior help and permitted to look through patient records when appropriate. One evening after placement, Alice is at the pub with her friends when one of them realises that their father is a patient where Alice is based at. They ask Alice if she has seen their father and if she can access his records to see if he has a certain allergy as he is unsure.

*How **important** to take into account are the following considerations for **Ellie** when deciding how to respond to the situation?*

25. Patient has not given consent
    a. Very important
    b. Important
    c. Of minor importance
    d. Not important at all

26. Alice does not want to make things awkward with her friend
    a. Very important
    b. Important
    c. Of minor importance
    d. Not important at all

27. Her friend only wants to check whether her father has an allergy.
    a. Very important
    b. Important
    c. Of minor importance
    d. Not important at all

28. Alice is not a qualified doctor yet.
    a. Very important
    b. Important
    c. Of minor importance
    d. Not important at all

Question Set 8

You are a medical student, completing a placement in an outpatient clinic. Your next patient, Rachel, needs to have monthly blood tests to ensure that she is taking the right amount of medication, as if not, this could have serious consequences. You see that there are no blood test results for the past 2 months in Rachel's notes. Rachel confirms that she missed the blood test appointments, because she "does not feel that they are necessary".

*How **appropriate** are each of the following responses in this situation?*

29. Ask Rachel If there is anything stopping her from going to get her blood taken
    a. A very appropriate thing to do
    b. Appropriate, but not ideal
    c. Inappropriate, but not awful
    d. A very inappropriate thing to do

30. Ask her why she feels it is unnecessary
    a. A very appropriate thing to do
    b. Appropriate, but not ideal
    c. Inappropriate, but not awful
    d. A very inappropriate thing to do

31. Tell her why it is so important that she get her bloods taken regularly
    a. A very appropriate thing to do
    b. Appropriate, but not ideal
    c. Inappropriate, but not awful
    d. A very inappropriate thing to do

32. Ask the doctor in charge of her care to explain the importance of having blood tests to her
    a. A very appropriate thing to do
    b. Appropriate, but not ideal
    c. Inappropriate, but not awful
    d. A very inappropriate thing to do

Question Set 9

Sophie is a dental student on placement in a dental practice. She is sat with the receptionist Levi when he gets up to use the toilet. Levi has been working at the practice for 6 weeks. Sophie uses the computer on the reception desk to check her shifts for next week, and sees a tab displaying Levi's personal social media account. The computer is only usually used by Levi. It is against practice policies to use work computers for personal reasons.

*How **appropriate** are each of the following responses by **Sophie** in this situation?*

33. Tell the practice manager what Levi has been doing whilst working.
    a. A very appropriate thing to do
    b. Appropriate, but not ideal
    c. Inappropriate, but not awful
    d. A very inappropriate thing to do

34. Talk to Levi in private to remind him of practice rules
    a. A very appropriate thing to do
    b. Appropriate, but not ideal
    c. Inappropriate, but not awful
    d. A very inappropriate thing to do

35. Ignore the findings unless it happens again
    a. A very appropriate thing to do
    b. Appropriate, but not ideal
    c. Inappropriate, but not awful
    d. A very inappropriate thing to do

36. Go through his social media while you wait for him to return to get to know him better
    a. A very appropriate thing to do
    b. Appropriate, but not ideal
    c. Inappropriate, but not awful
    d. A very inappropriate thing to do

Question Set 10

Ana is a medical student currently on a surgical rotation. Nikki, also a medical student, finds Ana in tears one lunchtime. Ana is finding this rotation very demanding and is struggling to cope especially because the consultant constantly asks difficult questions that she cannot answer.

*How **appropriate** are each of the following responses by **Nikki** in this situation?*

37. Tell Ana that she is sorry that she is struggling to cope and suggest that she may want to take some time off and work on her mental health.
    a. A very appropriate thing to do
    b. Appropriate, but not ideal
    c. Inappropriate, but not awful
    d. A very inappropriate thing to do

38. Empathise with her concerns and encourage her to discuss the issue with the doctors that are under the consultant as they will have dealt with the consultant.
    a. A very appropriate thing to do
    b. Appropriate, but not ideal
    c. Inappropriate, but not awful
    d. A very inappropriate thing to do

39. Explain to Ana that she may need to talk to the consultant directly and offer to go with her for support.
    a. A very appropriate thing to do
    b. Appropriate, but not ideal
    c. Inappropriate, but not awful
    d. A very inappropriate thing to do

40. Offer to assist Ana with some of the workload.
    a. A very appropriate thing to do
    b. Appropriate, but not ideal
    c. Inappropriate, but not awful
    d. A very inappropriate thing to do

Question Set 11

Ghambir is a junior doctor on a surgical training rotation. De does not find the work very challenging. He also has found that he gets all of his work done very quickly and has plenty of time to spare.

*How **appropriate** are the following responses by **Ghambir** in this situation?*

41. Ask a more senior doctor if he can offer to help other junior doctor who work on busier wards once he has spare time.
    a. A very appropriate thing to do
    b. Appropriate, but not ideal
    c. Inappropriate, but not awful
    d. A very inappropriate thing to do

42. Ask to be moved to a busier ward with more opportunities
    a. A very appropriate thing to do
    b. Appropriate, but not ideal
    c. Inappropriate, but not awful
    d. A very inappropriate thing to do

43. Tell the programme director that the position he is in is too quiet and future students would not benefit from it.
    a. A very appropriate thing to do
    b. Appropriate, but not ideal
    c. Inappropriate, but not awful
    d. A very inappropriate thing to do

Question Set 12

Ed, a junior doctor, has written prescription for a strong painkiller. A staff nurse with over 30 years of experience is challenging his decision to prescribe such a painkiller and refuses to give the medication to the patient in question. She claims that Ed should trust her judgment as she knows the patient well.

*How **appropriate** are the following responses by **Ed** in this situation?*

44. Listen to the nurses advice and cancel the prescription and prescribe a painkiller that she sees is suitable
    a. A very appropriate thing to do
    b. Appropriate, but not ideal
    c. Inappropriate, but not awful
    d. A very inappropriate thing to do

45. Ask a senior doctor for guidance and prescribe the painkiller you both feel is best even if it is the same as before
    a. A very appropriate thing to do
    b. Appropriate, but not ideal
    c. Inappropriate, but not awful
    d. A very inappropriate thing to do

46. Ask the nurse why she disagrees with him
    a. A very appropriate thing to do
    b. Appropriate, but not ideal
    c. Inappropriate, but not awful
    d. A very inappropriate thing to do

47. Tell the nurse that it is his decision to make as a doctor and that he is ordering her to administer the painkiller
    a. A very appropriate thing to do
    b. Appropriate, but not ideal
    c. Inappropriate, but not awful
    d. A very inappropriate thing to do

Question Set 13

Riley is a medical student shadowing Dr Pine, a junior GP. They are going on many home visits and the patients are spread over a wide region and Riley notices that on several occasions, Dr Pine drives well above the speed limit in order to get to the appointments on time and he is worried by this. He has warned Dr Pine about this several times, but nothing changes and he is considering raising the issue with his supervisor.

*How **important** are the following consideration for **Riley** when deciding how to respond to the situation?*

48. Dr Pine is an experienced driver
    a. Very important
    b. Important
    c. Of minor importance
    d. Not important at all

49. Riley could get a negative report from Dr Pine if he speaks up
    a. Very important
    b. Important
    c. Of minor importance
    d. Not important at all

50. Dr Pine is a danger to other road users
    a. Very important
    b. Important
    c. Of minor importance
    d. Not important at all

51. The supervisor might believe Dr Pine instead
    a. Very important
    b. Important
    c. Of minor importance
    d. Not important at all

52. Emergency vehicles are exempt from speed limits
    a. Very important
    b. Important
    c. Of minor importance
    d. Not important at all

53. It will be a hindrance to patients if they were late
    a. Very important
    b. Important
    c. Of minor importance
    d. Not important at all

Question Set 14

Darius, a junior doctor who is keen on a career as a surgeon, contacted the surgical unit many months ago to see if it would be possible for him to observe a few operations. They email back saying the only slot they have left is tomorrow at 9am to 1pm. But Darius is running a busy clinic at that time.

*How **appropriate** are the following responses by **Darius** in this situation?*

54. Ask the doctor in charge if he can leave for the last hour of clinic to attend a little bit of the surgery
    a. A very appropriate thing to do
    b. Appropriate, but not ideal
    c. Inappropriate, but not awful
    d. A very inappropriate thing to do

55. Call the doctor in charge early in the morning at 8am to say she is feeling unwell and then go to the surgery session.
   a. A very appropriate thing to do
   b. Appropriate, but not ideal
   c. Inappropriate, but not awful
   d. A very inappropriate thing to do

56. Call the patients due to be in clinic and ask if they would be okay to rebook for another day
   a. A very appropriate thing to do
   b. Appropriate, but not ideal
   c. Inappropriate, but not awful
   d. A very inappropriate thing to do

57. Ask another junior doctor to cover her clinic instead while she attends theatre and commit to covering that doctor's clinic session in return
   a. A very appropriate thing to do
   b. Appropriate, but not ideal
   c. Inappropriate, but not awful
   d. A very inappropriate thing to do

58. Go to her clinic session like planned and not go to theatre.
   a. A very appropriate thing to do
   b. Appropriate, but not ideal
   c. Inappropriate, but not awful
   d. A very inappropriate thing to do

Question Set 15

Jason, a medical student, has just finished a hectic day of placement. While he waits for his train to come he notices a man collapse on his platform. As a medical student he has some basic life saving training but not once has he applied this in a real life setting. He is not sure if he should get involved.

*How **important** are the following considerations for **Jason** when deciding how to respond?*

59. The patient is very close to the hospital
   a. Very important
   b. Important
   c. Of minor importance
   d. Not important at all

60. He knows there are lots of other healthcare workers on the same platform as him and the collapsed man
   a. Very important
   b. Important
   c. Of minor importance
   d. Not important at all

61. Someone has called 999 already
   a. Very important
   b. Important
   c. Of minor importance
   d. Not important at all

62. His boyfriend will be upset if he is late home for their evening meal
   a. Very important
   b. Important
   c. Of minor importance
   d. Not important at all

63. Jason assumes that train drivers are trained in CPR and so they can do it instead as he is very tired from his long day
   a. Very important
   b. Important
   c. Of minor importance
   d. Not important at all

Question Set 16

Mary is giving a lecture to final year medical students. One student she knows well somehow got access to a photocopy of the exam that they are due to sit next week. She asks Mary to cover all the topics that will come up. Mary finds out that a previous student gave her the copy because they think the paper is the same each year.

*How **appropriate** are the following responses by **Mary** in this situation?*

64. Take the paper away from the student and report her to the medical school
   a. A very appropriate thing to do
   b. Appropriate, but not ideal
   c. Inappropriate, but not awful
   d. A very inappropriate thing to do

65. Tell the student to not look at the paper as it will be unfair to other students
    a. A very appropriate thing to do
    b. Appropriate, but not ideal
    c. Inappropriate, but not awful
    d. A very inappropriate thing to do

66. Tailor the session so that all necessary topics are covered
    a. A very appropriate thing to do
    b. Appropriate, but not ideal
    c. Inappropriate, but not awful
    d. A very inappropriate thing to do

67. Convince the medical school to change the paper
    a. A very appropriate thing to do
    b. Appropriate, but not ideal
    c. Inappropriate, but not awful
    d. A very inappropriate thing to do

68. Find out who gave her the copy and report them to the GMC
    a. A very appropriate thing to do
    b. Appropriate, but not ideal
    c. Inappropriate, but not awful
    d. A very inappropriate thing to do

Question 69

Steven is a junior doctor working in an Obstetrics and Gynaecology department under the supervision of his consultant, Mr Fraser. Over the past few weeks, Steven notices several situations where he thinks Mr Fraser has failed to provide an adequate standard of care and is concerned that patient safety is at risk.

Choose **both** the one **most appropriate action** and the one **least appropriate action** that Steven should take in response to this situation.

You will not receive any marks for this question unless you select **both** the **most and least appropriate actions**.

Choose both the one most appropriate action and the one least appropriate action that Steven should take in response to this situation.

- *Most Appropriate*
- *Least Appropriate*

a. Report Mr Fraser to the GMC
b. Do nothing
c. Talk to Mr Fraser and raise his concerns

Answers: Situational Judgement Mock 1

Question Set 1

Question 1: A

Acting calmly is the most professional way to respond and may resolve the situation without jumping to stricter interventions.

Question 2: B

The patient is verbally abusing those in the department so calling security is reasonable, but it is not ideal as other attempt to calmly talk to the patient should be made first.

Question 3: D

This risks the patients safety. They came to A&E as they are clearly in need of medial help. Patient safety is the most important concept and is discussed regularly throughout our lessons as well on this page of the GMC good medical practice guidelines. https://www.gmc-uk.org/ethical-guidance/ethical-guidance-for-doctors/good-medical-practice/domain-2—-safety-and-quality

Question 4: D

This also puts patients at risk, both the patient in question and other patients in the area. Ignoring a patient that is acting violently toward staff and patients could only aggravate the situation.

Question Set 2

Question 5: A

This question tests your communication with colleagues. Doctors and medical students must always prioritise patient safety and optimise care when they can. It is best to speak to the colleague directly so that you can rectify any problems without going to someone else first. For this question you can refer to domain 3 of Good Medical Practice. https://www.gmc-uk.org/ethical-guidance/ethical-guidance-for-doctors/good-medical-practice/domain-3—communication-partnership-and-teamwork#paragraph-31

Question 6: C

C is the best option here. Other members of the team could be helpful in this situation in explaining protocol and the importance of infection control. It is not ideal to go straight higher authority as it does not involve the person who the issue is with.

Question 7: D

This is very inappropriate, as Marcus will have examined all the patients on the ward with dirty hands. This risks infection and endangers patient safety. https://www.gmc-uk.org/ethical-guidance/ethical-guidance-for-doctors/good-medical-practice/domain-2—-safety-and-quality

Question 8: C

This is inappropriate as it is and overreaction to something that can easily be solved locally by discussion with Marcus. Immediately informing infection control without even discussing the situation with Marcus is likely to put serious strain on the professional relationship between the pair. It is not awful however, because an effort was made to correct the situation.

Question Set 3

Question 9: C

By apologising on behalf of Harry, Jack would not be improving the situation as Harry could continue to be rude and sexist since no one has corrected him for his mistakes. It is not awful as Jack will likely make Molly feel slightly better and this action is unlikely to make the situation worse.

Question 10: A

Speaking Harry directly about his behaviour will likely ensure that he won't act this way again. GMC guidelines outline that the NHS have a zero-tolerance bullying policy and it is unacceptable and should not be ignored.

Question 11: C

The doctor they are working with will likely talk to Harry about his behaviour one to one. However it is not the most appropriate thing to do as no effort was made to talk to Harry directly first- and Harry should be spoken to first.

Question 12: D

Bullying and discrimination is not tolerated whatsoever and should not be ignored. The workplace should be a safe place for all employees.

Question Set 4

Question 13: A

The patient could be upset and angry because he does understand why he needs to have blood taken in the first place and he could even have a fear of needles. By talking calmly with him and explaining the reasoning behind the blood test and the procedure too, she could calm his nerves.

Question 14: D

Mr Brown is behaving in an unacceptable manner however, telling a patient to leave when they are in need of medical care is equally unacceptable and goes against the key principle of patient safety which is covered in our lessons and also the GMC guidelines.

Question 15: B

This does not solve the problem at hand. If she feels unsafe then it is understandable and she should call for security to help her but refusing to do the task she has been set without trying other avenues first is not the best way to act. Personal safety is an important issue regardless.

Question 16: D

By asking another student to do it she is not solving the situation and frankly shows a lack of commitment and poor teamwork. Mr Brown could continue being aggressive to the next medical student too and so something needs to be done to calm him down.

Question Set 5

Question 17: D

There might be some consequences of raising the concern with the doctor but the feelings of the patient should take precedent here. Patient safety and wellbeing should always be at the forefront of all decision making. Assessments should be marked objectively and so this is not an important consideration.

Question 18: A

Patient safety and wellbeing is the most important factor to keep in mind. https://www.gmc-uk.org/ethical-guidance/ethical-guidance-for-doctors/good-medical-practice/domain-2---safety-and-quality

Question 19: B

It is true that other patients could have heard him and could feel the same way and so it is important to consider as other patients safety could also be jeopardised. However it is not very important as it is based on an assumption not fact.

Question 20: C

Joshua has been told directly by a patient about his concerns and so should be more important and should be followed up regardless. It is not very important as the nurse also works on the ward and mentions a valid point about the patient not wanting to be in hospital in the first place. But, the patient's experience should be invalidated based on the experience the nurse has had with the doctor.

Question Set 6

Question 21: A

Patient confidentiality is principal to a doctor-patient relationship. Doctors and medical students should only ever access patient information if they are directly involved in the treatment and their care. Accessing patient information for any other reason breaches patient confidentiality, duty of candour as a doctor, is unethical, breaches data protection laws and would be viewed very poorly by the GMC.

Question 22: A

The most important thing is that Sal does not access those documents and give them to Gemma. A practical solution is provided here whilst also being sensitive to the fact that Gemma is worried about her friend.

Question 23: D

Accessing patient information for any other reason that being directly involved in their care breaches patient confidentiality, is unethical, breaches data protection laws could lead to disciplinary action from the medical school.

Question 24: D

As medical students they should understand that the doctor involved in the friends care will also not be allowed to give out confidential information without consent from the patient first. It would be more appropriate for Sal to tell Gemma that it is not possible to give out patient information from the beginning.

Question Set 7

Question 25: A

If a patient has capacity and has given consent for their information to be shared with someone, once this has been documented it is appropriate to do so. Breaching confidentiality is a serious offence and would likely lead to a fitness to practice investigation by the medical school and GMC.

Question 26: C

Alice should not do what is being asked of her but also has to handle the situation sensitively. Alice should explain why she cannot as is she will be doing the right thing that way.

Question 27: D

Regardless of what her friend wants to check, confidentiality should not be breached at all.

Question 28: D

Even as a medical student you will have the duty to protect patient confidentiality and so being a medical student does not change the scenario.

Question Set 8

Question 29: A

Speaking to the patient and finding out their concerns is a very reasonable and appropriate thing to do. It is also likely to allow her to feel safe to talk about her concerns so that they could be overcome. Further, allowing the patient to talk will improve the relationship she has with the healthcare system.

Question 30: A

By asking her and starting a discussion you will get to the bottom of her concerns and build better rapport with her.

Question 31: B

Simply telling her why she must go is unlikely to change her behaviour it would be more ideal to get her to explain to you why she is not attending in the first place, by exploring her ideas and concerns you will more likely change her mind.

Question 32: A

A senior member of the care team is likely to be able to explain the information to her better, as a medical student you might not have all the information to accurately and completely inform Rachel. Recognising this is important.

Question Set 9

Question 33: C

It is not awful as Sophie will be trying to solve the situation but it is inappropriate as she could tarnish the relationship she has with Levi. It is best to speak to the colleague directly so that you can rectify any problems without going to someone else first. For this question you can refer to domain 3 of Good Medical Practice. https://www.gmc-uk.org/ethical-guidance/ethical-guidance-for-doctors/good-medical-practice/domain-3—communication-partnership-and-teamwork#paragraph-31

Question 34: A

Talking to him directly is the most professional course of action. It will ensure that he is made aware of the rules and hopefully it won't happen again

Question 35: D

If it is not bought up, Levi will likely carry on doing it and could even be ignoring his duties which is inappropriate. By mentioning it to him she will at least be fixing the problem.

Question 36: D

Though he should not be looking up personal things on the work computer, it is inappropriate for Sophie to take advantage of what she has found as Levi likely thought it would only be him viewing that webpage.

Question Set 10

Question 37: C

Though her intentions are good, avoiding teaching is unprofessional. It is also unlikely that the situation will be resolved when ana returns. Since it won't make matters worse it is a C and not a D.

Question 38: A

Ana needs support from her friends and it can make a difference to her attitude and behaviour so offering. Talking to senior trainees who has experience of dealing with the consultant will help her understand the issue and find ways to resolve it.

Question 39: A

Addressing the issue with the consultant directly would be good for Ana. Being there to offer support is also appropriate as you know that Ana is scared of the consultant.

Question 40: D

Though it might seem like a nice thing to do, but it is important that Ana complete her own work as it will help make her a competent doctor in the future. It will not address any aspect of the fundamental problem. It will not show Ana how to cope in the future if the problem arose again.

Question Set 11

Question 41: A

Since he has already done what he was supposed to do it is very appropriate for him to help other junior doctors who may be struggling with their busy wards. This will help care for the patients and will also allow him to learn more.

Question 42: C

This might make sense at face value but the team currently works win needs him to care for its patients. So he will be leaving his ward and this is very inappropriate.

Question 43: A

This might seem rude but actually he is looking out for future doctors. If he feels that the post needs to be improved he should flag this up to the person in charge. This demonstrates that he is concerned about other people.

Question Set 12

Question 44: C

The prescription will be written based on his own clinical experience and knowledge. The nurse is experience and she should be able to contribute to that decision making process and point out any concerning issues but it will be Ed's decision ultimately. Changing a prescription because of an unexplained comment Is inappropriate. It is not awful and ranks a C because the passage says that a 'suitable' alternative is given and so we can infer that no harm was caused to the patient

Question 45: A

When unsure, it is always good to recognise your limitations and seek advice from senior colleagues in order to ensure that patient care is taken into account.

Question 46: A

The nurse has 30 years of experience and so must have a reason for disputing with Ed. She should explain her reasoning so Ed can learn for the future if he is indeed wrong.

Question 47: D

The nurse has the right to refuse to do something she deems inappropriate and Ed cannot force her to with an order. It is inappropriate to ignore the concern that the drug could be wrong.

Question Set 13

Question 48: D

Speeding is dangerous regardless of how experienced you. You can still be a danger to others and this behaviour is illegal.

Question 49: D

If Riley believes that he is a danger to other road user then his actions should not be dictated by possible revenge from Dr Pine.

Question 50: A

You have a duty of care to those around you and should not put people in danger regardless of status.

Question 51: D

It is possible that this could be a he said/ she said situation but that should not stop him from reporting the matter.

Question 52: D

He is not driving an emergency vehicle as he is going to routine house visits.

Question 53: D

Though it is important to consider how patients feel, there is no indication that this is an emergency and so being a bit late should not cause any serious harm to patients. Plus, by speeding just to get to their house on time, Dr Pine is risking his own life and also Riley's and anyone else that is on the road. So this factor should be irrelevant to the decision that Riley makes about reporting Dr Pine.

Question Set 14

Question 54: D

Cancelling several appointments with patients just to attend a theatre session that is not essential for you to go to is highly unprofessional. This is also inconvenient for patients as they likely waited a very long time just to get the appointment in the first place. He will putting patients care at risk and so this is very inappropriate.

Question 55: D

Lying is very wrong and should not be done and will not be tolerated at all.

Question 56: D

This is unfair for the patients because as a doctor Darius has some power over his patients and so they might feel they have to go along with having to rearrange another appointment even if they do not feel that it is okay. It is inconvenient for the patients and could put them in danger. Though Darius is not lying here and asking if the patients are okay with rearranging, his status makes us question how much power patients really have.

Question 57: C

This way at least clinic will not be cancelled and patients will still be seen to. By offering to cover the colleague's clinic session in return this becomes not awful. However it is still inappropriate as the colleague might not be familiar with any patients and might not have the knowledge to offer appropriate care. The theatre session is not essential and so missing clinic for it regardless is unprofessional.

Question 58: A

The clinic will be covered and so patients will be seen to.

Question Set 15

Question 59: D

The man has collapsed suddenly and so needs to be seen to immediately, it should not matter how close they are to the hospital when deciding if he should step into help. The proximity is irrelevant if no one takes the man there

Question 60: B

The stem states that Jason <u>knows</u> other healthcare staff are there and so are also trained enough to help. This should not stop Jason from intervening as his help is required. It is a B and not an A as the other healthcare workers are more qualified than him as he is a medical student.

Question 61: D

Knowing that the ambulance is on its way only informs us that the patient will be seen to eventually but does not help in that situation actively. We do not know how long the ambulance will take either. The man still needs assistance and this is the most important thing.

Question 62: D

The patient in question should be the first point considered not his boyfriend. Jason's decision to help should be based on the difference that he can make to the collapsed man.

Question 63: D

The stem states that Jason is waiting for the train to come so waiting till the train driver gets to the station could be too late. So though help might be given, we do not know how quickly it will come and it is only an assumption that the driver will actually be trained.

Question Set 16

Question 64: A

It is essential that the medical school find out what is going on so they can rectify the mistake in the future. Cheating is not fair and is a form of lying

Question 65: D

It would be foolish to believe the student will actually throw away the paper just because Mary asks her to. There could be other copies around and just getting rid of one might not actually solve the situation.

Question 66: D

Mary could have disciplinary action against her if she wants complicit in cheating too. It will not be good for the education of these students if they already knew all the answers. Competency is important and is highlighted in the GMC guidelines.

Question 67: B

This is appropriate as is it ensures that the students are all being tested fairly. However, it is not ideal as it does not prevent the same thing from happening with the newly set paper. It would be more ideal to discuss with the school how the paper gets leaked each year and put in defences from this happening again.

Question 68: D

Very inappropriate, as a medical student the maximum punishment should be the dean of the medical school rather than the GMC as med students are not registered

Question 69

Most appropriate = **C**, Least appropriate = **B**

Option A is neither the most appropriate nor the least appropriate option. This action would allow Steven to comply with his obligation to act his patient safety concerns which, is consistent with Good Medical Practice which states "[you must] Take prompt action if you think that patient safety, dignity or comfort is being compromised" (Good Medical Practice, p11). However, this option is **not** the most appropriate because Steven unnecessarily escalates the situation without first having a conversation with Mr Fraser about his concerns. Therefore, option 1 is **neither** the most appropriate **nor** the least appropriate option.

Option B is the least appropriate option. By doing nothing, Steven is failing to act on a patient safety issue. This violates Good Medical Practice which states "[you must] Take prompt action if you think that patient safety, dignity or comfort is being compromised" (Good Medical Practice, p11). Therefore, option 2 is the **least** appropriate option.

Option C is the most appropriate option. By talking to Mr Fraser before escalating his concerns, Steven is complying with his obligation to protect patient safety without escalating his concerns inappropriately. This is outlined in Good Medical Practice which states "[you must] Take prompt action if you think that patient safety, dignity or comfort is being compromised" (Good Medical Practice, p11) and "You must treat colleagues fairly and with respect" (Good Medical Practice, p14). Therefore, option 3 is the **most** appropriate option.

*Top Tip: Remember, patient safety **must** be your primary consideration.*

UCAT Mock 2

Verbal Reasoning Mock 2

Question Set 1

The cardiac drug digoxin, used indirectly for more than 200 years to treat heart conditions, stemmed from an herbal remedy rather than from laboratory chemistry. The active ingredient in digoxin is digitalis, a chemical which can be found in the foxglove plant.

English physician William Withering is credited with discovering in 1775 that the foxglove plant could help those suffering from abnormal fluid buildup, or dropsy, as it was called in those days. In a 1785 report, Withering writes that he was asked to evaluate a home remedy for dropsy compounded by Mrs. Hutton, an old woman in Shropshire. Her herbal concoction made cures after the more regular practitioners had failed, according to his report.

Withering quickly figured out that of the 20 or so herbs in the woman's remedy, foxglove was the key ingredient. He used dried foxglove leaves in his dropsy remedy and noted that foxglove was particularly helpful for his patients who developed dropsy after suffering from scarlet fever or bad sore throats. The leaves contain a number of glycosides that are all referred to by the umbrella term digitalis. The flowers, seeds, and sap also contain digitalis, but less than the leaves have.

(https://pubsapp.acs.org/cen/coverstory/83/8325/8325digoxin.html)

1. The leaves of the foxglove plant are still used today in the treatment of heart conditions.
    a. True
    b. False
    c. Can't tell

2. Mrs Hutton was able to cure dropsy in her patients.
    a. True
    b. False
    c. Can't tell

3. Digoxin may be useful in the treatment of scarlet fever or bad sore throats.
    a. True
    b. False
    c. Can't tell

4. When making digoxin from the foxglove plant, the leaves contain more of the active ingredient than the flowers.
   a. True
   b. False
   c. Can't tell

Question Set 2

Sandringham Time (ST) was the inspired idea of King Edward VII who altered the clocks on his estate at Sandringham in Norfolk to half an hour ahead of Greenwich Mean Time. This was the official time on the estate between 1901 and 1936. Sandringham was bought by the then Prince of Wales in 1862, as a private retreat away from London where he could indulge his passion for hunting.

The Prince of Wales loved outdoor sports and came up with the idea of Sandringham Time to make the most of the winter daylight hours for shooting.
He ordered all the clocks on the estate to be set half an hour ahead of Greenwich Mean Time. Sandringham Time was also adopted at Windsor Castle and Balmoral.

Even after his accession to the throne in 1901, Edward continued to make improvements to the house and estate. Following his death in 1910, Sandringham was left to Queen Alexandra, who continued to live there until her death in 1925.

The tradition of Sandringham Time, however, continued after Edward's death and throughout the reign of George V. This led to some confusion during the final hours of George's life (he died at Sandringham on 20th January 1936) and Edward VIII abolished ST on his accession in 1936.

(https://www.historic-uk.com/CultureUK/Sandringham-Time/)

5. King Edward VII:
   a. Invented Sandringham Time in order to maximise summer daylight hours.
   b. Was also known as the Prince of Wales.
   c. Was King between 1901 and 1936.
   d. Was the eldest son of Queen Victoria.

6. Sandringham Time:
   a. Was only implemented because Norfolk is in the East of England.
   b. Was only used in Sandringham Estate.
   c. Was abolished immediately after the death of King Edward VII.
   d. Displayed a later time than Greenwich Mean Time.

7. Which of the following statements is not true?
   a. King Edward VII must have been over 48 years old when he died.
   b. Shooting is considered an outdoor sport.
   c. King Edward VII was the only monarch to live in Sandringham.
   d. Sandringham Time only existed in the 20th century.

8. Which of the following statements is supported by the information in this passage?
   a. Sandringham Time was inspired by the concept of British Summer Time.
   b. Edward VII was the only monarch to make improvements to the house and estate.
   c. The death of George V may have been a catalyst to the abolition of Sandringham Time.
   d. King Edward VIII rose to the throne 25 years after King Edward VII.

Question Set 3

The Internet started in the 1960s as a way for government researchers to share information. Computers in the '60s were large and immobile and in order to make use of information stored in any one computer, one had to either travel to the site of the computer or have magnetic computer tapes sent through the conventional postal system.

Another catalyst in the formation of the Internet was the heating up of the Cold War. The Soviet Union's launch of the Sputnik satellite spurred the U.S. Defence Department to consider ways information could still be disseminated even after a nuclear attack. This eventually led to the formation of the ARPANET (Advanced Research Projects Agency Network), the network that ultimately evolved into what we now know as the Internet. ARPANET was a great success, but membership was limited to certain academic and research organisations who had contracts with the Defence Department. In response to this, other networks were created to provide information sharing.

January 1, 1983 is considered the official birthday of the Internet. Prior to this, the various computer networks did not have a standard way to communicate with each other. A new communications protocol was established called Transfer Control Protocol/Internetwork Protocol (TCP/IP). This allowed different kinds of computers on different networks to "talk" to each other. ARPANET and the Defence Data Network officially changed to the TCP/IP standard on January 1, 1983, hence the birth of the Internet.

(https://www.usg.edu/galileo/skills/unit07/internet07_02.phtml)

9. Before the development of the internet, government researchers could not share information without travelling to the site of a physical computer.
   a. True
   b. False
   c. Can't Tell

10. The looming threat of information being wiped out by a nuclear attack was partially responsible for the development of the Internet.
   a. True
   b. False
   c. Can't Tell

11. Before 1983, there was no way for different computer networks to communicate.
   a. True
   b. False
   c. Can't Tell

12. ARPANET ceased to exist after 1982.
   a. True
   b. False
   c. Can't Tell

Question Set 4

Córdoba's Mosque-Cathedral is a stunning monument to the two main religions and cultures that have shaped the Spanish autonomous community of Andalusia: Islam and Christianity. A Renaissance church squats right on top of what was once the most important mosque in the Islamic kingdom.

The site was originally home to a Roman temple, which was later replaced by a Christian church. In 711, when the Moors took Andalusia from the Christians, the structure was divided into two halves and used as a place of worship by both Muslims and Christians – a remarkable act of tolerance, given the fervour of the times. But the reign of religious pluralism in Córdoba didn't last; in 784, on the orders of the Emir Abd al-Rahman, the church was destroyed and work on a great mosque began. Construction lasted for over two centuries and, when the building was completed in 987 with the addition of the outer nave and courtyard, Córdoba's Mosque was the largest in the Islamic kingdom, save only for that of Kaaba in Arabia.

In 1236, Córdoba was recaptured by the Christians. King Ferdinand III immediately ordered the mosque's lanterns to be transported back to Santiago de Compostela, where they were converted back into bells for the city's cathedral. Subsequent Christian monarchs altered and added to – but never demolished – the mosque, resulting in the hybrid structure that remains.

(https://theculturetrip.com/europe/spain/articles/the-history-of-the-mosque-cathedral-of-cordoba-in-1-minute-2/)

13. The Mosque-Cathedral of Cordoba:
    a. Reflects Roman, Islamic and Christian influences in its architecture.
    b. Was used by Muslims and Christians throughout the 8th century.
    c. Was the largest mosque in the Islamic kingdom in the 10th century.
    d. Was considered to be the most important mosque in the Islamic kingdom.

14. Which of the following statements is true?
    a. Only two cultures have existed in Andalusian history.
    b. The church which exists today was built in the Renaissance period.
    c. The structure was divided into two halves in the 7th century AD.
    d. The church which exists today was built before 711 AD.

15. Which of the following statements is supported by information in the passage?
    a. Andalusia was under Christian rule prior to the year 711 AD.
    b. Religious tolerance was not unusual in the 8th century AD.
    c. Construction of the church took over 200 years to complete.
    d. The Kaaba in Arabia existed prior to the year 711 AD.

16. Which of the following is the most appropriate conclusion to this passage?
    a. The Mosque-Cathedral of Cordoba remains one of the largest mosques in the world.
    b. The Mosque-Cathedral of Cordoba is a hybrid structure influenced by Roman, Islamic and Christian rule.
    c. The Mosque-Cathedral of Cordoba demonstrates religious tolerance over many centuries in Andalusia.
    d. The Mosque-Cathedral of Cordoba is a reflection of the two cultures which have most influenced Andalusian history.

Question Set 5

Ninety-nine percent of exported bananas are a variety called the Cavendish—the attractive, golden-yellow fruit seen in the supermarket today.

But that wasn't always the case. There are many varieties of banana in the world, and until the latter half of the 19th century, the dominant one was called the Gros Michel. It was widely considered tastier than the Cavendish, and more difficult to bruise. But in the 1950s, the crop was swept by a strain of Panama disease, also known as banana wilt, brought on by the spread of a noxious, soil-inhabiting fungus. Desperate for a solution, the world's banana farmers turned to the Cavendish. The Cavendish was resistant to the disease and fit other market needs: it could stay green for several weeks after being harvested (ideal for shipments to Europe), it had a high yield rate and it looked good in stores. Plus, multinational fruit companies had no other disease-resistant variety available that could be ready quickly for mass exportation.

The switch worked. As the Gros Michel was ravaged by disease, the Cavendish banana took over the world's markets and kitchens. In fact, the entire banana supply chain is now set up to suit the very specific needs of that variety.

The Cavendish had now supplanted the Gros Michel, but—even though it had initially been selected for being disease-resistant—it was still at risk. Almost a decade ago, author Dan Koeppel warned in an interview that Panama Disease would return to the world's largest banana exporters, and this time with a strain that would hit the Cavendish hard.

(https://time.com/5730790/banana-panama-disease/)

17. Which of the following statements is supported by the information in this passage?
    a. The Gros Michel is an unattractive variety of banana.
    b. The Gros Michel has a better flavour than the Cavendish.
    c. A fungus from Panama was responsible for the death of the Gros Michel.
    d. The Cavendish is golden yellow when harvested.

18. The Cavendish banana:
    a. Is resistant to all fungal disease.
    b. Is the only variety of banana suitable for mass exportation.
    c. Is perfectly suited to the structure of the banana supply chain.
    d. Was the dominant variety of banana in the 1960s.

19. Which of the following is not a reason why banana farmers chose the Cavendish?
    a. The Cavendish was thought to be resistant to banana wilt.
    b. The green colour of the Cavendish after harvesting was desirable.
    c. The Cavendish was less likely to bruise on long journeys to Europe.
    d. There was no other choice as all other varieties were unsuitable.

20. Which of the following is the most appropriate conclusion to this passage?
    a. The bout of Panama disease in the 1950s is entirely responsible for the change in dominant banana variety worldwide.
    b. The Cavendish is a hardy variety of banana, chosen for its complete resistance to Panama disease.
    c. The Gros Michel was once the most popular variety of banana by far, until the 1950s when the Cavendish was discovered.
    d. There was a huge chain in the banana supply chain in the mid 20th century.

This statement is best supported by the passage. The other three statements are incorrect and there are contradictory statements within the passage.

Question Set 6

Homeopathy is a 200-year-old therapeutic system that uses small doses of various substances to stimulate autoregulatory and self-healing processes.

Medicines are prepared by serial dilution and shaking, which proponents claim imprints information into water. Although many conventional physicians find such notions implausible, homeopathy had a prominent place in 19th-century health care and has recently undergone a worldwide revival.

In the United States, patients who seek homeopathic care are more affluent and younger and more often seek treatment for subjective symptoms than those who seek conventional care. Homeopathic remedies were allowed by the 1939 Pure Food and Drug Act and are available over the counter. Some data, for example from randomised controlled trials and laboratory research, show effects from homeopathic remedies that contradict the contemporary rational basis of medicine.

There is also evidence that homeopathy may be effective for the treatment of influenza, allergies, postoperative ileus, and childhood diarrhoea. Evidence suggests that homeopathy is ineffective for migraine, delayed-onset muscle soreness, and influenza prevention.

There is a lack of conclusive evidence on the effectiveness of homeopathy for most conditions. Homeopathy deserves an open-minded opportunity to demonstrate its value by using evidence-based principles, but it should not be substituted for proven therapies.

21. Homeopathy was most popular in the 19th century and has since steadily decreased in popularity.
    a. True
    b. False
    c. Can't tell

22. In the United States, on average, income is higher in those who seek homeopathic treatment compared to those who seek conventional medical treatment.
    a. True
    b. False
    c. Can't tell

23. Homeopathy is effective in the treatment of pneumonia.
    a. True
    b. False
    c. Can't tell

24. Most doctors would agree that homeopathy should not be substituted for proven medical therapies.
   a. True
   b. False
   c. Can't tell

Question Set 7

In September 1944, trains in the Netherlands ground to a halt. Dutch railway workers were hoping that a strike could stop the transport of Nazi troops, helping the advancing Allied forces. But the Allied campaign failed, and the Nazis punished the Netherlands by blocking food supplies, plunging much of the country into famine. By the time the Netherlands was liberated in May 1945, more than 20,000 people had died of starvation.

The Dutch Hunger Winter has proved unique in unexpected ways. Because it started and ended so abruptly, it has served as an unplanned experiment in human health. Pregnant women, it turns out, were uniquely vulnerable, and the children they gave birth to have been influenced by famine throughout their lives.

When they became adults, they ended up a few pounds heavier than average. They also experienced much higher rates of such conditions as diabetes and schizophrenia. By the time they reached old age, those risks had taken a measurable toll.

It was found that the people who had been in the womb during the famine — known as the Dutch Hunger Winter cohort — died at a higher rate than people born before or afterward, with a 10 percent increase in mortality after 68 years.

(https://www.nytimes.com/2018/01/31/science/dutch-famine-genes.html)

25. Food supplies in the Netherlands in 1944 were delivered by railway.
   a. True
   b. False
   c. Can't tell

26. Based on the information in the passage, children of mothers starved during pregnancy are more likely to be overweight.
   a. True
   b. False
   c. Can't tell

27. The Dutch Hunger Winter cohort have a higher risk of developing schizophrenia than the rest of the population.
   a. True
   b. False
   c. Can't tell

28. The increase in mortality in the Dutch Hunger Winter cohort only occurs after the age of 68 years.
   a. True
   b. False
   c. Can't tell

Question Set 8

Coffee beans naturally contain caffeine. Although a jolt of caffeine is exactly what many people are looking for when they reach for a cup of coffee, the beans can be processed to remove most of the stimulant, creating a drink that can be enjoyed at night without losing sleep. There are several different methods used to rid the beans of their caffeine, all of which are done while they are still green. Decaffeination is often associated with less flavourful coffee because it is difficult to remove only the caffeine and not any of the numerous flavour chemicals, and decaffeinated beans are notoriously difficult to roast properly.

The most common methods of decaffeination involve the use of chemical solvents, usually ethyl acetate or methylene chloride. In the direct method, the coffee beans are steamed and then rinsed repeatedly with the chemical solvent to flush away the caffeine. In the indirect method, the chemical agent never touches the beans but treats the caffeine-laden water in which the beans have been soaked for hours. After the caffeine is removed from the water with the solvent, the bean-flavoured solution is reintroduced to the beans, allowing many of the oils and flavours to be reabsorbed. In both processes, the solvents are rinsed or evaporated out of the green beans and further vaporise upon roasting, meaning that only the tiniest trace amounts (which are deemed safe for consumption) are ever present in the decaffeinated beans you purchase.

(https://www.britannica.com/story/how-is-coffee-decaffeinated)

29. Coffee beans:
   a. Can be processed to remove all the caffeine stimulant.
   b. Are only decaffeinated while they are still green.
   c. Are most commonly used worldwide to make coffee.
   d. Always contain caffeine.

30. Which of the following is not part of a decaffeination method mentioned in the passage?
    a. Methylene chloride is used to rinse the coffee beans.
    b. Coffee beans are soaked for many hours in water.
    c. Ethyl acetate is reintroduced to the beans within the solution.
    d. Water containing caffeine and solvent is discarded.

31. The author of the passage most likely agrees that:
    a. Decaffeinated coffee has more health risks than its caffeinated counterpart.
    b. Most people do not enjoy decaffeinated coffee.
    c. Decaffeinated coffee has advantages over caffeinated at certain times of the day.
    d. The flavour of caffeinated and decaffeinated coffee is more or less equal.

32. Which of the following statements is true based on the information in this passage?
    a. Flavour chemicals can be washed away by rinsing or soaking beans in water.
    b. Steaming and rinsing coffee beans once is enough to remove caffeine.
    c. Methylene chloride has been deemed safe for consumption.
    d. Oils from coffee beans enhance the coffee flavour.

Question Set 9

The surprise discovery of gas that could be a sign of life on Venus has reignited scientific interest in Earth's closest neighbour. Researchers and space agencies worldwide are now racing to turn their instruments — both on Earth and in space — towards the planet to confirm the presence of the gas, called phosphine, and to investigate whether it could really be coming from a biological source.

Astrobiologists have flagged phosphine — a toxic compound of hydrogen and phosphorus — as a possible signature for life on other planets, and it is made by some organisms on Earth. "Anaerobic life produces it quite happily," says Clara Sousa-Silva, a molecular astrophysicist and lead of the phosphine-detection study.

But the gas should be broken down in Venus's harsh, highly acidic atmosphere. That led the discovery team to conclude that there must be some mechanism replenishing the gas, hinting at either biological production or an unknown chemical process that scientists cannot yet explain.

Not everyone is yet convinced by the team's observation. The researchers have identified only one absorption line for phosphine in their data, and the findings need to be confirmed by other researchers in line with good scientific practice.

Only data can settle the debate. "Maybe Earth and Venus are two different paths that habitable planets can take in their evolution," says another scientist. "To answer that, we need to get the fundamental data sets for Venus that we have for Mars and even Mercury."

(https://www.nature.com/articles/d41586-020-02785-5)

33. Scientists predicted that there was a possibility phosphine might be found on Venus.
    a. True
    b. False
    c. Can't tell

34. Phosphine is not produced by aerobic organisms on Earth.
    a. True
    b. False
    c. Can't tell

35. In accordance with good scientific practice, researchers other than Clara Sousa-Silva need to replicate the same findings.
    a. True
    b. False
    c. Can't tell

36. We have more information overall about Mercury than Venus.
    a. True
    b. False
    c. Can't tell

Question Set 10

The ancient Maya people were clever and hardworking farmers who used a variety of techniques to raise enough food to feed the large populations in Maya cities. Their sophistication can be compared to other ancient empires such as the Egyptians. Corn, or maize, was the main staple crop. Maize was grown together with beans and squash as each of the three provide support to the others. In order to deal with difficult terrain, the Maya had to engineer a variety of farming methods.

Aerial photography provides evidence of raised beds alongside canals. Like the Aztecs, the Maya also farmed field raised up from low, swampy areas. They created these fertile farm areas by digging up the mud from the bottom and placing it on mats made of woven reeds two feet above the water level.

In mountainous areas, the Maya made terraces on the steep hillsides, which make the most productive use of mountainous or hilly land by creating a series of steps to reduce water runoff and erosion.

They also used forest gardening, planting trees that provided economic benefit for them as food or firewood. Cacao and gum trees were encouraged to grow, for example.

(https://www.historyonthenet.com/mayan-farming)

37. The Maya people:
    a. Were similar in number to the ancient Egyptians.
    b. Had three staple crops.
    c. Resided in modern-day Mexico.
    d. Relied on agriculture as a main practice.

38. Which of the following is not part of a farming method used by the Maya?
    a. Creating raised farming areas within swamps.
    b. Planting multiple types of crops together.
    c. Carving steps into steep mountains.
    d. Planting trees which are cheap to maintain.

39. Which of the following is the best conclusion for this passage?
    a. The farming practices of the Maya people maximised the suboptimal circumstances.
    b. Farming practices from the ancient Maya culture can be applied even today.
    c. The ancient Maya people were superior to other cultures in their innovation.
    d. The Maya and the Aztecs were both able to farm in hilly areas.

40. Which of the following statements is the author of this passage most likely to agree with?
    a. The techniques used by the Maya people can be applied to other civilisations.
    b. The Maya people were among the most sophisticated of their time.
    c. The Aztecs were equal to the Maya people in their sophistication.
    d. The farming practices used by the Maya were only possible due to the number of farmers.

Question Set 11

Ice acts like a protective cover over the Earth and our oceans. These bright white ice spots reflect excess heat back into space and keep the planet cooler. In theory, the Arctic remains colder than the equator because more of the heat from the sun is reflected off the ice, back into space.

Glaciers around the world can range from ice that is several hundred to several thousand years old and provide a scientific record of how climate has changed over time. Through their study, we gain valuable information about the extent to which the planet is rapidly warming. They provide scientists a record of how climate has changed over time.

Today, about 10% of land area on Earth is covered with glacial ice. Almost 90% is in Antarctica, while all of the remaining is in the Greenland ice cap.

Rapid glacial melt in Antarctica and Greenland also influences ocean currents, as massive amounts of very cold glacial-melt water entering warmer ocean waters is slowing ocean currents. And as ice on land melts, sea levels will continue to rise.

(https://www.worldwildlife.org/pages/why-are-glaciers-and-sea-ice-melting)

41. Which of the following statements is the author of this passage most likely to agree with?
    a. True
    b. False
    c. Can't tell

42. By studying glaciers, we can see how the climate has changed over hundreds and thousands of years.
    a. True
    b. False
    c. Can't tell

43. There is no glacial ice on Earth outside of Antarctica and the Greenland ice cap.
    a. True
    b. False
    c. Can't tell

44. A sudden change in oceanic temperature is likely to increase the speed of ocean currents and worsen the rising of the sea levels.
    a. True
    b. False
    c. Can't tell

Answers: Verbal Reasoning Mock 2

Question Set 1

Question 1: C

We know that digoxin is derived from this herbal remedy, but the passage does not say whether it has completely replaced its role.

Question 2: A

The passage states that her concoction made cures after the more regular practitioners had failed, so this statement is true.

Question 3: C

This is not supported by the passage and there is no evidence to contradict this, so the correct answer is C.

Question 4: A

The passage states that the active ingredient in digoxin is digitalis. At the end of the passage, it states that more digitalis is found in the leaves than the flowers.

Question Set 2

Question 5: B

The passage states that Sandringham Time was the idea of King Edward VII, and later refers to the Prince of Wales coming up with the idea of Sandringham Time. Therefore, this statement is true.

Question 6: D

This is the only option which is supported by the passage – all other statements are contradicted.

Question 7: C

We are told in the passage that both Queen Alexandra and King George V lived in Sandringham after King Edward VII's death.

Question 8: C

The passage states that there was some confusion surrounding the death of King George V and that ST was abolished soon after. Therefore, this statement is true.

Question Set 3

Question 9: B

The passage states that there was also the option to have magnetic computer tapes sent through the postal system.

Question 10: A

The passage mentioned that the U.S. Defence Department had to consider ways in which information could be disseminated even after a nuclear attack, and that the Cold War was a catalyst for the formation of the internet. Therefore, this statement is true.

Question 11: C

The passage states that there was no 'standard' way to communicate, but we do not know whether there were different forms of communication between computer networks that were not universal.

Question 12: A

The passage states that ARPANET and the Defence Data Network changed to the TCP/IP standard on January 1, 1983. Therefore, this statement is true.

Question Set 4

Question 13: D

We know that this is true from the end of the first paragraph.

Question 14: B

From the first paragraph, we can deduce that statement B is true.

Question 15: A

From the passage, we know that the Moors took Andalusia from the Christians in the year 711, so we can deduce that this statement is true.

Question 16: D

Option D is best supported by the passage and is the main message that the passage is trying to get across.

Question Set 5

Question 17: B

The passage states that the Gros Michel was widely considered to be tastier than the Cavendish. This statement is therefore true.

Question 18: C

From the passage we know that the banana supply chain is set up to suit the needs of the Cavendish, so statement C is true.

Question 19: C

The Gros Michel was considered 'more difficult to bruise', and this statement is not supported by the passage.

Question 20: A

This statement is best supported by the passage. The other three statements are incorrect and there are contradictory statements within the passage.

Question Set 6

Question 21: B

The passage states that it has recently undergone a 'worldwide revival', supporting option B as the correct answer.

Question 22: A

The passage states that those who seek homeopathic care are more affluent, so this statement is true.

Question 23: C

The passage does not mention pneumonia, so the correct answer is C.

Question 24: C

Although this is what the author of the passage is most likely to agree with, we do not know whether this is what all doctors are likely to think. Therefore, the correct answer is C.

Question Set 7

Question 25: C

Although it is mentioned that the railway workers were on strike, we do not know from the passage whether the food supplies were delivered by railway. Therefore, the correct answer is C.

Question 26: A

From the passage, we know that these children ended up 'a few pounds heavier than average'.

Question 27: A

This is supported by the passage, as is states that these children were more likely to develop diabetes and schizophrenia in adulthood.

Question 28: C

Although the passage says that there is a 10% increase in mortality after 68 years, it does not mention the increase in mortality in this cohort before this age. Therefore, the correct answer is C.

Question Set 8

Question 29: B

The passage states that the decaffeination methods are all done while the beans are still green.

Question 30: C

Option C is the only one not supported by the second paragraph of the passage.

Question 31: C

In the first paragraph, the passage states that decaffeinated coffee can be drunk at night without losing sleep. Therefore, option C is correct.

Question 32: A

From the passage, we can see that adding the solution back to the beans reintroduces the flavour. Therefore, we can deduce that A is the correct answer.

Question Set 9

Question 33: B

The start of the passage states that the discovery was a 'surprise'.

Question 34: C

Although the passage states that anaerobic life produces phosphine happily, we do not know about aerobic life. Therefore, the correct answer is C.

Question 35: A

This statement is supported by the fourth paragraph of the passage.

Question 36: C

Although the final statement suggests that there are more basic datasets on Mercury, we do not know about the amount of overall information.

Question Set 10

Question 37: D

This is the only statement supported by the passage ("clever and hardworking farmers').

Question 38: D

The purpose of growing these trees is to provide economic benefit by producing useful substances, such as food or firewood. Therefore, this statement is false.

Question 39: A

This is the most appropriate conclusion to the passage, as the other statements are either contradicted or unsupported by the passage.

Question 40: B

The passage states that their sophistication can be compared to ancient empires, such as the Egyptians. Therefore, this statement is true.

Question Set 11

Question 41: C

The passage states that more heat is reflected off the ice in the Arctic but does not deny that there is ice at the equator. Therefore, the correct answer is C.

Question 42: A

This is supported by the second paragraph, where it mentions that ice in glaciers can be several hundred to several thousands of years old.

Question 43: A

This is supported by the third paragraph, where the passage states that 'almost 90% is in Antarctica' and that 'all of the remaining is in the Greenland ice cap'.

Question 44: B

In the final paragraph, we are told that the change in temperature will slow ocean currents, so this statement is false.

Decision Making Mock 2

Question 1

Of all the skirts in stock at the local boutique this season, none are made from silk and cotton. Some of the skirts are made entirely from linen.

Place "Yes" if the conclusion does follow. Place "No" if the conclusion does not follow.
   a. Some of the skirts in stock at the boutique are made from silk (but not cotton).
   b. Only cotton skirts are in stock at the boutique.
   c. The boutique does not stock cotton skirts which also contain silk.
   d. Silk skirts in the boutique cannot also contain linen.
   e. All the skirts stocked at the boutique are made from a blend of silk and cotton.

Question 2

Six sixth-form students are to be arranged by height, with the tallest person in the front of the line. No two students are the same height.
Nelly is taller than Elisha, who is taller than Priya but not taller than Ani.
Joel is taller than Henri, but not taller than Ani.
When correctly arranged, exactly three students are situated between Joel and Henri.

Who must be the tallest?
   a. Ani
   b. Joel
   c. Nelly
   d. Priya
   e. Elisha

Question 3

There were 200 students in my anatomy lecture. Not all the students in attendance were medical students, but all the medical students wanted to be paediatricians. Most of the students were female.

Place "Yes" if the conclusion does follow. Place "No" if the conclusion does not follow.
   a. All female students want to be paediatricians.
   b. Not all students studying medicine attending the anatomy lecture wanted to be a paediatrician.
   c. Every medical student attending the lecture was also male.
   d. All the lecture attendees who wanted to be paediatricians were also medical students.
   e. Not all students attending the anatomy lecture were female and studying medicine.

Question 4

The four friends Bob, Dylan, George, and Michael went on holiday together to Mauritius. One day, each opted for a different activity out of jet skiing, skydiving, surfing or snorkelling. The fees for these activities were £30, £40, £65, and £75 (not in any order).
Bob did not spend the highest amount on his activity but he spent £10 more than Michael.
George did not participate in skydiving but his activity cost less than Dylan's activity.
Michael opted for snorkelling; Dylan did not select surfing as his beach activity.
Snorkelling was the cheapest activity.

Who paid £75 for their activity?
  a. Bob
  b. Dylan
  c. George
  d. Michael

Question 5

A lioness has a litter of cubs. The likelihood of any one cub being female is 50%.
The first cub born is female.

If four more cubs are born, will the probability of all cubs in the litter being female be 50%?
  a. No, because the probability of all cubs being female after the first is 1 in 16.
  b. Yes, because the probability of any one cub being female is 50%.
  c. No, because the chances of another female cub being born decrease with each further birth.
  d. Yes, because each cub is equally likely to be male or female.

Question 6

At present, the newest two treatments for disease X are undergoing clinical trials.
Treatment B has been shown to effectively treat the condition in 75% of patients.
8 of every 9 patients successfully treated with medication B do not have a relapse in disease X.
Treatment A is effective in treating disease X in all but one-quarter of patients.
Only 21% of those successfully treated with treatment A encounter a relapse in the condition.

With justification based only on the effectiveness of treating disease X without relapse, is treatment B the better treatment?
  a. Yes, because treatment B treats disease X successfully in 92% of patients.
  b. No, because patients treated with treatment A were less likely to encounter a relapse of the condition.
  c. No, because treatment A has treated a greater proportion of patients successfully.
  d. Yes, because 10% more patients were treated successfully without a relapse of the condition with treatment B.

Question 7

Should secondary schools abolish issuing homework altogether, to allow pupils more time to independently determine their learning progress?

Select the strongest argument from the statements below.
   a. Yes, because the homework set by teachers nowadays is too difficult and stressful for parents to track their children's progress.
   b. Yes, because many students spend too much time answers from the internet to complete their assignments.
   c. No, because students enjoy their homework and abolishing it would adversely affect their mental health.
   d. No, because the underlying purpose of homework is to support students' understanding of their own knowledge and progress.

Question 8

Should the British public be encouraged to farm their own fruit, since eating fresh fruit every day brings many health benefits?

Select the strongest argument from the statements below.
   a. Yes, because most people nowadays do not have access to a greengrocer's selling fresh fruit.
   b. No, because not every Briton has access to a garden to grow their own produce in.
   c. Yes, because fresh fruit is more aesthetically-pleasing than frozen fruit.
   d. No, because the cost of gardening tools is too expensive, given the recent shipping disruptions.

Question 9

Would lower student intakes mean that universities are raising their entry requirements?

Select the strongest argument from the statements below.
   a. Yes, because the national birth rates of recently have surged, meaning that there will be more university students in the future to accommodate.
   b. No, because whilst lower intakes are definitely associated with higher entry requirements, these requirements still vary between different-sized higher education institutions.
   c. Yes, because people would not respect university degrees if the entry requirements were too low.
   d. No, because student intake numbers have been reduced as a result of government capping on university student numbers across the country.

Question 10

The diagram below shows the outlines of some companies.

The pentagon represents companies which have sustainable production methods.

The triangle represents companies which are run by female entrepreneurs.

The rectangle represents companies which have factories in Cambodia.

The circle represents companies mentioned in the news headlines this week.

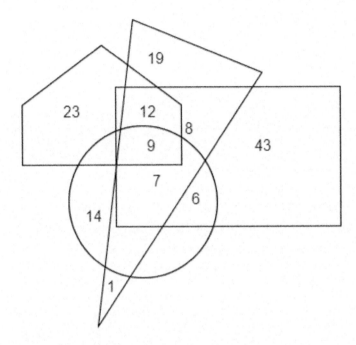

Based on the diagram, what is the proportion of companies run by female entrepreneurs which have sustainable production methods?

    a. 61%

    b. 64%

    c. 68%

    d. 69%

    e. 70%

Question 11

This Venn diagram shows the numbers of students taking classes in three different languages.

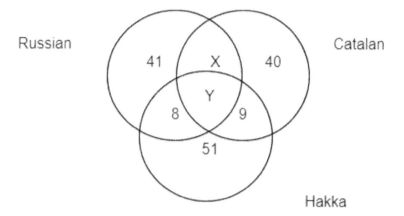

Based on this diagram, which of the following must be true?
   a. Russian is the least popular language out of these three classes.
   b. More students are taking classes in Catalan than in Hakka.
   c. These students prefer to learn two languages at once, rather than learn one language.
   d. Catalan is the most popular language out of these three classes.
   e. If Y is equal to or less than 19, Hakka is the least popular language.

Question 12

A busy takeaway is preparing the orders for 68 of its customers. Of these, 39 ordered chips, 19 ordered a curry, and 19 ordered a doner kebab. 16 have ordered both curry and chips, and of these, 4 have also ordered a doner kebab.

Which of the following diagrams best represents the above data?

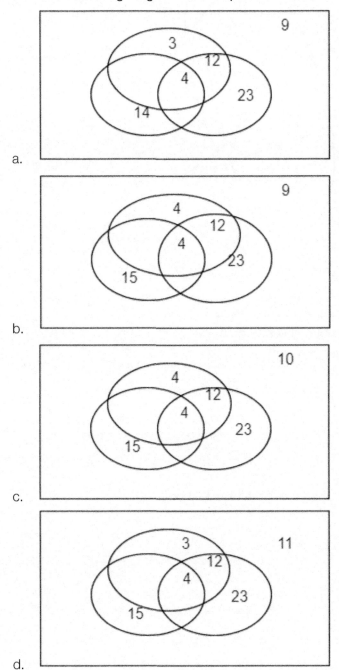

Question 13

The diagram below shows some information about Zogs and Bontles.

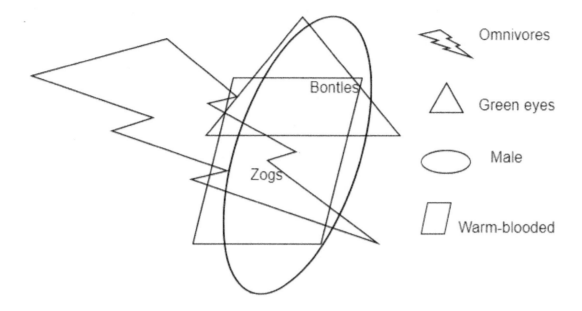

Which of the following statements is true?
a. Zogs are male and green-eyed.
b. Bontles are warm-blooded, male, and green-eyed.
c. Zogs are warm-blooded, but not male omnivores.
d. Bontles are cold-blooded, but not green-eyed.

Question 14

In the Helvetica region, there are 42 schools, a third of which have a mixed-gender intake. 26 schools admit girls.

How many more schools admit girls than those which admit boys?
a. 8
b. 9
c. 10
d. 11
e. 12

Question 15

Janice flips a coin four times in a row. Being unbiased, her coin has an even chance of landing on heads or tails.

Given that the first coin flip comes up as tails, the probability that all four flips will land on tails is 1 in 16.
   a.   Yes, because 1/2 to the power of four is 1/16.
   b.   Yes, because each coin flip out of the four has a 50% probability of landing on tails.
   c.   No, the probability is 1 in 2, as the coin has an even chance of landing on tails or heads.
   d.   No, the probability is 1 in 8, because Janice now has to flip the coin three more times.

Question 16

A prize draw is being held for a school charity raffle, in which one winner will be selected at random. Each entrant can only buy one entry ticket. Of the 100 entries, 45 were bought by people in Year 11, 25 by people in Year 13, and 30 by people in Year 12.

If 5 people from each year group withdraw their entries, will this increase the chance of someone from Year 11 winning the raffle?
   a.   Yes, the chances of someone from Year 11 winning increase when the number of Year 14 entries decreases.
   b.   Yes, the chances of someone from Year 11 winning increase when there is a bigger decrease in the total number of entries than the number of Year 11 entries.
   c.   No, the chances of someone from Year 11 winning remain the same when 5 people from each year group withdraw their entries.
   d.   No, the chances of someone from Year 11 winning decrease when the total number of entries decreases.

Question 17

The diagram below shows four buildings, which are located in the corners of a city square.

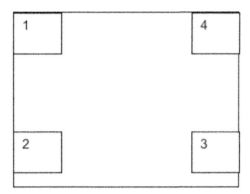

The square is occupied by (not in order) a bank, a cathedral, a school, and a government office building.
The government office building is diagonally opposite to the school.
The bank is not on on the same side of the square as the cathedral, and is adjacent to the government office building.
The school is in the lower right corner.

Which of the following is false?
   a. The bank is in the top right corner.
   b. The government office building is in the top left corner.
   c. The cathedral is diagonally opposite to the school.
   d. The school is on the same side as the bank.

Question 18

The diagram below shows the characteristics of the snacks stored in Kelly's tin.

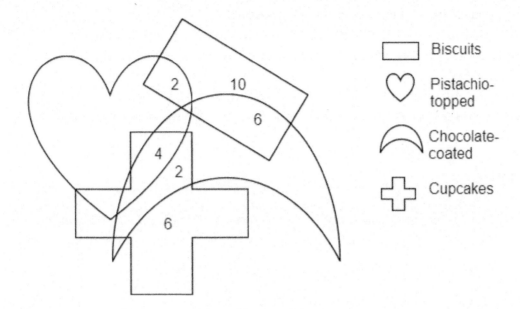

Biscuits

Pistachio-topped

Chocolate-coated

Cupcakes

Which of the following statements is incorrect?
   a. The ratio of biscuits to cupcakes is 3 to 12.
   b. Half of the cupcakes are not coated with chocolate.
   c. The probability of a pistachio-topped biscuit being selected at random is half the probability of a pistachio-topped cupcake being selected at random.
   d. Less than half of the biscuits are not topped with pistachios.

Question 19

Should every citizen be legally required to perform military service, to physically protect this nation from hostile foreign forces?

Select the strongest argument from the statements below.
   a. Yes, the prospects of a violent nuclear war with totalitarian states have been steadily increasing for the past ten years.
   b. Yes, it is the civil obligation of every citizen to develop personally by training for national defence.
   c. No, because conscription is fundamentally a form of servitude forced on individuals who may not agree with the ruling government's policies.
   d. No, because not every citizen is able to physically defend the country in the armed forces – for example, due to disability or serious illness.

Question 20

Should smacking be legally allowed for parents towards their children?

Select the strongest argument from the statements below.
 a. Yes, because corporal punishment by teachers was allowed in the Victorian era.
 b. Yes, because children can become unruly and uncivil, if proper discipline is not enforced.
 c. No, because it could greatly harm children physically and psychologically.
 d. No, because people are less motivated to do the right thing when penalised than when praised.

Question 21

The diagram shows where these five people went on holiday last year during the summer.

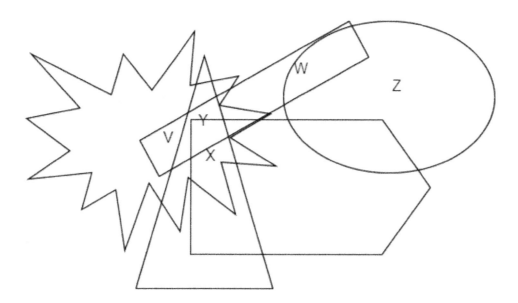

Last summer, Alex interrailed across Hungary, Croatia, Italy, and Switzerland, for a total of four countries.
 a. V
 b. W
 c. X
 d. Y
 e. Z

Question 22

Athalia is looking at investing her savings in either property or a business.
There is a 6 in 10 chance of the property earning a return of 12% or less.
The return for business has a 4 in 10 likelihood of being greater than 12%.
There is a 1 in 5 likelihood of the property earning a return of 50% or more.
The probability of the business earning a return between 12% and 50% is 1 in 20.

When considering only the return, is the business a better investment option?
- a. Yes, the chance of the returns being 50% or more is higher for business.
- b. Yes, the chance of the returns being 12% or less is lower for business.
- c. No, the return for property is 50% higher.
- d. No, the return for property is 12% higher.
- e. Can't tell

Question 23

This fruit is nutritious. All nutritious foods are in short supply.

Place 'Yes' if the conclusion does follow. Place 'No' if the conclusion does not follow.
- a. All fruits are nutritious.
- b. All fruits are in short supply.
- c. Some nutritious fruits are in short supply.
- d. All foods which are in short supply are nutritious.
- e. Some foods in short supply are fruits.

Question 24

On Saturday afternoon, Annie, Ben, Carl and Dan are playing cricket in the park. A ball batted by one of them smashes the windscreen of Mr. Danvers' car.

Annie says, 'It was Ben'.
Ben says, 'It was Carl'.
Carl says, 'It was not me'.
Dan says, 'It was not me'.

Given the information above, who must be the only one lying?
- a. Annie
- b. Ben
- c. Carl
- d. Dan
- e. Can't tell

Question 25

The firm Betts International produces two types of machines, Machine P and Machine Q. One single unit of Machine P can be produced in 50 hours. One single unit of Machine Q can be produced in 25 hours. The sole limiting factor in this production process is the labour available to the firm, in hours per month. The table below shows certain combinations of the number of units of each machine that the company can produce during a month, when using all the available labour.

Production of machines

Machine P (units)	Machine Q (units)
700	0
500	500
350	800
250	1,000

Place 'Yes' if the conclusion does follow. Place 'No' if the conclusion does not follow.
   a. A target requiring 1,500 units of Machine Q alone in one month can be met.
   b. A target requiring 300 units of Machine P and 950 units of Machine Q respectively in one month can be met.
   c. A target requiring 600 units of Machine P and 100 units of Machine Q respectively in one month may leave production equipment underused.
   d. A target requiring 400 units of Machine P and 750 units of Machine Q respectively in one month may cause worker burnout.
   e. Within a production system running competently, if 700 units of Machine Q are produced in a month, then the number of units produced of Machine P must be lower.

Question 26

At an outdoor swimming pool in Miami, there are 52 people using the pool, including both adults and children. Whilst there are 2 more males than females, 10 of the 22 adults are male.

How many more boys than girls are there in this pool?
   a. 3
   b. 4
   c. 5
   d. 6
   e. 7

Question 27

Before a cross-country race, the team of seven from Rayner High School are asked to line up for the coach, Mrs. Sheridan, to take a photograph. They line up in a row, as shown in the diagram below.

	Freddie					

Left-hand side

Right-hand side

Marcus stands next to Julia.

Harry stands as close to Rosie as possible, at the far right.

Paul is standing between two boys, but neither of them is Harry.

The runner who is standing furthest from the right is Anna, who is five places away from Rosie.

Which of the following must be true?
a. Harry is standing on the far left.
b. Julia is standing between Marcus and Paul.
c. Freddie is standing between Paul and Marcus.
d. Rosie is standing between Julia and Harry.
e. Paul is standing between Freddie and Julia.

Question 28

This democracy and human rights think tank, Liberté Hall International, produces annual reports on the degree of political freedom in every political system of the world. Its analysts score each political system out of 50 for civil rights, individual and national freedoms, and independent rule of law. All political systems with a score of 40 or more out of 50 are considered a "completely free" system. Those scoring above 25, but below 40, out of 50, are called "semi-free"; whilst those scoring under 25 are considered "restricted". This political system has a score of 39 out of 50 this year.

Place 'Yes' if the conclusion does follow. Place 'No' if the conclusion does not follow.
a. This political system is restricted.
b. Last year, some political systems were semi-free.
c. This political system was completely free a year ago.
d. This think tank has scored every political system of the world this year.
e. This political system has been scored by every think tank this year.

Question 29

Kington High School for Boys and Kington High School for Girls are looking at the educational attainment of their pupils in mathematics, in the oldest and youngest year groups. After data collection, tracking the same cohort of students from Year 7 up to Year 13, they produce the following diagrams:

Year 7 - Kington High School for Boys

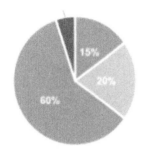

■ 80-100%   ▨ 70-80%   ■ 50-70%   ■ Below 50%

Year 13 - Kington High School for Boys

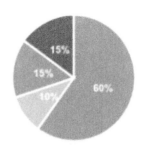

■ 80-100%   ▨ 70-80%   ■ 50-80%   ■ Below 50%

Year 7 - Kington High School for Girls

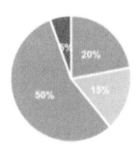

■ 80-100%   ▨ 70-80%   ■ 50-70%   ■ Below 50%

Year 13 - Kington High School for Girls

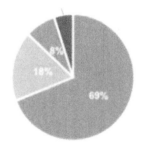

■ 80-100%   ▨ 70-80%   ■ 50-70%   ■ Below 50%

Place 'Yes' if the conclusion does follow. Place 'No' if the conclusion does not follow.

a. The proportion of students scoring 80-100% in mathematics at Kington High School for Boys, increased by 4 times between Years 7 and 13.

b. At both schools, the combined rates of achieving grades in the top two highest-scoring categories in mathematics, increased between Years 7 and 13.

c. Students in Year 7 at both schools were more likely to score below 70% in mathematics, than they were to score above it.

d. The Year 13 students at Kington High School for Boys were, on average, higher-achieving in maths, than their counterparts at Kington High School for Girls.

e. The proportion of students scoring 50-70% in maths at Kingston High School for Girls, decreased more slowly between Years 7 and 13, than their counterparts at Kington High School for Boys.

Answers: Decision Making Mock 2

Question 1

A. Some of the skirts in stock at the boutique are made from silk (but not cotton).
No. We do not know if these skirts are made entirely from silk, as we are only told that none are made from both silk and cotton.

B. Only cotton skirts are in stock at the boutique.
No. We are told that some of the skirts are made entirely from linen. Therefore, we can deduce that there are other skirts made from different materials, in addition to cotton skirts.

C. The boutique does not stock cotton skirts which also contain silk.
No. For the same reasons as the first statement, we cannot make this conclusion.

D. Silk skirts in the boutique cannot also contain linen.
No. We are not given any explicit information in the passage about the boutique stocking skirts made from both silk and linen, so we cannot draw this conclusion.

E. All the skirts stocked at the boutique are made from a blend of silk and cotton.
No. The last sentence tells us that some of the skirts stocked are made entirely from linen.

Question 2: A

In this logic puzzle, we place each student in height order, from tallest to smallest.

We can begin with Nelly > Elisha > Priya.

We are then told that Ani > Elisha.

We know that Joel > student > student > student > Henri.

Ani is taller than Joel. Therefore, Ani > Joel > student > student > student > Henri.

As Ani > Elisha, and there are six students in total, we can therefore conclude that Ani must be the tallest person in the group.

Question 3

A. **No.** We are told that most of the students were female, but we do not know if all of the female students want to be paediatricians, and/or study medicine.

B. **No.** We are told that all of the medical students want to be paediatricians.

C. **No.** We are not told anything about the gender of the medical students in the lecture, only the career aspiration they all share.

D. **No.** We are told that all of the medical students attending the lecture wanted to be paediatricians. However, we do not know if there were students studying other subjects who also wanted to be paediatricians.

E. **Yes.** We are told that most of the students in attendance were female, and not all were studying medicine – with the inference that some are male and/or studying other subjects.

Question 4: B

From the information given, we can deduce that Michael opted for snorkelling, which cost either £30 or £65. Bob's activity cost either £40 or £75.

Dylan did not select surfing, and neither did Michael, so either Bob or George surfed. George did not select skydiving, so either Bob or Dylan skydived.

As surfing was the cheapest activity, Michael must have paid £30, so Bob must have paid £40.

This leaves George and Dylan. As George's activity cost less than Dylan's, we can therefore conclude that Dylan paid £75.

Question 5: A

- We can see that one cub being born female is an event independent of any other cubs being born female.
- Only one of the five cubs has already been born, with a gender of female. Therefore, the probability of all cubs being female = probability that the 4 other yet-unborn cubs are female.
- Every cub out of the unborn 4 has a 50% chance of being female.

Hence, we can say that the probability that all 4 are female = $0.5 \times 0.5 \times 0.5 \times 0.5 = 1/2 \times 1/2 \times 1/2 \times 1/2 = 1/16$

The other options (B, C, D) do not address the independence of the event where one cub being born as female.

Question 6: D

Treatment A is effective in treating the condition in three quarters of patients ("all but one-quarter"), or 75% to the nearest integer. Treatment B is effective in treating the condition in 75% of patients.

Approximately 89% (88.9%) of patients successfully treated with treatment B do not have a relapse in disease X.

100 − 21 = 79% of patients successfully treated with treatment A do not have a relapse.

Hence, we can eliminate options B and C. We know that treatment B has treated approximately 10% (=89 − 79) more patients successfully without relapse, so D is the correct option.

Question 7: D

A broadens the terms of the argument to include pupils' parents.

B shifts the terms of the argument from the time students spend on estimating their own progress, to the time students spend on completing their homework (in a specific, morally-questionable manner!).

C makes a conclusion on students' mental health – irrelevant to the original question focus.

Only **D** focuses on the original terms of the argument. If homework supports students' understanding of their own knowledge and progress, abolishing it would stop pupils from determining their learning progress, which addresses the question most clearly.

Question 8: A

Looking at the options, **A** addresses the focus of the question most directly. People cannot access fresh fruit (and so the health benefits associated) if they can't buy them locally. Hence, they are more likely to have a source of fresh fruit, with the health benefits, if they can grow their own.

B shifts the terms of the argument from the health benefits of personal fruit farming, to the opportunity/conditions needed for it. This is not the same as health.

C shifts the terms of the argument from health benefits to the aesthetic/artistic benefits of fresh fruit. This is also not equivalent to health.

D broadens the terms of the argument to the tools required for farming fruit, but the question does not stipulate how the fruit would be grown. It is one of the weaker arguments, because it is not a good enough reason – for example, people could access garden tools by borrowing them from neighbours.

Question 9: D

D highlights another reason for lower student intakes, which is that the universities are responding to government capping on student numbers, and not to applicants' academic standards.

A shifts the terms of the argument to the birth rates associated with the future intake numbers, away from the academic ability associated in the original question.

C refers to the respect gauged from university degrees which is the consequence, but not the cause of, a change in entry requirements.

D implies that, whilst higher entry requirements is linked with lower intakes, the requirements still differ with universities of differing sizes. Given that it contradicts itself, D is a weak argument.

Question 10: B

There are $19 + 12 + 9 + 8 + 7 + 1 = 56$ female entrepreneur-run companies in total.

Out of these, $19 + 1 = 20$ companies are not in the sustainable production rectangle, and $56 - 20 = 36$ companies have sustainable production methods.

$(36 / 56) \times 100 = 64.28(...) = 64\%$

Question 11: E

Whilst Hakka has $68 + Y$ students, Catalan and Russian both have $49 + X + Y$ students. If Y is 19 or fewer, the number of students taking Hakka will be less than those taking Catalan or Russian.

Question 12: D

There are 16 – 4 = 12 orders for curry and chips with no doner kebab.

There are 19 – 4 = 15 orders for a doner kebab only.

There are 19 – 16 = 3 orders for a curry only.

There are 39 – 16 = 23 orders for chips only.

These are all correctly shown in D.

The numbers in options A and B do not add up to 68.

C shows, incorrectly, that 4 + 4 + 12 = 20 people ordered a curr

Question 13: B

Bontles lie in the overlap between "Green eyes", "Warm-blooded", and "Male", but do not lie in the "Omnivore" category.

Question 14: C

We know that 26 schools admit girls.

42 – 26 = 16 schools admit boys.

Therefore, 26 – 16 = 10 more schools admit girls.

Question 15: D

The first coin flip has already happened, but we are focusing on the probability of the remaining three uncompleted flips. A and B assume that the flips have been completed, so must be eliminated.

D is the correct probability, as each of the three flips is an independent event – the probability we are asked about = 1/2 x 1/2 x 1/2, which is 1/8.

Question 16: B

Originally before this withdrawal, the chances of selecting an entry from someone in Year 11 was 45%.

If 5 people from each year group withdraw their entries, there will now be 100 – 15 = 85 entries.

The chances of selecting an entry from someone in Year 11 will now be (40/85) x 100 = 47% (nearest whole number).

Therefore, the chances of Year 11 selection will be higher.

Question 17: C

We are told that the school is in square 3. As the government office building is diagonally opposite to the school, the government office building is in square 1. We can eliminate B.

The bank and cathedral are not on the same side, and so must be in squares 2 and 4. The bank is adjacent to the government office building, so it must be in square 4. Therefore, we can eliminate A.

We can now visualise the positions as below:

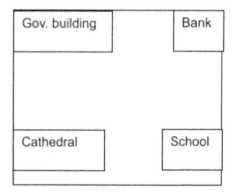

The school (square 3) must be adjacent to the bank (square 4), so we can eliminate D. The cathedral must be in square 2, and is adjacent, not diagonally opposite, to the school, so C is false.

Question 18: C

10/18 = 5/9 of the biscuits are not topped with pistachios. 5/9 = 55.555(...)%, which is more than half of the biscuits.

All the other options are correct.

Question 19: D

A broadens the argument to focus on the hostile foreign forces mentioned in the question stem. However, it does not explain enough how these forces justify citizens' having to perform military service.

B shifts the focus to the personal, citizen-level benefits of national military service, away from its original motive, to defend the country.

C shifts the original terms of the argument from the purpose of military conscription, to its associated and consequential human rights problems.

D provides a strong argument, by explaining the ineffectiveness of mandatory conscription, based on how not all citizens can physically defend the nation.

Question 20: C

A is a weak argument, as it does not address or justify the role of parents in disciplining children by smacking.

B does not explicitly address smacking, or link it with the idea of "proper discipline", and so is a vague argument.

D is weak, because it broadens the argument focus to all people in general, and shifts it to alternative methods of discipline, without clearly addressing smacking.

C is the strongest argument, because it explicitly addresses how justifiable smacking is, if it has serious adverse consequences.

Question 21: D

Only Y is in the overlap between Hungary (rectangle), Croatia (star), Italy (arrow/pentagon), and Switzerland (triangle).

Question 22: A

We know that both investments have the same chance of earning a return of 12% or less – 60%.

However, investing in property has a 20% chance of earning a return of 50% or more. Investing in business has a 35% chance of earning the same return.

Question 23

A. All fruits are nutritious.
No. Although this fruit is nutritious, we do not know anything about whether other fruits, or all fruits in general, are nutritious.

B. All fruits are in short supply.
No. We do not know if all fruits are nutritious foods – we are only told that this particular fruit is nutritious. Therefore, we cannot conclude that all fruits are in short supply.

C. Some nutritious fruits are in short supply.
Yes. We know that all nutritious foods, are in short supply, and this extends to fruits.

D. All foods which are in short supply are nutritious.
No. Although all nutritious foods are in short supply, we are not told anything about all the foods in short supply. Hence, we do not know anything about all foods in short supply.

E. Some foods in short supply are fruits.
Yes. We are told that this fruit is a nutritious food, and all nutritious foods are in short supply. Therefore, some of the foods in short supply must be fruits.

Question 24: B

If Annie is lying, then Ben would not have smashed the windscreen, and it might have been Carl who did. So Ben or Carl (or both) would also be lying.

If Ben is lying, then Carl wouldn't have been the one to smash the windscreen. It also wouldn't have been Dan. Hence, Carl and Dan would both be telling the truth. If Annie is also telling the truth, Ben must be lying. So Ben must be the correct option.

If Carl is lying, he would have smashed the windscreen himself, so Annie would also be lying.

If Dan is lying, he would have smashed the windscreen himself, so Ben would also be lying.

Question 25

From the first row of the table, we can see that the firm spends (700 x 50 =) 35, 000 hours per month producing these machines.

A. **No.** This would require [1,500 x 25=] 37,500 hours. This exceeds the maximum number of hours the firm spends on production – 35,000.

B. **No.** This would require [(300 x 50) + (950 x 25)=] 38, 750 hours to produce, which exceeds the firm's maximum amount of time spent on production. This would be more likely to lead to machines being overused.

C. **Yes.** This would require [(600 x 50) + (100 x 25)=] 32, 500 hours to produce, which is less than the firm's maximum amount of time spent on production.

D. **Yes.** This would require [(400 x 50) + (750 x 25)=] 38, 750 hours to produce, which exceeds the firm's maximum amount of time spent on production – which would cause burnout.

E. **Yes.** [700 x 25=]17,500 hours would be spent on making the units of Machine Q. This would leave 17,500 hours for Machine P, making 350 units of Machine P at most.

Question 26: B

We are told that 10 of the 22 adults are male, so there must be 12 female adults. There must also be 30 children in total.

Let the total number of females be f, making the number of males (f + 2). We can solve this like a mathematical equation: 52 = f + f + 2, so f = 25 = total number of females. Hence, there are 27 males in total.

There must be [27-10=]17 boys, and [25-12=]13 girls – so there are 4 more boys than girls.

We can note everything down on a two-way table, such as below:

	Females	Males	Total
Adults	12	10	22
Children	13	17	30
Total	25	27	52

Question 27: D

From the information given, we know that Harry is standing on the far right, so we can eliminate A.

Paul must be standing between Freddie and Marcus – from the diagram, we can see this standing order must be Freddie/Paul/Marcus. Hence, we can eliminate B and C. We can also eliminate E (given the above deduction) as well as the given information that Marcus is standing next to Julia.

Hence, we are left with D. This statement makes sense, as Harry stands at the far right, with Rosie on his left. With all the conclusions reached before, the space to Rosie's left must be left for Julia.

Question 28

A. **No.** We can see that 39/50 goes in the "semi-free" range of Liberté Hall International's indexing.

B. **No.** We are not told anything about the freedom classifications of any political systems last year.

C. **No.** For the same reason as (2), we are not told anything about this political system a year ago.

D. **Yes.** This is clearly stated in the paragraph of information given.

E. **No.** We are not told anything about other think tanks, or how they might relate to this political system.

Question 29

A. **Yes.** We can see from the pie charts that this was 15% in Year 7, but then increased to 60% in Year 13.

B. **Yes.** We can see that the segments for the two categories take up more space in the Year 13 pie charts, than in the Year 7 pie charts.

C. **Yes**. We can see that the two segments for the scores below 70% are bigger than those for the scores above 70%. Therefore, a higher proportion of Year 7 students at both schools have scored below 70%.

D. **No.** We can see that the top two attainment categories (80-100 and 70-80) take up a greater proportion of the Year 13 pie chart for Kington High School for Girls.

E. **No.** At Kington High School for Girls, the rate decreased from 50% to 8% (by factor of 6.25), whereas at Kington High School for Boys, the rate decreased from 60% to 15% (by factor of 4).

Quantitative Reasoning Mock 2

Question Set 1

Mrs Taylor purchases a bakery. A floor plan of the shop is shown below.

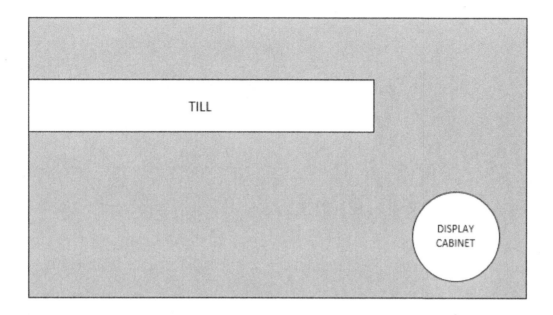

9 metres

1. The width of the shop is 9 metres. If the area of the shop is equal to (two thirds of the width)^2, what is the length of the shop?
   a.   3 metres
   b.   4 metres
   c.   5 metres
   d.   6 metres
   e.   7 metres

2. The area of the circular display cabinet is 2m^2. What is the diameter of the display cabinet? Take π to equal 3.14.
   a.   0.6m
   b.   0.8m
   c.   1.2m
   d.   1.6m
   e.   2.0m

3. The area of the till is 6.3m². Given that the width of the till is at least half the 9-metre width of the shop, what is the largest possible length of the short side of the till?

    a. 0.7 metres
    b. 1.4 metres
    c. 2.3 metres
    d. 3.2 metres
    e. Can't Tell

4. The bakery across the street has an identical layout and identical floor plan but is slightly larger than Mrs Taylor's.

The shaded area on the floor plan represents the shop floor and has an area of 37.8m2. Due to fire safety regulations, there is a maximum of 2 people per square metre at any given time.

What is the maximum number of people able to be contained within this bakery at any given time?

    a. 18
    b. 19
    c. 38
    d. 75
    e. 76

Question Set 2

The table below displays the 2021 quarterly sales from a vintage clothing company, categorised by type of item.

Term	Sweatshirts	Jeans	Hats	Shoes
January – March	1820	2390	1010	180
April – June	1470	1870	890	160
July – September	2080	2460	910	240
October – December	2120	2880	990	190

On average, sweatshirts cost £24.50 throughout the year.
The average price of a pair of jeans was £36.00 from January to March 2021.
The price of a hat was, on average, one ninth of the price of a pair of shoes throughout the year.

5. In the January-March term, what proportion of total sales did the hats contribute across all four item types, to the nearest whole percentage?

    a. 3%

    b. 9%

    c. 13%

    d. 19%

    e. 23%

6. What was the income generated in 2021 by sweatshirts alone?

    a. £7490

    b. £18350

    c. £74905

    d. £137905

    e. £183505

7. The price of a pair of jeans rose by 5% in each of the terms. What was the total income generated in 2021 by jeans alone?

    a. £334733

    b. £343773

    c. £374373

    d. £374337

    e. £374773

8. The average price of a pair of shoes was £50 in the first term, which rose by 8% in the second term. What was the average price of a hat in April-June 2021?

    a. £5

    b. £6

    c. £7

    d. £8

    e. £9

Question Set 3

Robert buys an ice-cream machine, which is capable of making 2 litres of ice-cream per hour. He also buys three ice lolly moulds, which can hold up to 16 ice lollies each. Ice lollies take two hours to make.

9. What is the maximum number of ice lollies Robert can make in a single day?

    a. 288

    b. 576

    c. 864

    d. 1152

    e. 1440

10. Robert wants to sell the ice-cream for £3.75 per litre. If he works for 12 hours every day, what is the maximum income he can generate from the ice cream produced in a week?

    a. £90

    b. £180

    c. £360

    d. £630

    e. £1260

11. Robert sells the ice-cream initially for £3.75 per litre. If he now wishes to sell the ice-cream for £4.50 per litre, what will be the percentage increase in his revenue from ice-cream sales?

    a. 10%

    b. 15%

    c. 20%

    d. 25%

    e. 30%

12. Ice lolly moulds cost £26.40 each. If each ice lolly is sold for £1.50, how many lollies will be needed to repay the cost of the moulds alone?

    a. 17

    b. 18

    c. 35

    d. 52

    e. 53

Question Set 4

A group of friends are discussing interest rates on savings accounts from different banks.
Bank A has compound interest of 1.2% annually on savings accounts. There is no additional charge on money withdrawn at any time.
Bank B has compound interest of 1.4% annually on all savings accounts. There is a 5% charge on all sums taken out of the savings account in the first three years.

13. Amelia deposits £1200 into her account with Bank A. After 5 years, what would be her balance to the nearest pond, assuming she makes no withdrawals?

    a. £1214

    b. £1229

    c. £1244

    d. £1259

    e. £1274

14. Billy puts £900 into his savings account with Bank B. After a year, he wishes to withdraw all the money he has put in. How much money will he be able to withdraw, to the nearest pound?
   a. £855
   b. £873
   c. £913
   d. £955
   e. £1013

15. Charlie deposits £2100 into a savings account with bank A. What is the minimum number of years it will take for the saved total to reach over £2250?
   a. 3 years
   b. 4 years
   c. 5 years
   d. 6 years
   e. 7 years

16. Delilah puts £500 into a savings account with bank A and £500 into a savings account with bank B. She withdraws both of these sums entirely after two years. What will be the change in Delilah's earnings overall?
   a. £4.60 decrease
   b. £0.46 decrease
   c. There is no change overall
   d. £0.46 increase
   e. £4.60 increase

Question Set 5

There are 90 students reading Mathematics at University. A fifth of these students have blonde hair, 60% have black hair and the remainder of the students, bar one, have brown hair. The mean age of this cohort is 20.8, where the highest age is 26 and the lowest age is 19. Male students outnumber female students in the ratio 1.5:1.

17. How many male students are there within this cohort?
   a. 36
   b. 45
   c. 54
   d. 63
   e. 72

18. What percentage of the students have brown hair?
    a. 19%
    b. 20%
    c. 21%
    d. 22%
    e. 23%

19. The professor of this class is aged 68. If his age were to be taken into account when calculating the mean age of this class, what would be the percentage change in the mean age for this class?
    a. 2.5%
    b. 2.8%
    c. 3.1%
    d. 3.3%
    e. 3.6%

20. What is the minimum number of male students in this cohort with black hair?
    a. 0
    b. 9
    c. 12
    d. 18
    e. 24

Question Set 6

The table below shows the income tax paid by the residents of Worthington.

Annual taxable income (£)	Tax rate (%)
0-15,000	5
15,000-30,000	10
30,000-45,000	15
45,000-60,000	20
60,000-75,000	25
75,000 and over	30

21. Mrs Jones has an annual salary of £50,000. How much money does she pay in income tax annually?
    a. £4500
    b. £5500
    c. £6000
    d. £7500
    e. £10000

22. Natalie gets a promotion, and her annual salary increases from £29,000 to £35,000. What will be the percentage increase in the amount of income tax Natalie has to pay?
    a. 21%
    b. 39%
    c. 72%
    d. 121%
    e. 139%

23. Andrew pays £2772 in income tax annually. How much does he earn in a year?
    a. £30500
    b. £30430
    c. £33080
    d. £33480
    e. £34080

24. Nadia has an average weekly salary of £1270. She sets aside some of this money every month to cover her income tax. How much money will she have to save every month, to the nearest pound?
    a. £749
    b. £750
    c. £751
    d. £752
    e. £753

Question Set 7

Julie is redecorating her kitchen. She is looking at retiling a rectangular area of the kitchen measuring 8 metres by 14 metres. The table below shows the costs of installation.

Type	Flooring cost (£/m2)	Installation cost (£/m2)
Wood	64	10.20
Vinyl tile	37	5.70
Porcelain tile	54	8.80
Marble	78	10.80

25. How much would it cost Julie to replace the flooring in the area of the kitchen with wood flooring, to the nearest pound?
   a. £7168
   b. £7480
   c. £7960
   d. £8108
   e. £8310

26. One of Julie's friends suggests using the vinyl tile. The other recommends porcelain tile. What would be the difference in overall cost between the two options for this area, to the nearest pound?
   a. £1323
   b. £1897
   c. £2363
   d. £2897
   e. £3203

27. Julie extends the area to be tiled to 10 metres by 15 metres. How much more expensive is it to install marble tiles in this new area compared to the old area?
   a. £3374.40
   b. £3474.80
   c. £3484.40
   d. £3744.80
   e. £3784.40

28. Julie opts for the porcelain tile but decides to install it herself so that she does not have to pay an installation fee. What is the percentage decrease in overall cost if Julie does not need to pay for installation?
   a. 14%
   b. 15%
   c. 16%
   d. 17%
   e. 18%

Question Set 8

A factory produces boxes of paper using 6 identical machines.
The machines begin production at 8am and work continuously until 5pm from Monday to Saturday.
One machine can produce 90 boxes per hour.
Each box is closed. The dimensions of one box are 36 x 25 x 20 centimetres.

29. What is the maximum number of boxes the factory can produce in a working week?
   a. 4860
   b. 5670
   c. 26740
   d. 29160
   e. 34020

30. One of the machines breaks down while there are still 1100 boxes remaining for the day. How long will it take for the remaining machines to make 1100 boxes?
   a. 2 hours and 4 minutes
   b. 2 hours and 22 minutes
   c. 2 hours and 27 minutes
   d. 2 hours and 44 minutes
   e. 2 hours and 47 minutes

31. These boxes are shipped in a large box with dimensions 2.43 x 0.72 metres. What is the maximum number of smaller boxes that may be able to be contained within one large box?
   a. 96
   b. 97
   c. 98
   d. 99
   e. 100

32. The paper company wishes to print its logo on all surfaces of the box. The cost of printing the logo is £1.20 per square metre. How much will it cost to print the logos on all the boxes produced in the factory in one day, to the nearest pound?
    a. £1832
    b. £2086
    c. £2473
    d. £2578
    e. £2890

Question Set 9

The diagram below represents the distances between five towns in miles.

Parston	Parston				
Quailand	3.6	Quailand			
Rownley	4.4	6.1	Rownley		
Stepfield	7.9	3.8	3.2	Stepfield	
Talcester	3.9	5.4	4.5	6.2	Talcester

33. How much shorter is a direct trip from Parston to Stepfield, compared to a journey from Parston to Stepfield via Talcester?
    a. 2.1 miles
    b. 2.2 miles
    c. 2.3 miles
    d. 2.4 miles
    e. 2.5 miles

34. Anya travels from her home in Rownley to Stepfield directly. On her way home, she visits a friend in Quailand. She travels in her car at an average speed of 31 miles per hour. How long does Anya spend driving, to the nearest minute?
    a. 24 minutes
    b. 25 minutes
    c. 26 minutes
    d. 27 minutes
    e. 28 minutes

35. A direct journey from Quailand takes exactly 6 minutes at an average speed of 38 miles per hour. What is the destination?
   a. Parston
   b. Rownley
   c. Stepfield
   d. Talcester
   e. Can't Tell

36. The road which leads directly from Parston to Talcester has an average speed limit of 30 miles per hour. On the train, this journey takes exactly 6 minutes. What is the percentage reduction in time when taking the train from Parston to Talcester, compared to taking the car?
   a. 21%
   b. 22%
   c. 23%
   d. 24%
   e. 25%

Answers: Quantitative Reasoning Mock 2

Question Set 1

Question 1: B

1. Calculate the area of the shop:
2/3 x 9 = 6
6 x 6 = 36

2. Calculate the length of the shop:
36/9 = 4 metres

Question 2: D

1. Substitute numbers into the formula for area:
Area = πr^2
$2 = 3.14r^2$
$r^2 = (2/3.14) = 0.637$
$r = = 0.798$

2. Find the diameter from the radius:
0.798 x 2 = 1.596
Diameter = 1.6m

Top Tip: read the question carefully to ensure you work out the correct value. Some candidates may select option B after working out the radius, but the question asks for the diameter.

Question 3: B

1. Calculate the smallest possible length of the long side of the till:
9/2 = 4.5 metres

2. Calculate the short length of the till:
6.3/4.5 = 1.4 metres

Question 4: D

1. Calculate the maximum number of people:
$37.8 \times 2 = 75.6$

Rounding down gives a maximum of 75 people.

Question Set 2

Question 5: D

1. Calculate the total number of sales:
$1820 + 2390 + 1010 + 180 = 5400$

2. Calculate the proportion contributed by hats:
$1010/5400 \times 100 = 18.7\%$

Question 6: E

1. Calculate the total number of sweatshirts sold:
$1820 + 1470 + 2080 + 2120 = 7490$

2. Calculate the income generated:
$24.5 \times 7490 = 183505$

Timing tip: with calculations such as these, try and maximise your efficiency by familiarising yourself with the online UCAT calculator. Keyboard shortcuts and the use of certain buttons may be useful to learn prior to the exam.

Question 7: C

1. Calculate the prices of the jeans:
January – March: £36.00
$36 \times 1.05 = 37.8$
April – June = £37.80
$37.8 \times 1.05 = 39.69$
July – September = £39.69
$39.69 \times 1.05 = 41.67$
October – December = £41.67

2. Calculate the income for each term:

$36 \times 2390 = 86040$

$37.8 \times 1870 = 70686$

$39.69 \times 2460 = 97637.40$

$41.67 \times 2880 = 120009.60$

3. Calculate the total income:

$86040 + 70686 + 97637.40 + 120009.60 = 374373$

Question 8: B

1. Calculate the new cost of a pair of shoes:

$50 \times 1.08 = 54$

2. Calculate the cost of a hat:

$54/9 = 6$

Question Set 3

Question 9: B

1. Calculate the maximum number of ice lollies per two hours:

$3 \times 16 = 48$

2. Work out how many ice lollies can be made in a day:

$24/2 = 12$

$12 \times 48 = 576$

Question 10: D

1. Calculate the amount of ice-cream produced in 12 hours:

$12 \times 2 = 24$ litres

2. Calculate the income generated over a week:

$24 \times 7 = 168$

$168 \times 3.75 = 630$

Question 11: C

1. Calculate the percentage increase:

$450/375 \times 100 = 120$

$120 - 100 = 20\%$ increase

Question 12: E

1. Calculate the total cost of the moulds:
26.40 x 3 = 79.20

2. Calculate the number of ice lollies needed:
79.20/1.50 = 52.8

So 53 lollies will need to be sold.

Question Set 4

Question 13: E

1. Calculate the balance after 5 years:
1200 x 1.0125 = 1273.75

So to the nearest pound, Amelia will have £1274.

Top Tip: learn the difference between simple and compound interest. In this question, the savings accounts are all subject to compound interest, so the gain increases every year, unlike simple interest where the gain is the same for every year.

Question 14: A

1. Calculate the compound interest:
900 x 1.014 = £912.60

2. Calculate the money deducted:
912.60 x 0.95 = £855

Question 15: D

Through trial and error:
2100 x 1.0124 = 2202.63
2100 x 1.0125 = 2229.06
2100 x 1.0126 = 2255.80

So it will take at least 6 years.

Top Tip: *learn the formula for compound interest, as this will speed up your working considerably.*

Question 16: D

1. Calculate the money from bank A:
500 x 1.0122 = 512.07

2. Calculate the money from bank B:
500 x 1.0142 = 514.10
514.10 x 0.95 = 488.39

3. Calculate the total:
488.39 + 512.07 = 1000.46

4. Calculate the increase:
1000.46 – 1000 = 0.46

Question Set 5

Question 17: C

1. Calculate the number of male students:
1.5 + 1 = 2.5
90/2.5 = 36
36 x 1.5 = 54

Question 18: C

1. Calculate the number of students with brown hair:
100 – 20 – 60 = 20
20 – 1 = 19 students

2. Calculate the proportion of students with brown hair:
19/90 x 100 = 21%

Question 19: A

1. Calculate the new total:
20.8 x 90 = 1872
1872 + 68 = 1940

2. Calculate the new mean:
1940/91 = 21.32

3. Calculate the percentage change:

1.32/20.8 x 100 = 102.5

102.5 – 100 = 2.5%

Question 20: D

1. Calculate the number of female students:

90/2.5 = 36

2. Calculate the number of students with black hair:

0.6 x 90 = 54

3. Calculate the number of male students with black hair:

54 – 36 = 18

Question Set 6

Question 21: B

1. Calculate the amount of income tax Mrs Jones pays:

15000 x 0.05 = 750

15000 x 0.10 = 1500

15000 x 0.15 = 2250

5000 x 0.20 = 1000

Total = 750 + 1500 + 2250 + 1000 = 5500

Top Tip: with income tax questions, it might be useful to make a note of the tax paid at the top of each income band, as these frequently come up in the questions.

Question 22: B

1. Calculate the original income tax:

15000 x 0.05 = 750

14000 x 0.10 = 1400

Total = 2150

2. Calculate the new income tax:

15000 x 0.05 = 750

15000 x 0.1 = 1500

5000 x 0.15 = 750

Total = 3000

3. Calculate the percentage increase:

3000/2150 x 100 = 139.53

139.53 – 100 = 39% increase

Question 23: D

1. Work out which bracket he is in:

15000 x 0.05 = 750

15000 x 0.10 = 1500

Total = 2250

Therefore, he must be in the third income bracket (30,000-45,000).

2. Calculate the amount of tax paid within this bracket:

2772 – 2250 = 500

3. Carry out a reverse percentage calculation:

522/0.15 = 3480

4. Calculate his total income:

30000 + 3480 = 33480

Question 24: C

1. Calculate her annual income:

1270 x 52 = 66040

2. Calculate the annual income tax:

15000 x 0.05 = 750

15000 x 0.10 = 1500

15000 x 0.15 = 2250

15000 x 0.20 = 3000

6040 x 0.25 = 1510

Total = 9010

3. Calculate the monthly cost:

9010/12 = 750.83

So £751 to the nearest pound.

Question Set 7

Question 25: E

1. Calculate the cost per metre squared:
64 + 10.20 = 74.20

2. Calculate the area:
8 x 14 = 112m2

3. Calculate the total cost:
112 x 74.20 = 8310.40

Question 26: C

1. Calculate the cost per metre squared for both:
Vinyl = 37 + 5.70 = 42.70
Porcelain = 54 + 8.80 = 62.80

2. Calculate the difference in cost per metre squared:
62.80 − 42.70 = 21.10

3. Calculate the difference in cost:
21.10 x 112 = 2363.20

Question 27: A

1. Calculate the difference between new and old areas:
Old area = 112 metres squared
New area = 10 x 15 = 150 metres squared.
Difference = 150 − 112 = 38 metres squared

2. Calculate the total cost per metre squared:
78 + 10.80 = 88.80

3. Calculate the total cost:
88.80 x 38 = 3374.40

Question 28: A

1. Calculate the percentage decrease:
54 + 8.80 = 62.80
54/62.80 x 100 = 86
100 − 86 = 14%

Question Set 8

Question 29: D

1. Calculate the total number of boxes produced by one machine:
Number of working hours = 9
Number of boxes in a day by one machine = 9 x 90 = 810
Number of boxes in a day by six machines = 810 x 6 = 4860
Number of boxes produced in a week = 4860 x 6 = 29160

Question 30: C

1. Calculate the remaining time:
1100/5 = 220
220/90 = 2.444
0.444 x 60 = 26.7

So it will take 2 hours and 27 minutes.

Question 31: B

1. Calculate the volume of the large box:
2.43 x 0.72 = 1.7496

2. Calculate the volume of the smaller boxes:
0.36 x 0.25 x 0.2 = 0.018

3. Calculate the maximum number:
1.7496/0.018 = 97.2

So the maximum number is 97.

Question 32: C

1. Calculate the surface area of the boxes:
0.36 x 0.25 = 0.09
0.25 x 0.2 = 0.05
0.2 x 0.36 = 0.072
0.09 + 0.05 + 0.072 = 0.212
0.212 x 2 = 0.424 metres squared

2. Calculate the cost per box:
0.424 x 1.20 = 0.5088

3. Calculate the number of boxes produced in one day:
9 x 6 x 90 = 4860

4. Calculate the cost in one day:
4860 x 0.5088 = 2472.77

Timing Tip: if a question involves multiple steps and is beginning to take too long to complete, flag it and move on to the next question.

Question Set 9

Question 33: B

1. Calculate the difference:
Journey 1: 7.9 miles
Journey 2: 3.9 + 6.2 = 10.1 miles
10.1 – 7.9 = 2.2 miles

Question 34: B

1. Calculate the distance:
3.2 + 3.8 + 6.1 = 13.1 miles

2. Calculate the time:
Time = distance/speed
Time = 13.1/31 = 0.42258 hours
0.42258 x 60 = 25.4 minutes

So 25 minutes to the nearest minute.

Question 35: C

1. Calculate the distance:
Time = 6/60 = 0.1 hours
Distance = speed x time = 38 x 0.1 = 3.8 miles

Since Stepfield is 3.8 miles away, this must be the correct answer.

Timing Tip: try and do sums in your head where possible, as using the UCAT calculator can be a relatively slow process.

Question 36: C

1. Calculate the time taken in the car:
Time = distance/speed
Time = 3.9/30 = 0.13 hours
0.13 x 60 = 7.8 minutes

2. Calculate the percentage reduction:
6/7.8 x 100 = 76.92
100 – 76.92 = 23.08%

Abstract Reasoning Mock 2

Question Set 1

Set A   *Set B*

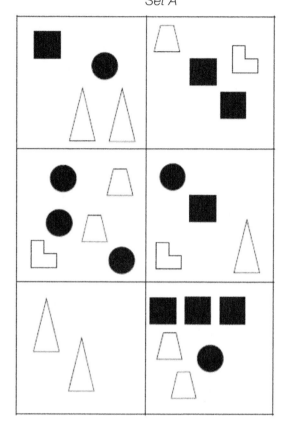 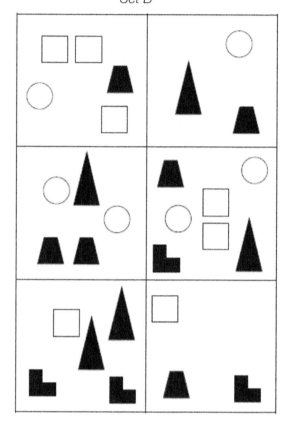

Question 1

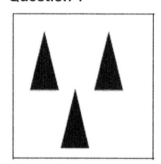

a. Set A
b. Set B
c. Neither

Question 2

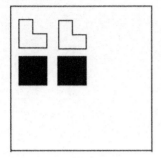

    a.   Set A
    b.   Set B
    c.   Neither

Question 3

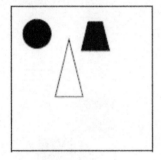

    a.   Set A
    b.   Set B
    c.   Neither

Question 4

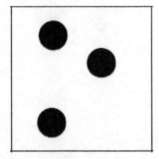

    a.   Set A
    b.   Set B
    c.   Neither

Question 5

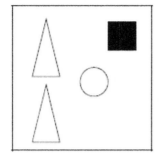

   a. Set A
   b. Set B
   c. Neither

Question Set 2

Set A   *Set B*

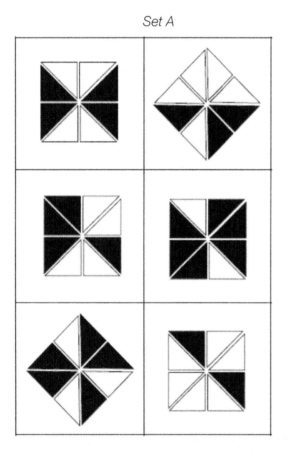

Question 6

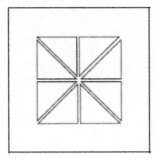

    a. Set A
    b. Set B
    c. Neither

Question 7

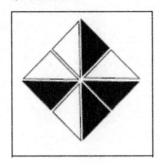

    a. Set A
    b. Set B
    c. Neither

Question 8

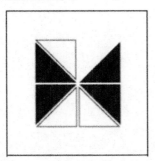

    a. Set A
    b. Set B
    c. Neither

Question 9

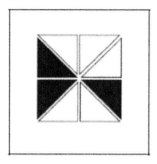

   a. Set A

   b. Set B

   c. Neither

Question 10

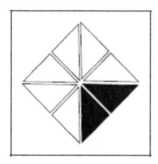

   a. Set A

   b. Set B

   c. Neither

Question Set 3

Set A *Set B*

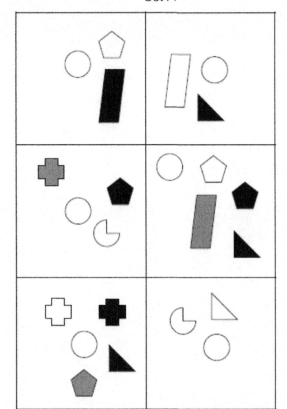 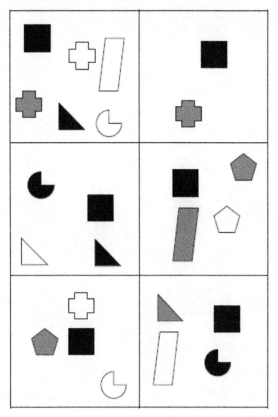

Question 11

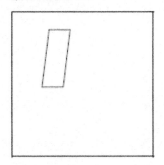

a. Set A
b. Set B
c. Neither

Question 12

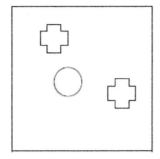

a. Set A
b. Set B
c. Neither

Question 13

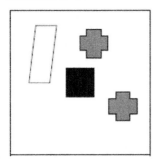

a. Set A
b. Set B
c. Neither

Question 14

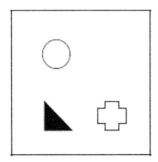

a. Set A
b. Set B
c. Neither

Question 15

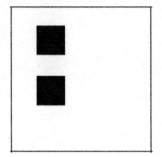

a. Set A
b. Set B
c. Neither

Question Set 4

Set A   *Set B*

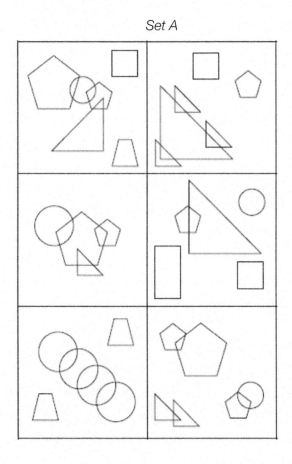   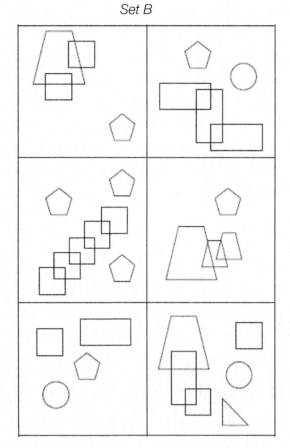

Question 16

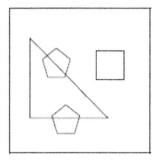

a. Set A
b. Set B
c. Neither

Question 17

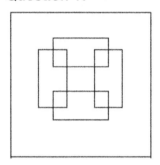

a. Set A
b. Set B
c. Neither

Question 18

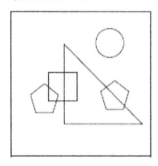

a. Set A
b. Set B
c. Neither

Question 19

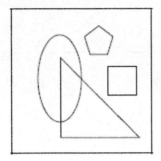

    a. Set A
    b. Set B
    c. Neither

Question 20

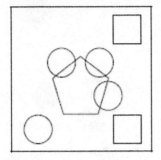

    a. Set A
    b. Set B
    c. Neither

Question Set 5

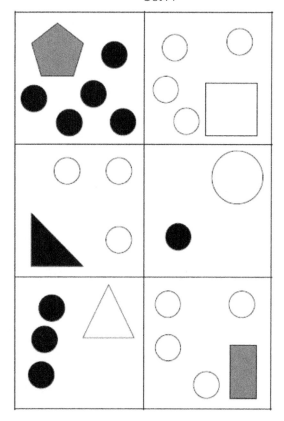

Set A

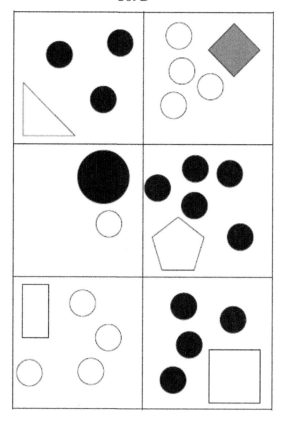

Set B

Question 21

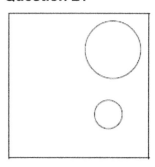

a. Set A
b. Set B
c. Neither

Question 22

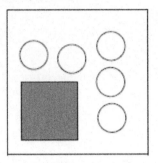

a. Set A
b. Set B
c. Neither

Question 23

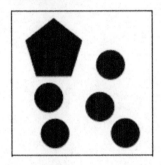

a. Set A
b. Set B
c. Neither

Question 24

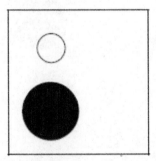

a. Set A
b. Set B
c. Neither

Question 25

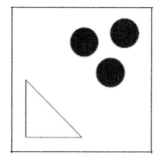

    a. Set A
    b. Set B
    c. Neither

Question Set 6

Set A

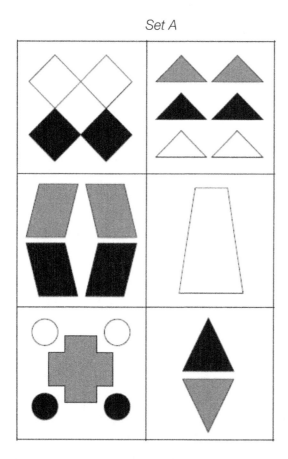

Set B

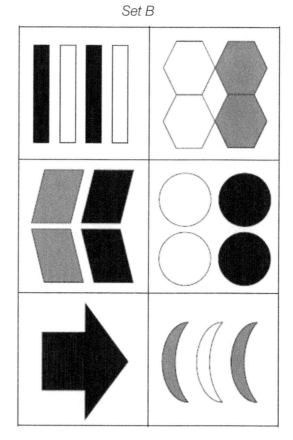

Question 26

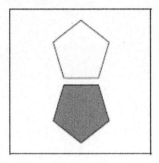

a. Set A
b. Set B
c. Neither

Question 27

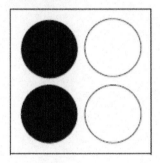

a. Set A
b. Set B
c. Neither

Question 28

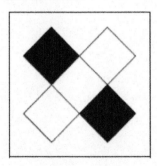

a. Set A
b. Set B
c. Neither

Question 29

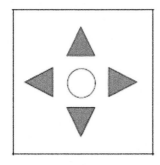

   a. Set A
   b. Set B
   c. Neither

Question 30

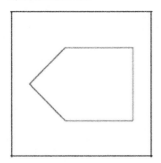

   a. Set A
   b. Set B
   c. Neither

Question Set 7

Set A   *Set B*

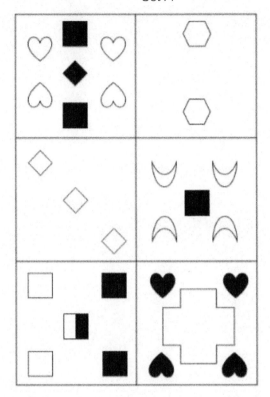 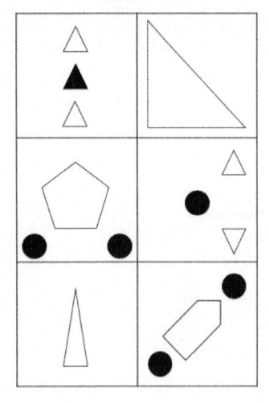

Question 31

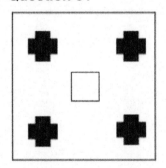

   a. Set A
   b. Set B
   c. Neither

Question 32

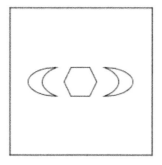

a. Set A
b. Set B
c. Neither

Question 33

a. Set A
b. Set B
c. Neither

Question 34

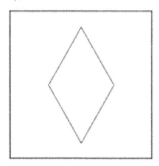

a. Set A
b. Set B
c. Neither

Question 35

   a. Set A
   b. Set B
   c. Neither

Question Set 8

Set A

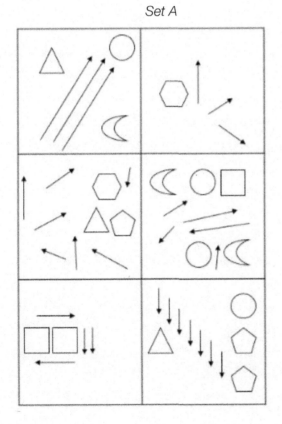

Set B

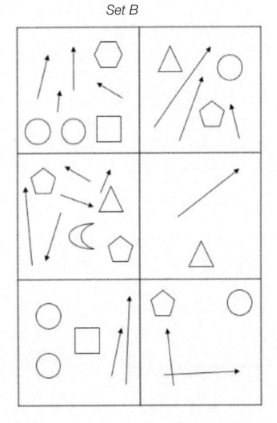

Question 36

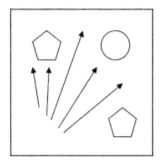

a. Set A
b. Set B
c. Neither

Question 37

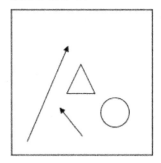

a. Set A
b. Set B
c. Neither

Question 38

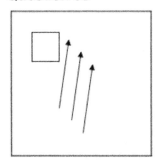

a. Set A
b. Set B
c. Neither

Question 39

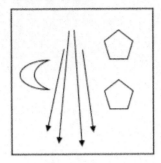

a. Set A
b. Set B
c. Neither

Question 40

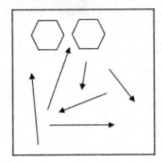

a. Set A
b. Set B
c. Neither

Question Set 9

Set A   *Set B*

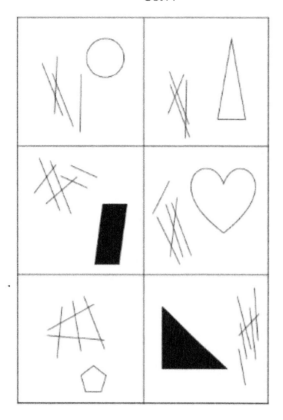 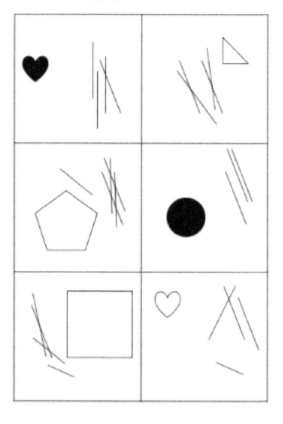

Question 41

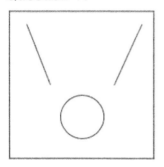

a. Set A
b. Set B
c. Neither

Question 42

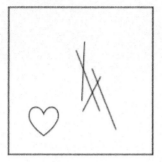

a. Set A
b. Set B
c. Neither

Question 43

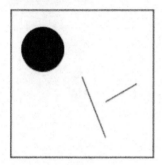

a. Set A
b. Set B
c. Neither

Question 44

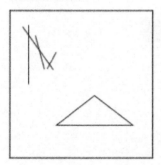

a. Set A
b. Set B
c. Neither

Question 45

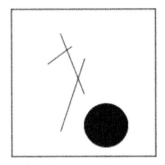

    a. Set A

    b. Set B

    c. Neither

Question 46

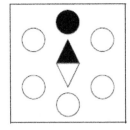 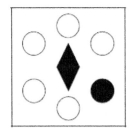 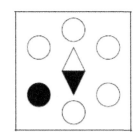 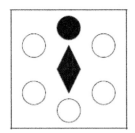

Which figure completes the series?

a.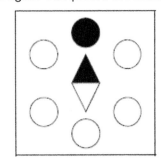

b.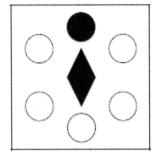

c.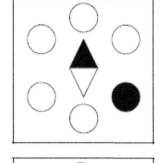

d.

Question 47

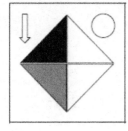 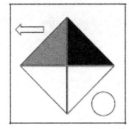 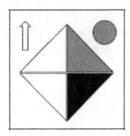 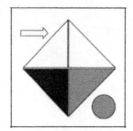

Which figure completes the series?

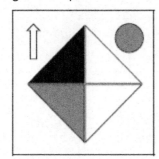

a.

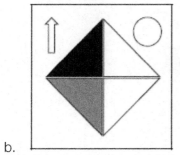

b.

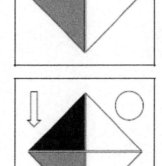

c.

d.

Question 48

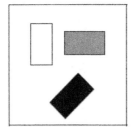 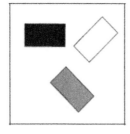 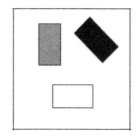 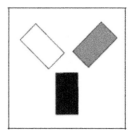

Which figure completes the series?

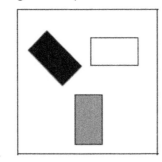

a.

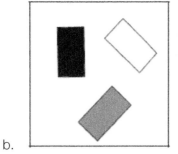

b.

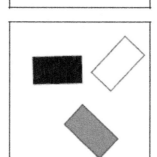

c.

d.

Question 49

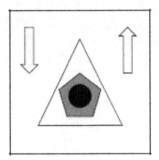

is to

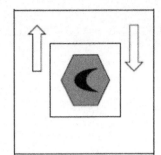

as

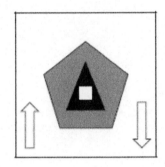

is to

Which figure completes the series?

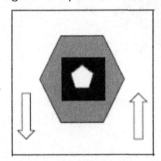

a.

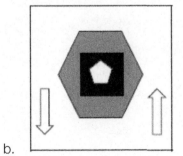

b.

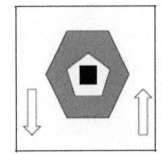

c.

d.

Question 50

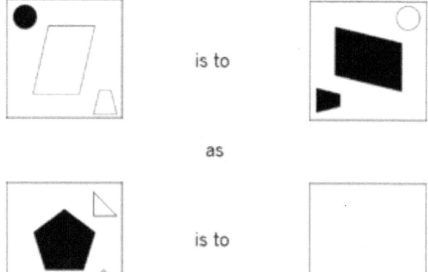

Which figure completes the series?

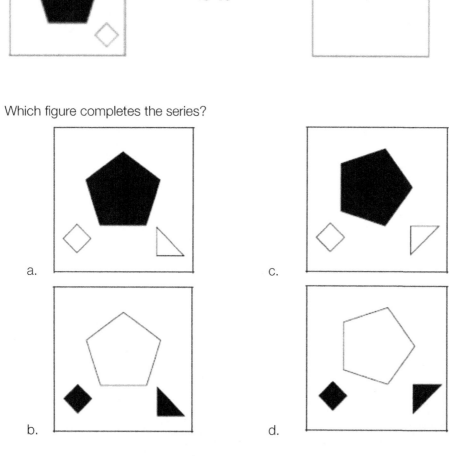

1:1 UCAT TUTORING

 Delivered by UCAT experts, who scored in the top 10% of the exam

 A personalised 1:1 approach, tailored to your unique needs

 Proven success, with Medic Mind students achieving an average score of 2810 (top 10% nationally)

Book your FREE consultation now

Visit the link or scan the QR code below for more information:
www.medicmind.co.uk/ucat-tutoring

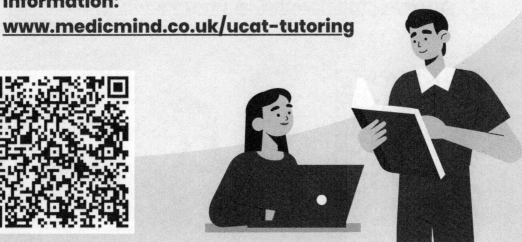

UCAT ONLINE COURSE

 100+ tutorials, designed by our UCAT experts, to guide you through every section of the exam

 Access to our UCAT Question Bank, with 8,000+ practice questions to use in your revision

 Invites to regular UCAT webinars, live classes and interactive sessions

Buy Now!

Visit the link or scan the QR code below for more information:
https://www.medicmind.co.uk/ucat-online-course/

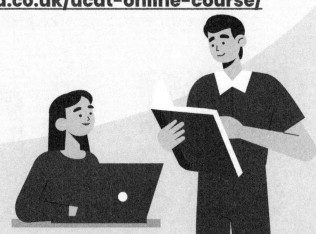

1:1 MEDICINE INTERVIEW TUTORING

 Delivered by Medicine Interview experts, who scored in the top 10% of the exam

 A personalised 1:1 approach, tailored to your unique needs

 Proven success, with Medic Mind students acing their Medicine Interview.

Book your FREE consultation now

Visit the link or scan the QR code below for more information:
www.medicmind.co.uk/interview-tutoring/

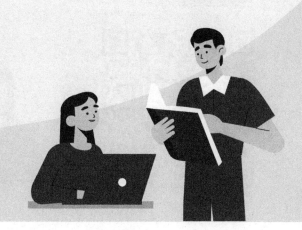

MEDICINE INTERVIEW ONLINE COURSE

 100+ tutorials, and 200+ MMI stations , designed by our Medicine interview experts

 Learn how to answer questions on motivation for Medicine, personal skills, work experience, hot topics, and more

 A range of packages available, including a live day of teaching and 1:1 tutoring

Buy Now!

Visit the link or scan the QR code below for more information:
www.medicmind.co.uk/interview-online-course/

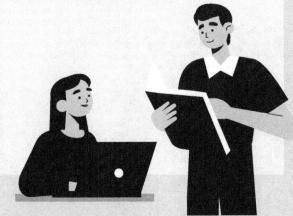

Answers: Abstract Reasoning Mock 2

Question Set 1

Question 1: B

SET A: There is an even number of shapes. All shapes with two or more lines of symmetry are shaded, while shapes with one line of symmetry are unshaded.

SET B: There is an odd number of shapes. All shapes with two or more lines of symmetry are unshaded, while shapes with one line of symmetry are shaded.

All three shapes have one line of symmetry and therefore they are all shaded.

Top Tip: Always start with the simplest box first to work out the pattern. The greater the number of shapes, the greater the number of potential patterns, so start with the simplest visually.

Question 2: A

SET A: There is an even number of shapes. All shapes with two or more lines of symmetry are shaded, while shapes with one line of symmetry are unshaded.

SET B: There is an odd number of shapes. All shapes with two or more lines of symmetry are unshaded, while shapes with one line of symmetry are shaded.

There are four shapes. The squares have more than 1 line of symmetry and are shaded, while shapes with one line of symmetry only are unshaded.

Question 3: C

SET A: There is an even number of shapes. All shapes with two or more lines of symmetry are shaded, while shapes with one line of symmetry are unshaded.

SET B: There is an odd number of shapes. All shapes with two or more lines of symmetry are unshaded, while shapes with one line of symmetry are shaded.

The trapezium and triangle have different shading, even though they both have one line of symmetry.

Question 4: C

SET A: There is an even number of shapes. All shapes with two or more lines of symmetry are shaded, while shapes with one line of symmetry are unshaded.

SET B: There is an odd number of shapes. All shapes with two or more lines of symmetry are unshaded, while shapes with one line of symmetry are shaded.

There are three shapes, but this cannot be in Set B since the circles (with infinite lines of symmetry) are shaded.

Question 5: C

SET A: There is an even number of shapes. All shapes with two or more lines of symmetry are shaded, while shapes with one line of symmetry are unshaded.

SET B: There is an odd number of shapes. All shapes with two or more lines of symmetry are unshaded, while shapes with one line of symmetry are shaded.

There are four shapes, but this cannot belong to Set A as the circle is unshaded.

Question Set 2

Question 6: A

SET A: There are eight triangles. If an even number of triangles is shaded, then it will be arranged in a square shape. If an odd number of triangles is shaded, it will be arranged in a diamond shape.

SET B: There are eight triangles. If an odd number of triangles is shaded, then it will be arranged in a square shape. If an even number of triangles is shaded, it will be arranged in a diamond shape.

An even number of triangles is shaded and the shape is arranged in a square, so this belongs to set A.

Timing Tip: Try to work out how long each question should take you for each section. This is particularly important for the AR section, because you should be spending around 1 minute on each set of 5 questions. If it is taking too long to work out, flag the questions and move on.

Question 7: B

SET A: There are eight triangles. If an even number of triangles is shaded, then it will be arranged in a square shape. If an odd number of triangles is shaded, it will be arranged in a diamond shape.

SET B: There are eight triangles. If an odd number of triangles is shaded, then it will be arranged in a square shape. If an even number of triangles is shaded, it will be arranged in a diamond shape.

An even number of triangles is shaded and it is arranged in a diamond shape, so this belongs to set B.

Question 8: C

SET A: There are eight triangles. If an even number of triangles is shaded, then it will be arranged in a square shape. If an odd number of triangles is shaded, it will be arranged in a diamond shape.

SET B: There are eight triangles. If an odd number of triangles is shaded, then it will be arranged in a square shape. If an even number of triangles is shaded, it will be arranged in a diamond shape.

This belongs to neither set as there are only seven triangles.

Question 9: B

SET A: There are eight triangles. If an even number of triangles is shaded, then it will be arranged in a square shape. If an odd number of triangles is shaded, it will be arranged in a diamond shape.

SET B: There are eight triangles. If an odd number of triangles is shaded, then it will be arranged in a square shape. If an even number of triangles is shaded, it will be arranged in a diamond shape.

There is an odd number of shaded triangles and it is arranged in a square shape. Therefore this belongs to set B.

Question 10: B

SET A: There are eight triangles. If an even number of triangles is shaded, then it will be arranged in a square shape. If an odd number of triangles is shaded, it will be arranged in a diamond shape.

SET B: There are eight triangles. If an odd number of triangles is shaded, then it will be arranged in a square shape. If an even number of triangles is shaded, it will be arranged in a diamond shape.

An even number of triangles is shaded, and this is arranged in a diamond shape. Therefore, this belongs to set A.

Question Set 3

Question 11: C

SET A: Each figure contains only one white circle. There is an odd number of shapes within the set.

SET B: Each figure contains only one black square. There is an even number of shapes within the set.

There is neither a white circle nor a black square within the figure, so this belongs to neither set.

Question 12: A

SET A: Each figure contains only one white circle. There is an odd number of shapes within the set.

SET B: Each figure contains only one black square. There is an even number of shapes within the set.

There is an odd number of shapes and a white circle, so this belongs to set A.

Question 13: B

SET A: Each figure contains only one white circle. There is an odd number of shapes within the set.

SET B: Each figure contains only one black square. There is an even number of shapes within the set.

There is an even number of shapes and a black square, so this belongs to set B.

Question 14: A

SET A: Each figure contains only one white circle. There is an odd number of shapes within the set.

SET B: Each figure contains only one black square. There is an even number of shapes within the set.

There is an odd number of shapes and a white circle, so this belongs to set A.

Question 15: C

SET A: Each figure contains only one white circle. There is an odd number of shapes within the set.

SET B: Each figure contains only one black square. There is an even number of shapes within the set.

There are two black squares, so this cannot belong to set B. Therefore, this belongs to neither set.

Question Set 4

Question 16: C

SET A: There is an odd number of shapes that are intersecting. All intersections are between shapes with an odd number of sides.

SET B: There is an even number of shapes that are intersecting. All intersections are between shapes with an even number of sides.

There is an even number of shapes intersecting, but these are between shapes with an odd number of sides, so this belongs to neither set.

Top Tip: Try to memorise some 'triggers' for certain patterns. For example, the presence of lines should trigger you to think about the number of intersections or enclosed spaces as a possible pattern.

Question 17: B

SET A: There is an odd number of areas of intersections. All intersections are between shapes with an odd number of sides.

SET B: There is an even number of areas of intersections. All intersections are between shapes with an even number of sides.

There is an even number of intersections between shapes with an even number of sides, so this belongs to set B.

Question 18: C

SET A: There is an odd number of intersections. All intersections are between shapes with an odd number of sides.

SET B: There is an even number of intersections. All intersections are between shapes with an even number of sides.

The intersections are between shapes with even and odd numbers of sides, so this belongs to neither set.

Question 19: A

SET A: There is an odd number of intersections. All intersections are between shapes with an odd number of sides.

SET B: There is an even number of intersections. All intersections are between shapes with an even number of sides.

There is one intersection between two shapes with odd numbers of sides, so this belongs to set A.

Question 20: A

SET A: There is an odd number of intersections. All intersections are between shapes with an odd number of sides.

SET B: There is an even number of intersections. All intersections are between shapes with an even number of sides.

There are three intersections between shapes with an odd number of sides, so this belongs to set A.

Question Set 5

Question 21: B

SET A: There is a shape in the top or bottom half of the figure. The number of circles in each figure corresponds to the number of sides of the shape. If the shape is in the top half of the figure, the circles will be shaded. If the shape is in the bottom half of the figure, the circles will be unshaded.

SET B: There is a shape in the top or bottom half of the figure. The number of circles in each figure corresponds to the number of sides of the shape. If the shape is in the top half of the figure, the circles will be unshaded. If the shape is in the bottom half of the figure, the circles will be shaded.

There is a large circle in the top half of the figure, and a smaller unshaded circle, so this belongs to set B.

Common Trap: Many candidates will only spot half the pattern – in this case we have number of sides and position. Try to work through all the possible patterns using SPONCS, because many AR sets in the UCAT will have multiple elements to the patterns.

Question 22: C

SET A: There is a shape in the top or bottom half of the figure. The number of circles in each figure corresponds to the number of sides of the shape. If the shape is in the top half of the figure, the circles will be shaded. If the shape is in the bottom half of the figure, the circles will be unshaded.

SET B: There is a shape in the top or bottom half of the figure. The number of circles in each figure corresponds to the number of sides of the shape. If the shape is in the top half of the figure, the circles will be unshaded. If the shape is in the bottom half of the figure, the circles will be shaded.

This belongs to neither set as there is a square with four sides and five circles which do not correspond to the number of sides.

Question 23: A

SET A: There is a shape in the top or bottom half of the figure. The number of circles in each figure corresponds to the number of sides of the shape. If the shape is in the top half of the figure, the circles will be shaded. If the shape is in the bottom half of the figure, the circles will be unshaded.

SET B: There is a shape in the top or bottom half of the figure. The number of circles in each figure corresponds to the number of sides of the shape. If the shape is in the top half of the figure, the circles will be unshaded. If the shape is in the bottom half of the figure, the circles will be shaded.

There are five circles corresponding to five sides on the pentagon. These circles are shaded since the pentagon is in the top half of the shape. Therefore this belongs to set A.

Question 24: A

SET A: There is a shape in the top or bottom half of the figure. The number of circles in each figure corresponds to the number of sides of the shape. If the shape is in the top half of the figure, the circles will be shaded. If the shape is in the bottom half of the figure, the circles will be unshaded.

SET B: There is a shape in the top or bottom half of the figure. The number of circles in each figure corresponds to the number of sides of the shape. If the shape is in the top half of the figure, the circles will be unshaded. If the shape is in the bottom half of the figure, the circles will be shaded.

There is one smaller circle corresponding to one side of the bigger circle. This is unshaded since the larger shape is in the bottom half. Therefore, this belongs to set A.

Question 25: B

SET A: There is a shape in the top or bottom half of the figure. The number of circles in each figure corresponds to the number of sides of the shape. If the shape is in the top half of the figure, the circles will be shaded. If the shape is in the bottom half of the figure, the circles will be unshaded.

SET B: There is a shape in the top or bottom half of the figure. The number of circles in each figure corresponds to the number of sides of the shape. If the shape is in the top half of the figure, the circles will be unshaded. If the shape is in the bottom half of the figure, the circles will be shaded.

There are three circles corresponding to three sides of the triangle. These are shaded since the triangle is in the bottom half, so this belongs to set B.

Question Set 6

Question 26: A

SET A: There is a vertical line of symmetry only.

SET B: There is a horizontal line of symmetry only.

There is a vertical line of symmetry only.

Question 27: B

SET A: There is a vertical line of symmetry only.

SET B: There is a horizontal line of symmetry only.

There is a horizontal line of symmetry only.

Question 28: C

SET A: There is a vertical line of symmetry only.

SET B: There is a horizontal line of symmetry only.

There is neither a horizontal nor a vertical line of symmetry.

Question 29: C

SET A: There is a vertical line of symmetry only.

SET B: There is a horizontal line of symmetry only.

There is both a horizontal and vertical line of symmetry.

Question 30: B

SET A: There is a vertical line of symmetry only.

SET B: There is a horizontal line of symmetry only.

There is a horizontal line of symmetry only.

Question Set 7

Question 31: C

SET A: All shapes have an even number of sides. There are two lines of symmetry.

SET B: All shapes have an odd number of sides. There is one line of symmetry.

All shapes have an even number of sides, however, there are more than two lines of symmetry. Therefore, this cannot belong to set A.

Question 32: A

SET A: All shapes have an even number of sides. There are two lines of symmetry.

SET B: All shapes have an odd number of sides. There is one line of symmetry.

All shapes have an even number of sides. There are two lines of symmetry, so this belongs to set A.

Question 33: B

SET A: All shapes have an even number of sides. There are two lines of symmetry.

SET B: All shapes have an odd number of sides. There is one line of symmetry.

The shape has seven sides, and there is one vertical line of symmetry within the box, so this belongs to set B.

Question 34: A

SET A: All shapes have an even number of sides. There are two lines of symmetry.

SET B: All shapes have an odd number of sides. There is one line of symmetry

The shape has four sides, and there are two lines of symmetry (one horizontal and one vertical) within the box, so this belongs to set A.

Question 35: C

SET A: All shapes have an even number of sides. There are two lines of symmetry.

SET B: All shapes have an odd number of sides. There is one line of symmetry

There are an even number of sides in all the shapes, however, the box has no lines of symmetry. Therefore, this belongs to neither set.

Common Trap: Many candidates will only spot half the pattern – in this case even and odd. Try to work through all the possible patterns just to rule them out, because many AR sets in the UCAT will have multiple elements to the patterns.

Question Set 8

Question 36: C

SET A: The number of arrows in the box is equal to half the number of sides of the shapes.

SET B: The number of arrows in the box is equal to a third of the number of sides of the shapes.

The total number of sides is 11. This is not divisible by 2 or 3, so this cannot belong to either set.

Question 37: A

SET A: The number of arrows in the box is equal to half the number of sides of the shapes.

SET B: The number of arrows in the box is equal to a third of the number of sides of the shapes.

The total number of sides is 4. There are two arrows, so this belongs to set A.

Question 38: C

SET A: The number of arrows in the box is equal to half the number of sides of the shapes.

SET B: The number of arrows in the box is equal to a third of the number of sides of the shapes.

There are four sides on the shape and only three arrows. Therefore, this belongs to neither set A nor set B.

Question 39: B

SET A: The number of arrows in the box is equal to half the number of sides of the shapes.

SET B: The number of arrows in the box is equal to a third of the number of sides of the shapes.

The total number of sides is 12. There are 4 arrows, equal to a third of the number of the sides. Therefore, this belongs to set B.

Question 40: A

SET A: The number of arrows in the box is equal to half the number of sides of the shapes.

SET B: The number of arrows in the box is equal to a third of the number of sides of the shapes.

There are 12 sides in total and 6 arrows, so this belongs to set A.

Timing Tip: Try to work out how long each question should take you for each section. This is particularly important for the AR section, because you should be spending around 1 minute on each set of 5 questions. If it is taking too long to work out, flag the questions and move on.

Question Set 9

Question 41: B

SET A: The number of intersections is one more than the number of sides on the shape.

SET B: The number of intersections is one less than the number of sides on the shape.

There are no intersections, and the number of sides of the shape is 1. Therefore, this belongs to set B.

Question 42: A

SET A: The number of intersections is one more than the number of sides on the shape.

SET B: The number of intersections is one less than the number of sides on the shape.

There are three intersections and two sides on the shape, so this belongs to set A.

Question 43: B

SET A: The number of intersections is one more than the number of sides on the shape.

SET B: The number of intersections is one less than the number of sides on the shape.

There are no intersections and one side on the shape, so this belongs to B.

Question 44: C

SET A: The number of intersections is one more than the number of sides on the shape.

SET B: The number of intersections is one less than the number of sides on the shape.

There are three intersections and three sides on the shape, so this cannot belong to either set.

Question 45: A

SET A: The number of intersections is one more than the number of sides on the shape.

SET B: The number of intersections is one less than the number of sides on the shape.

There are two intersections and only one side on the shape. Therefore, this belongs to set A.

Top Tip: Try to memorise some 'triggers' for certain patterns. For example, the presence of lines should trigger you to think about the number of intersections or enclosed spaces as a possible pattern.

Question 46: C

The triangles alternate with shading – every four turns, the top and bottom triangles become unshaded, with spacing of two turns apart. The black circle moves clockwise by 2 spaces for each turn.

Question 47: D

The arrow moves 90 degrees clockwise with each turn. The shading of the triangles also moves one space right with each turn. The position of the circle alternates between the top and the bottom, and the shading of the circle is the same as that of the triangle nearest to it.

Question 48: C

The position of each of the shapes shifts clockwise with each turn. With each turn, the shapes are all rotated 45 degrees clockwise.

Question 49: A

The arrows are rotated by 180 degrees. Each of the shapes 'gains' one side while keeping the same shading.

Question 50: D

The entire image is rotated by 90 degrees in a clockwise direction. The shading of all shapes is inverted.

Situational Judgement Mock 2

Question Set 1

Dr Hopson is a junior doctor working in an Accident and Emergency (A&E) department. Over, the past week she has noticed that the A&E managers seem to be pushing to discharge elderly patient prematurely. She feels the unit is not complying with the NICE guidelines. Dr Hopson is seriously concerned that the standard of care being offered to elderly patients is inadequate.

How **appropriate** are each of the following responses by **Dr Hopson** in this situation?

1. Do nothing
    a. A very appropriate thing to do
    b. Appropriate, but not ideal
    c. Inappropriate but not awful
    d. A very inappropriate thing to do

2. Inform the consultant in charge of her concerns
    a. A very appropriate thing to do
    b. Appropriate, but not ideal
    c. Inappropriate but not awful
    d. A very inappropriate thing to do

3. Report her concerns to the hospital's regulator
    a. A very appropriate thing to do
    b. Appropriate, but not ideal
    c. Inappropriate but not awful
    d. A very inappropriate thing to do

4. Seek advice from a senior colleague
    a. A very appropriate thing to do
    b. Appropriate, but not ideal
    c. Inappropriate but not awful
    d. A very inappropriate thing to do

5. Report her concerns via the hospital's reporting procedure
    a. A very appropriate thing to do
    b. Appropriate, but not ideal
    c. Inappropriate but not awful
    d. A very inappropriate thing to do

6. Anonymously inform the media of her concerns
   a. A very appropriate thing to do
   b. Appropriate, but not ideal
   c. Inappropriate but not awful
   d. A very inappropriate thing to do

Question Set 2

Jack is a 2nd-year medical student. Following, his exams, Jack goes out to a pub with several friends. Outside the pub, Jack gets into a fight with another student and punches him in the face. When the police arrive, Jack is arrested on suspicion of assault. The next morning, Jack is charged with assault and released on bail. He is unsure whether he needs to inform the medical school.

How **appropriate** are each of the following responses by **Jack** in this situation?

7. Wait to see if he is found guilty before informing the medical school
   a. A very appropriate thing to do
   b. Appropriate, but not ideal
   c. Inappropriate but not awful
   d. A very inappropriate thing to do

8. Do not inform the medical school
   a. A very appropriate thing to do
   b. Appropriate, but not ideal
   c. Inappropriate but not awful
   d. A very inappropriate thing to do

9. Ask his advisor for advice
   a. A very appropriate thing to do
   b. Appropriate, but not ideal
   c. Inappropriate but not awful
   d. A very inappropriate thing to do

10. Inform the medical school a few weeks later
    a. A very appropriate thing to do
    b. Appropriate, but not ideal
    c. Inappropriate but not awful
    d. A very inappropriate thing to do

Question Set 3

Dr Bercow is a junior doctor working an on-call night shift. He is asked by the nurses on a general surgery ward to prescribe pain relief to an elderly woman recovering from major surgery. After he has written the prescription, one of the senior nurses tells Dr Bercow that she thinks he has prescribed the wrong dose of the painkiller. She is worried the patient may suffer an overdose, which could be lethal.

*How **appropriate** are each of the following responses by **Dr Bercow** in this situation?*

11. Check the dose but reprimand the nurse for questioning a doctor
    a. A very appropriate thing to do
    b. Appropriate, but not ideal
    c. Inappropriate but not awful
    d. A very inappropriate thing to do

12. Ask one of the medical students to change the prescription
    a. A very appropriate thing to do
    b. Appropriate, but not ideal
    c. Inappropriate but not awful
    d. A very inappropriate thing to do

13. Check the prescription and correct the dosage if necessary
    a. A very appropriate thing to do
    b. Appropriate, but not ideal
    c. Inappropriate but not awful
    d. A very inappropriate thing to do

14. Shout at the nurse for questioning his authority
    a. A very appropriate thing to do
    b. Appropriate, but not ideal
    c. Inappropriate but not awful
    d. A very inappropriate thing to do

15. Do nothing
    a. A very appropriate thing to do
    b. Appropriate, but not ideal
    c. Inappropriate but not awful
    d. A very inappropriate thing to do

Question Set 4

Dr Harding is a newly qualified junior doctor working on a surgical ward. It is her first job as a doctor, and she is still nervous about doing certain practical procedures as she is concerned that she may harm her patients. One of the nurses asks her to insert a catheter into one of her patients. This is a procedure Dr Harding does not feel confident performing. Dr Harding is unsure what to do.

*How **appropriate** are each of the following responses by **<u>Dr Harding</u>** in this situation?*

16. Ask the nurse for advice on how to perform the procedure
    a. A very appropriate thing to do
    b. Appropriate, but not ideal
    c. Inappropriate but not awful
    d. A very inappropriate thing to do

17. Do not perform the procedure
    a. A very appropriate thing to do
    b. Appropriate, but not ideal
    c. Inappropriate but not awful
    d. A very inappropriate thing to do

18. Perform the procedure
    a. A very appropriate thing to do
    b. Appropriate, but not ideal
    c. Inappropriate but not awful
    d. A very inappropriate thing to do

19. Ask the nurse to help her perform the procedure
    a. A very appropriate thing to do
    b. Appropriate, but not ideal
    c. Inappropriate but not awful
    d. A very inappropriate thing to do

Question Set 5

Zubin is a third-year medical student undertaking his cardiac surgery placement. Today, he is shadowing a consultant surgeon Mr Pain. Today, Mr Pain is due to perform a surgery on a 31-year-old patient, Mr Jones. Whilst scrubbing into the surgery with Mr Pain, Zubin smells alcohol on Mr Pain's breath.

*How **appropriate** are each of the following responses by **Zubin** in this situation?*

20. Confront Mr Pain in front of the other theatre staff
    a. A very appropriate thing to do
    b. Appropriate, but not ideal
    c. Inappropriate but not awful
    d. A very inappropriate thing to do

21. Do nothing
    a. A very appropriate thing to do
    b. Appropriate, but not ideal
    c. Inappropriate but not awful
    d. A very inappropriate thing to do

22. Inform Mr Pain's registrar
    a. A very appropriate thing to do
    b. Appropriate, but not ideal
    c. Inappropriate but not awful
    d. A very inappropriate thing to do

23. Privately approach Mr Pain and raise his concern
    a. A very appropriate thing to do
    b. Appropriate, but not ideal
    c. Inappropriate but not awful
    d. A very inappropriate thing to do

Question Set 6

Kim is a junior doctor working on the Obstetrics and Gynaecology ward. At 1am, she is called to help perform an emergency Caesarean Section. During the delivery, Kim accidentally cuts the baby's cheek with her scalpel. The cut is small, and the baby is otherwise healthy. Kim feels terrible as she knows this should not happen but is unsure what to tell the mother.

*How **appropriate** are each of the following responses by **Kim** in this situation? Assume that each of the following responses would be said politely.*

24. Inform the mother about the cut but tell her it is a common side effect
    a. A very appropriate thing to do
    b. Appropriate, but not ideal
    c. Inappropriate but not awful
    d. A very inappropriate thing to do

25. Ask her senior colleague to apologise to the mother for the mistake
    a. A very appropriate thing to do
    b. Appropriate, but not ideal
    c. Inappropriate but not awful
    d. A very inappropriate thing to do

26. Inform the mother about the mistake and give an apology
    a. A very appropriate thing to do
    b. Appropriate, but not ideal
    c. Inappropriate but not awful
    d. A very inappropriate thing to do

27. Seek advice from her clinical supervisor about the situation
    a. A very appropriate thing to do
    b. Appropriate, but not ideal
    c. Inappropriate but not awful
    d. A very inappropriate thing to do

28. Report the incident through the hospital's procedures
    a. A very appropriate thing to do
    b. Appropriate, but not ideal
    c. Inappropriate but not awful
    d. A very inappropriate thing to do

Question Set 7

A group of nine first-year medical students are undertaking a group project which forms part of their final grade. One of the group members, Michael, has turned up 20 minutes late to their fifth team meeting. He has been late to every single meeting so far. Alfie, the team leader is becoming increasingly frustrated as he feels Michael's lack of punctuality is disrupting the group's progress. He is worried how it will impact his grade.

*How **appropriate** are each of the following responses by **Alfie** in this situation? Assume that each of the following responses would be said politely.*

29. At the next team meeting, remind everyone of the importance of turning up on time
    a. A very appropriate thing to do
    b. Appropriate, but not ideal
    c. Inappropriate but not awful
    d. A very inappropriate thing to do

30. Shout at Michael for turning up late
    a. A very appropriate thing to do
    b. Appropriate, but not ideal
    c. Inappropriate but not awful
    d. A very inappropriate thing to do

31. Speak with Michael in private and ask why he is turning up late
    a. A very appropriate thing to do
    b. Appropriate, but not ideal
    c. Inappropriate but not awful
    d. A very inappropriate thing to do

32. Wait and see if Michael turns up on time for the next meeting
    a. A very appropriate thing to do
    b. Appropriate, but not ideal
    c. Inappropriate but not awful
    d. A very inappropriate thing to do

33. Report Michael to their tutor
    a. A very appropriate thing to do
    b. Appropriate, but not ideal
    c. Inappropriate but not awful
    d. A very inappropriate thing to do

Question Set 8

Jeremy is a fifth-year medical student. He is on a train going home to Edinburgh to visit his parents as he has a week off from medical school. Just after departing Newcastle station, lots of people start gathering around a seat a few rows in front of him after a man has collapsed. Whilst he has some medical knowledge, he is not sure if he will be able to help the patient in this situation as he is not a qualified doctor yet. He is unsure whether he should volunteer to help.

*How **important** to take into account are the following considerations for **Jeremy** when deciding how to respond to the situation?*

34. He might face legal action if he makes a mistake
    a. Very important
    b. Important
    c. Of minor importance
    d. Not important at all

35. His level of competence
    a. Very important
    b. Important
    c. Of minor importance
    d. Not important at all

36. Whether there are any other medical professionals on board that might come forward
    a. Very important
    b. Important
    c. Of minor importance
    d. Not important at all

37. He has only had three hours of sleep the night before
    a. Very important
    b. Important
    c. Of minor importance
    d. Not important at all

Question Set 9

Ali is a senior doctor who sits on the board of a CCG (Clinical Commissioning Group), a group which makes decisions about funding for the hospitals in the area. He has to decide whether to provide funding for one of two new treatments for the patients in his area. One treatment has the potential to save around one thousand lives per year by preventing stroke. The other treatment would allow sufferers of a life-limiting lung disease to live 10 to 15 more years, potentially helping around 60 people a year.

*How **important** to take into account are the following considerations for **Ali** when deciding which treatment to choose?*

38. The age of each treatment group
    a. Very important
    b. Important
    c. Of minor importance
    d. Not important at all

39. Stroke risk is associated with lifestyle factors e.g. smoking
    a. Very important
    b. Important
    c. Of minor importance
    d. Not important at all

40. The number of patients affected by each treatment
    a. Very important
    b. Important
    c. Of minor importance
    d. Not important at all

41. Any legal obligations Ali has
    a. Very important
    b. Important
    c. Of minor importance
    d. Not important at all

42. The proportion of ethnic minority in each target treatment groups
    a. Very important
    b. Important
    c. Of minor importance
    d. Not important at all

Question Set 10

Sarah is a doctor working in a GP practice. The first patient in the clinic is a 21-year-old student called Mike who has been diagnosed with a sexually transmitted disease. Mike tells Sarah that he has had unprotected sex with another student called Mary but does not wish to inform Mary. Sarah knows it is important for Mary to be informed as she will require treatment.

*How **important** is it to take into account are the following considerations for **Sarah** when deciding how to respond to the situation?*

43. Mike's right to confidentiality
    a. Very important
    b. Important
    c. Of minor importance
    d. Not important at all

44. Whether Mary's health is at risk
    a. Very important
    b. Important
    c. Of minor importance
    d. Not important at all

45. Mike is a student
    a. Very important
    b. Important
    c. Of minor importance
    d. Not important at all

46. That the infection is sexually transmitted
    a. Very important
    b. Important
    c. Of minor importance
    d. Not important at all

47. Mary's age
    a. Very important
    b. Important
    c. Of minor importance
    d. Not important at all

Question Set 11

Tim is a 15-year-old boy. He has been involved in a car accident and suffered significant injuries. He has been informed that he will require surgery to save his life. However, Tim has recently joined several online forums and now believes modern medicine is a scam. Timmy tells the surgeon, Ms Smith, that he does not want the surgery, but Ms Smith knows the surgery is in Tim's best interests.

*How **important** is it to take into account are the following considerations for **Ms Smith** when deciding how to respond to the situation?*

48. Tim is 15 years old
    a. Very important
    b. Important
    c. Of minor importance
    d. Not important at all

49. The risks of not having the surgery
    a. Very important
    b. Important
    c. Of minor importance
    d. Not important at all

50. Tim's wishes
    a. Very important
    b. Important
    c. Of minor importance
    d. Not important at all

51. The risks of the surgery
    a. Very important
    b. Important
    c. Of minor importance
    d. Not important at all

Question Set 12

Dr Neil is a GP working in a Glasgow GP practice. His third patient of the day is a 32-year-old woman called Theresa. Theresa explains she is pregnant and informs Dr Neil that she wants to have an abortion as she does not feel ready to have a baby. However, Dr Neil is a devout Christian who has a deeply held belief that abortion is morally wrong.

*How **important** to take into account are the following considerations for **<u>Dr Neil</u>** when deciding how to respond to the situation?*

52. Theresa's wish to have an abortion
    a. Very important
    b. Important
    c. Of minor importance
    d. Not important at all

53. Theresa is 32 years old
    a. Very important
    b. Important
    c. Of minor importance
    d. Not important at all

54. Dr Neil's beliefs about abortion
    a. Very important
    b. Important
    c. Of minor importance
    d. Not important at all

55. Whether other doctors are available to see Theresa
    a. Very important
    b. Important
    c. Of minor importance
    d. Not important at all

Question Set 13

Rishi is a fifth-year medical student undertaking a project in a research lab. He is assisting a senior research doctor, Dr Johnson, with research into a new cancer drug. Rishi discovers that Dr Johnson is purposefully omitting the negative findings from his research to allow the drug to progress to the next phase of trials.

*How **important** to take into account are the following considerations for **Rishi** when deciding how to respond to the situation?*

56. The potential patient safety issue
    a. Very important
    b. Important
    c. Of minor importance
    d. Not important at all

57. Dr Johnson has to mark his project
    a. Very important
    b. Important
    c. Of minor importance
    d. Not important at all

58. Dr Johnson is committing research fraud
    a. Very important
    b. Important
    c. Of minor importance
    d. Not important at all

59. Dr Johnson's action may undermine trust in the medical profession
    a. Very important
    b. Important
    c. Of minor importance
    d. Not important at all

Question Set 14

Dr Connell is a GP partner working in an Edinburgh GP Practice. One of his long-term patients is a young woman called Melania. Whilst she recovered, she was left in chronic pain. Dr Connell has helped Melania to recover and manage her chronic pain. As a sign of appreciation, Melania buys Dr Connell a few bottles of wine as a Christmas present. Dr Connell is unsure whether he should accept this gift.

*How **important** is it to take into account are the following considerations for **Dr Connell** when deciding how to respond to the situation?*

60. How refusing the gift would affect his relationship with Melania
    a. Very important
    b. Important
    c. Of minor importance
    d. Not important at all

61. Dr Connell is a wine enthusiast
    a. Very important
    b. Important
    c. Of minor importance
    d. Not important at all

62. The monetary value of the wine
    a. Very important
    b. Important
    c. Of minor importance
    d. Not important at all

63. That Dr Connell prescribes strong painkillers to Melania
    a. Very important
    b. Important
    c. Of minor importance
    d. Not important at all

64. What was said during the previous consultation
    a. Very important
    b. Important
    c. Of minor importance
    d. Not important at all

Question Set 15

Jane is an ST4 surgical registrar working in a general surgery department. Whilst she is operating on a 42-year-old man called Nick, she makes a mistake which leads to Nick losing blood and requiring a blood transfusion and a longer hospital stay. Jane feels bad about the mistake but is unsure how to tell Nick about the mistake.
How appropriate are each of the following responses by Jane in this situation?

65. Do not tell Nick about the mistake
    a. A very appropriate thing to do
    b. Appropriate, but not ideal
    c. Inappropriate but not awful
    d. A very inappropriate thing to do

66. Apologise for the complications but do not admit any mistake
    a. A very appropriate thing to do
    b. Appropriate, but not ideal
    c. Inappropriate but not awful
    d. A very inappropriate thing to do

Question 67

Sarah is a GP trainee working within a large GP Practice. The first patient in the clinic is an 18-year-old called Fraser who has recently been diagnosed with epilepsy. Sarah informs Fraser that he will have to stop driving for now. At their next consultation, Fraser tells Sarah that he is still driving.

Choose both the **one most appropriate** action and the **one least appropriate** action that **Sarah** should take in response to this situation.

You will not receive any marks for this question unless you select both the most and least appropriate actions.
- Most Appropriate
- Least Appropriate

    a. Report Fraser to the DVLA, which could get his licence revoked.
    b. Do nothing
    c. Talk to Fraser and explain how he must stop driving

Question 68

Brenda is a third-year medical student who is partaking in a medical school performance. When reading the script, she notices a joke about international medical graduates working in the NHS in her lines and is worried that the joke is offensive.

You will not receive any marks for this question unless you select both the most and least appropriate actions.

- Most Appropriate
- Least Appropriate

a. Do nothing
b. Talk to the director of the performance
c. Not say the joke during the performance

Question 69

Colin is a 2nd year medical student attending a lecture on diet and obesity. During the lecture, the lecturer makes comments about the weight of another student called Ruth. Ruth looks visibly upset by the remarks.

You will not receive any marks for this question unless you select both the most and least appropriate actions.

- Most Appropriate
- Least Appropriate

a. Do nothing
b. Talk to the lecturer after the lecture and explain his concerns
c. Report the lecturer to their supervisor

Answers: Situational Judgement Mock 2

Question 1: D

Very Inappropriate – if there is inadequate staffing, this may jeopardise patient safety and therefore, you **must** act on your concerns. This is outlined in Good Medical Practice which states "You must take prompt action if you think that patient safety, dignity or comfort is or may be seriously compromised. If patients are at risk because of inadequate premises, equipment or other resources, policies or systems, you should put the matter right if that is possible. You must raise your concern in line with our guidance and your workplace policy. You should also make a record of the steps you have taken" (Good Medical Practice, p11). Therefore, by doing nothing, Dr Hopson would be violating Good Medical Practice, so this action is **very inappropriate**.

Top Tip: Remember, you are not ranking options, multiple options can be very appropriate or very inappropriate.

Question 2: A

Very Appropriate – if there is inadequate staffing, this may jeopardise patient safety and therefore, you **must** act on your concerns. This is outlined in Good Medical Practice which states "You must take prompt action if you think that patient safety, dignity or comfort is or may be seriously compromised. If patients are at risk because of inadequate premises, equipment or other resources, policies or systems, you should put the matter right if that is possible. You must raise your concern in line with our guidance and your workplace policy. You should also make a record of the steps you have taken" (Good Medical Practice, p11). Therefore, by raising her concerns with a senior colleague, Dr Hopson would be complying with Good Medical Practice, so this action is **very appropriate**.

Question 3: C

Inappropriate but not awful – if there is inadequate staffing, this may jeopardise patient safety and therefore, you **must** act on your concerns. This is outlined in Good Medical Practice which states "You must take prompt action if you think that patient safety, dignity or comfort is or may be seriously compromised. If patients are at risk because of inadequate premises, equipment or other resources, policies or systems, you should put the matter right if that is possible. You must raise your concern in line with our guidance and your workplace policy. You should also make a record of the steps you have taken" (Good Medical Practice, p11). This action would allow Dr Hopson to act on her concerns however, it is inappropriate as it unnecessarily escalates the situation without utilising internal hospital procedures. Generally, it is inappropriate to unnecessarily escalate concerns. However, due to the significant patient safety issues, this action is **not** very inappropriate. Therefore, this action is **inappropriate but not awful**.

Question 4: A

Very Appropriate – it will always be appropriate to **seek advice from a senior colleague** or mentor if you have concerns about patient safety. This is outlined in GMC guidance which states "If you're not sure whether you should raise a concern formally, you should ask your medical school or an experienced healthcare professional for advice" (Achieving Good Medical Practice: Guidance for Medical Students, p22). Therefore, this action is **very appropriate**.

Question 5: A

Very Appropriate – if there is inadequate staffing, this may jeopardise patient safety and therefore, you **must** act on your concerns. This is outlined in Good Medical Practice which states "You must take prompt action if you think that patient safety, dignity or comfort is or may be seriously compromised. If patients are at risk because of inadequate premises, equipment or other resources, policies or systems, you should put the matter right if that is possible. You must raise your concern in line with our guidance and your workplace policy. You should also make a record of the steps you have taken" (Good Medical Practice, p11). Therefore, by raising her concerns through the hospital's reporting procedures, Dr Hopson would be complying with Good Medical Practice, so this action is **very appropriate**.

Question 6: D

Very Inappropriate – by speaking to the media, Dr Hopson is unlikely to rectify the potential patient safety issue as she does not use official channels to raise her concerns and therefore violates Good Medical Practice which states "You must take prompt action if you think that patient safety, dignity or comfort is or may be seriously compromised. If patients are at risk because of inadequate premises, equipment or other resources, policies or systems, you should put the matter right if that is possible. You must raise your concern in line with our guidance and your workplace policy. You should also make a record of the steps you have taken" (Good Medical Practice, p11). Furthermore, there is no evidence as yet that the unit is not compliant with NICE guidelines. Therefore, this action is **very inappropriate**.

Question Set 2

Question 7: D

Very inappropriate – it is your professional responsibility to inform your medical school or the GMC if you are charged with or convicted of a crime. This is outlined in Good Medical Practice which states "You must tell us without delay if, anywhere in the world: you have been charged with or found guilty of a criminal offence" (Good Medical Practice, p23). Therefore, if Jack was to wait until he was found guilty, this would violate Good Medical Practice and therefore, this action would be **very inappropriate**.

Question 8: D

Very inappropriate – it is your professional responsibility to inform your medical school or the GMC if you are charged with or convicted of a crime. This is outlined in Good Medical Practice which states "You must tell us without delay if, anywhere in the world: you have been charged with or found guilty of a criminal offence" (Good Medical Practice, p23). Therefore by failing to inform the medical school Jack is violating Good Medical Practice. Therefore, this action would be **very inappropriate**.

Question 9: A

Very appropriate – seeking advice from your advisor would enable you to get advice and ensure you were supported in any investigation. This is outlined in GMC guidelines which state "If you have any questions about what you should declare to the GMC or to your medical school, you can get advice from your medical school, a medical defence organisation or the British Medical Association (BMA)" (Achieving Good Medical Practice: Guidance for Medical Students, p46). Therefore this action would be **very appropriate**.

Question 10: C

Inappropriate but not awful – it is your professional responsibility to inform your medical school or the GMC if you are charged with or convicted of a crime. This is outlined in Good Medical Practice which states "You must tell us without delay if, anywhere in the world: you have been charged with or found guilty of a criminal offence" (Good Medical Practice, p23). Therefore, by waiting to inform the medical school, Jack is not informing them 'without delay', so this action violates Good Medical Practice. However, as Jack is still informing the medical school, this action is **not** very inappropriate. Therefore, this action is **inappropriate but not awful**.

Question Set 3

Question 11: C

Inappropriate but not awful – this action would allow Dr Bercow to address the patient safety issue as the dose would be checked. This complies with Good Medical Practice which states "[you must] Take prompt action if you think that patient safety, dignity or comfort is being compromised" (Good Medical Practice, p11). Therefore, this action would **not be** very inappropriate. However, by telling the nurse not to question a doctor, Dr Bercow is creating an environment where it is difficult to raise concerns which violates Good Medical Practice which states "You must promote and encourage a culture that allows all staff to raise concerns openly and safely" (Good Medical Practice, p11). Therefore, this action would be **inappropriate but not awful.**

Top Tip: All members of the healthcare team have their own specific by equally important role. Therefore, regardless of their profession, their concerns must always be listened to.

Question 12: D

Very inappropriate – medical students **are not** allowed to write prescriptions, only doctors can prescribe medications. Therefore, by allowing a medical student to change the prescription, Dr Bercow would be breaking the law and therefore, this action would be **very inappropriate**.

Question 13: A

Very appropriate – this action would allow Dr Bercow to protect patient safety as it ensures the correct dose of the drug is given and would therefore comply with Good Medical Practice which states "[you must] Take prompt action if you think that patient safety, dignity or comfort is being compromised" (Good Medical Practice, p11). Furthermore, by acting on the concerns of the nurse, Dr Bercow is promoting an open environment which is consistent with Good Medical Practice which states "You must promote and encourage a culture that allows all staff to raise concerns openly and safely" (Good Medical Practice, p11). Therefore, this action would be **very appropriate.**

Question 14: D

Very inappropriate – If any colleague, regardless of their profession, raises a concern about a patient or a course treatment you **must** consider that concern. Dr Bercow does not necessarily have to agree with the nurse's concern however, in the interests of her patient, Dr Bercow must consider it. This is outlined in Good Medical Practice which states "You **must** work collaboratively with colleagues, respecting their skills and contributions" (Good Medical Practice, p14). Furthermore, this action would create a culture where concerns are not raised openly which violates Good Medical Practice which states "You must promote and encourage a culture that allows all staff to raise concerns openly and safely" (Good Medical Practice, p11). This action does not address the patient safety issue and would be extremely disrespectful to his colleague therefore, this action would be **very inappropriate**.

Question 15: D

Very inappropriate – by doing nothing, Dr Bercow would be jeopardising patient safety as it could allow an incorrect dose to be given. This would violate Good Medical Practice which states "[you must] Take prompt action if you think that patient safety, dignity or comfort is being compromised" (Good Medical Practice, p11). Therefore, this action would be **very inappropriate**.

Question Set 4

Question 16: A

Very Appropriate– this action would allow Dr Harding to seek advice from a more experienced colleague which protects patient safety. This is in line with Good Medical Practice which states "In providing clinical care you must: consult colleagues where appropriate" (Good Medical Practice, p8). The reason this action is very appropriate because Dr Harding is proactively attempting to improve her clinical skills. Therefore this action is **very appropriate**.

Top Tip: Whilst patient safety is always the primary consideration, when attempting these questions you must also consider secondary considerations e.g. professional development.

Question 17: C

Inappropriate but not awful – this action would protect patient safety as Dr Harding is not performing the procedure which is consistent with Good Medical Practice which states "[you must] Take prompt action if you think that patient safety, dignity or comfort is being compromised" (Good Medical Practice, p11). Therefore, this action is **not** very inappropriate. However, by **not** performing the procedure, Dr Harding is potentially leaving the patient in pain and therefore this action is not Therefore, this action is **inappropriate but not awful**.

Question 18: D

Very inappropriate – by performing the procedure when she does not feel competent doing so, Dr Harding is jeopardising patient safety. This violates Good Medical Practice which states "You must recognise and work within the limits of your competence." (Good Medical Practice, p7) and "Patients need good doctors. Good doctors make the care of their patients their first concern: they are competent, keep their knowledge and skills up to date" (Good Medical Practice, p4). Therefore, this action is **very inappropriate**.

Question 19: C

Inappropriate but not awful – this action would allow Dr Harding to protect patient safety by allowing a competent individual to perform the procedure. The reason this action is **not** appropriate is because Dr Harding is not attempting to improve his clinical skills. This violates Good Medical Practice which states "You must regularly take part in activities that maintain and develop your competence and performance" (Good Medical Practice, p6). Therefore, this action is **inappropriate but not awful**.

Question Set 5

Question 20: D

Very Inappropriate – this action would be confrontational and disrespectful to Mr Pain. This violates Good Medical Practice which states "You must treat colleagues fairly and with respect" (Good Medical Practice, p14). Therefore, this action would be **very inappropriate**.

Top Tip: You should always try and address any concerns with the individual first before escalating your concerns.

Question 21: D

Very Inappropriate – if a surgeon is under the influence the alcohol, they could be jeopardising patient safety. Remember, your primary concern **must always** be the **patient's safety** as outlined in Good Medical Practice which states "[you must] Take prompt action if you think that patient safety, dignity or comfort is being compromised" (Good Medical Practice, p11). Therefore, by doing nothing Zubin would be knowingly jeopardising patient safety so, this action would be **very inappropriate**.

Question 22: B

Appropriate, but not ideal – by taking this action, Zubin would be protecting patient safety and therefore complying with his responsibility to protect patients. This is in line with Good Medical Practice which states "[you must] Take prompt action if you think that patient safety, dignity or comfort is being compromised" (Good Medical Practice, p11). However, Zubin is involving another member of staff before talking to the surgeon and therefore is potentially distributing sensitive information about the surgeon. Generally, you should always try and address the issue with the person concerned before escalating your concerns. Therefore, this action would be **appropriate but not ideal**.

Question 23: A

Very appropriate – by taking this action, Zubin would be protecting patient safety and so is complying with his responsibility to protect patients. This is in line with Good Medical Practice which states "[you must] Take prompt action if you think that patient safety, dignity or comfort is being compromised" (Good Medical Practice, p11). Zubin is also being sensitive regarding the surgeon's drinking, this will allow him to ascertain whether the surgeon may require help which is in line with Good Medical Practice which states "You must treat colleagues fairly and with respect" (Good Medical Practice, p14). Therefore, this action would be **very appropriate**.

Question Set 6

Question 24: D

Inappropriate – this action would involve lying to the mother by telling her it is a common side effect. This violates Good Medical Practice which states "You must be open and honest with patients if things go wrong. If a patient under your care has suffered harm or distress, you should: a) put matters right (if that is possible) b) offer an apology c) explain fully and promptly what has happened and the likely short-term and long-term effects" (Good Medical Practice, p18). Therefore, this action is **inappropriate**.

Top Tip: Remember, actions are not taken in isolation. Multiple actions can be appropriate.

Question 25: D

Inappropriate – the duty of candour is a key principle in medical ethics. The duty of candour requires doctors to inform patients if they have made a mistake. This duty is outlined in Good Medical Practice which states "You must be open and honest with patients if things go wrong. If a patient under your care has suffered harm or distress, you should: a) put matters right (if that is possible) b) offer an apology c) explain fully and promptly what has happened and the likely short-term and long-term effects" (Good Medical Practice, p18). The key term in the guidance is "**you**", as Kim has made the mistake, she should make every effort to explain the mistake herself. Furthermore, it is usually inappropriate to delegate these difficult conversations to more junior colleagues without direct supervision. Therefore, this action is **inappropriate**.

Question 26: A

Appropriate – by informing the patient about the mistake and offering an apology, Kim is complying with the duty of candour. This is outlined in Good Medical Practice which states "You must be open and honest with patients if things go wrong. If a patient under your care has suffered harm or distress, you should: a) put matters right (if that is possible) b) offer an apology c) explain fully and promptly what has happened and the likely short-term and long-term effects" (Good Medical Practice, p18). Therefore, this action is **appropriate**.

Question 27: A

Appropriate – by seeking advice from her clinical supervisor Kim is trying to learn from her mistakes and improve her clinical practice. This is outlined in Good Medical Practice which states "You must keep your professional knowledge and skills up to date. You must regularly take part in activities that maintain and develop your competence and performance" (Good Medical Practice, p6). Therefore, this action is **appropriate**.

Question 28: A

Appropriate – if any mistakes are made or you notice any clinical incidents you should report them through the appropriate procedures for your hospital. This is outlined in Good Medical Practice which states "To help keep patients safe you must: contribute to adverse event recognition". Therefore, by reporting the incident you are complying with Good Medical Practice, so this action is **appropriate**.

Question Set 7

Question 29: D

Inappropriate – this action would address the issue of Michael's punctuality by reminding him to turn up to the meetings on time. However, this is not addressing any underlying issues Michael may be facing which is disrespectful to him. This violates Good Medical Practice which states "You must treat colleagues fairly and with respect" (Good Medical Practice, p14). Therefore, this action is **inappropriate**.

Top Tip: In these types of questions, Appropriate means you should take the action whereas Inappropriate means you should not take the action.

Question 30: D

Inappropriate – this action would be overly aggressive and disrespectful to Michael. This violates Good Medical Practice which states "You must treat colleagues fairly and with respect" (Good Medical Practice, p14). Therefore, this action is **inappropriate**.

Question 31: A

Appropriate – this would be the ideal course of action as it allows Alfie to address the issue of Michael's lack of punctuality whilst still being respectful to him. This is in line with GMC guidance which states "Persistent inappropriate attitude or behaviour [for a medical student includes] poor time management [and] non-attendance]" (Achieving Good Medical Practice: Guidance for Medical Students, p48) and "You must treat colleagues fairly and with respect" (Good Medical Practice, p14). Therefore, this action would be **appropriate**.

Question 32: D

Inappropriate – by taking no action, Alfie is not addressing the issue of Michael's lack of punctuality. This violates GMC guidance which states "It can be difficult to raise concerns about fellow students, who may be people you work with on projects or placements or your friends.

But as a student choosing to join a regulated profession, it is your duty to put patients first and this includes patients you see on placements and those treated by your fellow students in the future." (Achieving Good Medical Practice: Guidance for Medical Students, p21). Therefore, this action would be **inappropriate**.

Question 33: D

Inappropriate – by reporting Michael to their tutor before trying to address the issue, Alfie is unnecessarily escalating the situation. Remember, you should always try and address the issue with the individual concerned before escalating it further. Therefore, this action would be **inappropriate**.

Question Set 8

Question 34: D

Not Important – no factors about the patient other than their clinical need should ever affect the treatment you give to them. This is outlined in Good Medical Practice which states "You must not unfairly discriminate against patients or colleagues by allowing your personal views to affect your professional relationships or the treatment you provide or arrange " (Good Medical Practice, p20). Furthermore, all doctors are required by the GMC to be covered by indemnity or insurance as stated in Good Medical Practice: "You must make sure you have adequate insurance or indemnity cover so that your patients will not be disadvantaged if they make a claim about the clinical care you have provided in the UK." (Good Medical Practice, p20). Therefore, this factor **should not** be considered.

*Top Tip: In these types of questions, Important means you **should** consider the factor whereas Not Important means you **should not** consider the factor.*

Question 35: B

Important – Jeremy's level of competence is an important consideration, as you **MUST** never treat a patient outside your competence. This is outlined in Good Medical Practice which states "You **must** recognise and work within the limits of your competence." (Good Medical Practice, p7). Therefore this factor must be considered.

Question 36: D

Not Important – regardless of whether there are any other medical professionals on the train, Jeremy still has an obligation to offer assistance as outlined in Good Medical Practice which states "You must offer help if emergencies arise in clinical settings or in the community, taking account of your own safety, your competence and the availability of other options for care" (Good Medical Practice, p11). Therefore, this factor **should not** be considered.

Question 37: B

Important – Jeremy's capacity to provide medical treatment may be impaired if he has had insufficient sleep. His sleep deprivation may cause his competence to be reduced and so he **should** consider this factor.

Question Set 9

Question 38: B

Important – the age of the patients may affect how many extra years of life a treatment can provide to the patients and therefore this **should usually** be considered. The reason this factor is **not** a very important consideration is because age does not directly correlate to the number of extra years of life provided by a treatment. Therefore, this factor **should** be considered.

Top Tip: Any discrimination will **always** *be inappropriate unless the factor is clinically relevant.*

Question 39: D

Not important at all – doctors **must never** discriminate based a patient's lifestyle as this violates Good Medical Practice which states "You must not unfairly discriminate against patients or colleagues by allowing your personal views [This includes your views about a patient's or colleague's lifestyle, culture or their social or economic status, as well as the characteristics protected by legislation: age, disability, gender reassignment, race, marriage and civil partnership, pregnancy and maternity, religion or belief, sex and sexual orientation] to affect your professional relationships or the treatment you provide or arrange" (Good Medical Practice, p20). Therefore, this factor **must not** be considered.

Question 40: A

Very Important – the principle of justice is one of the four core pillars of medical ethics. Justice is the principle of ensuring doctor's actions are lawful, respect patient's rights and are fair. Part of this principle of fairness is ensuring that resources in a healthcare system are distributed effectively to ensure the most benefit can be derived by the population. Therefore, Ali must consider how many patients will benefit from each treatment, so he can comply with the principle of Justice. Therefore, this factor **must** be considered.

Question 41: A

Very Important – part of the pillar of Justice is that doctors must comply with the law. This principle is also outlined in Good Medical Practice which states "Patients need good doctors. Good doctors... act with integrity and within the law" (Good Medical Practice, p4). Therefore, Ali **must** consider his legal obligations and so this factor **must** be considered.

Question 42: D

Not Important at all – the proportion of ethnic minorities affected by the treatments **must not** be considered as it is not clinically relevant and would likely be discriminatory. If Ali considered this factor, he would be acting in a discriminatory way which violates Good Medical Practice which states "You must not unfairly discriminate against patients or colleagues by allowing your personal views [This includes your views about a patient's or colleague's lifestyle, culture or their social or economic status, as well as the characteristics protected by legislation: age, disability, gender reassignment, race, marriage and civil partnership, pregnancy and maternity, religion or belief, sex and sexual orientation] to affect your professional relationships or the treatment you provide or arrange" (Good Medical Practice, p20). Therefore, this factor **must not** be considered.

Question Set 10

Question 43: A

Very Important – Confidentiality is a key principle of medical ethics, this principle is also found in Good Medical Practice which states "You must treat information about patients as confidential. This includes after a patient has died." (Good Medical Practice, p17). The reason confidentiality is important is because it forms the basis of the trust required for the doctor-patient relationship, this is outlined in GMC guidelines which states "Trust is an essential part of the doctor-patient relationship and confidentiality is central to this. Patients may avoid seeking medical help, or may under-report symptoms, if they think their personal information will be disclosed by doctors without consent, or without the chance to have some control over the timing or amount of information shared." (GMC Confidentiality Guidelines, p10). Therefore, this consideration is **very important**.

Top Tip: There should be a strong presumption against breaking confidentiality, confidentiality should only ever be broken if it can be justified.

Question 44: A

Very Important – whilst confidentiality is a very important consideration, doctors also have an obligation to disclose information where someone else may be at risk. This is outlined in GMC guidelines which states "But there can be a public interest in disclosing information to protect individuals or society from risks of serious harm, such as from serious communicable diseases or serious crime… Other examples of situations in which failure to disclose information may expose others to a risk of death or serious harm include when a patient is not fit to drive, or has been diagnosed with a serious communicable disease, or poses a serious risk to others through being unfit for work." (GMC Confidentiality Guidelines, p10). Therefore, this consideration is **very important**.

Question 45: D

Not Important at All – the patient's student status is irrelevant to the situation. You must never discriminate against patients based on any characteristics other than clinical factors. This is outlined in Good Medical Practice which states "You must not deny treatment to patients because their medical condition may put you at risk. If a patient poses a risk to your health or safety, you should take all available steps to minimise the risk before providing treatment or making other suitable alternative arrangements for providing treatment" (Good Medical Practice, p19). Therefore, this factor is **not important at all**.

Question 46: C

Of minor Importance – the method of transmission for the patient's infection should not affect your treatment of the patient unless clinically relevant. This is outlined in Good Medical Practice which states "You must not deny treatment to patients because their medical condition may put you at risk. If a patient poses a risk to your health or safety, you should take all available steps to minimise the risk before providing treatment or making other suitable alternative arrangements for providing treatment" (Good Medical Practice, p19). Therefore, this factor **is not** However, the reason this factor is **not** not important at all is because the transmission risk may affect whether any contacts need to be notified. Therefore, this factor **could** be considered so, this factor is of **minor importance**.

Question 47: B

Important – **Mary's age** will usually be irrelevant to the situation as you must never discriminate against patients based on any characteristics other than clinical factors. This is outlined in Good Medical Practice which states "You must not deny treatment to patients because their medical condition may put you at risk. If a patient poses a risk to your health or safety, you should take all available steps to minimise the risk before providing treatment or making other suitable alternative arrangements for providing treatment" (Good Medical Practice, p19).

However, if Mary is underage, this could pose a safeguarding issue and therefore, **in some cases Mary's age would** warrant Therefore, this factor is **important**.

Question Set 11

Tim is a 15-year-old boy. He has been involved in a car accident and suffered significant injuries. He has been informed that he will require surgery to save his life. However, Tim has recently joined several online forums and now believes modern medicine is a scam. Timmy tells the surgeon, Ms Smith, that he does not want the surgery, but Ms Smith knows the surgery is in Tim's best interests.

*How **important** is it to take into account are the following considerations for **Ms Smith** when deciding how to respond to the situation?*

Question 48: A

Very important – the age of the patient will always be a **very important** consideration when considering consent. A 15-year-old can consent to treatment if they have capacity, this is outlined in GMC guidance which states "a young person under 16 may have the capacity to consent, depending on their maturity and ability to understand what is involved." (0–18 years: guidance for all doctors, p12). The age of the patient has a significant impact on the patient's maturity and ability to consent and so **must** be considered.

Top Tip: The rules around consent in under 18s are complex, you are not expected to understand all the legal nuance. You should just attempt to apply the principles of medical ethics and the principles laid out in Good Medical Practice to determine your answers.

Question 49: A

Very important – your primary concern must be your patient's best interest. Therefore, if Tim may die as a result of not getting treatment, Ms Smith must consider this factor. This is outlined in Good Medical Practice which states "They treat each patient as an individual. They do their best to make sure all patients receive good care and treatment that will support them to live as well as possible, whatever their illness or disability." (Good Medical Practice, p4). Therefore, this factor **must** be considered.

Question 50: B

Important – you **must** always consider a patient's beliefs and respect them when providing clinical case as outlined in Good Medical Practice which states "You must treat patients fairly and with respect whatever their life choices and beliefs" (Good Medical Practice, p16). However, considering his age, there is a possibility that he does not have the competence to make an informed decision.

Question 51: B

Important – the risks of any medical intervention must be considered before it is performed. However, the reason this factor is **not** very important is because, Tim will die without the surgery and Ms Smith knows the surgery is in Tim's best interest. Therefore, this factor **should** be considered.

Question Set 12

Question 52: A

Very Important – you **must** always consider a patient's wishes and respect their right to autonomy. Autonomy is the right of a patient to control their own medical decisions. This principle is also outlined in Good Medical Practice which states "Respect patients' right to reach decisions with you about their treatment and care." (Good Medical Practice, p1). Therefore, this factor **must** be considered.

*Top Tip: Doctors are allowed to have a conscientious objection to a specific procedure however, they **must** ensure this does not affect the patient's care.*

Question 53: D

Not Important at all – Theresa's age is irrelevant and therefore should not be considered as this would violate Good Medical Practice which states "You must not unfairly discriminate against patients or colleagues by allowing your personal views [This includes your views about a patient's or colleague's lifestyle, culture or their social or economic status, as well as the characteristics protected by legislation: age, disability, gender reassignment, race, marriage and civil partnership, pregnancy and maternity, religion or belief, sex and sexual orientation] to affect your professional relationships or the treatment you provide or arrange" (Good Medical Practice, p20). Therefore, this factor **must not** be considered.

Question 54: B

Important – If you have a conscientious objection to a procedure (for example abortion), you must ensure that the patient understands you are making no judgement on them. This is outlined in Good Medical Practice which states "You must explain to patients if you have a conscientious objection to a particular procedure. You must tell them about their right to see another doctor and make sure they have enough information to exercise that right. In providing this information you must not imply or express disapproval of the patient's lifestyle, choices or beliefs. If it is not practical for a patient to arrange to see another doctor, you must make sure that arrangements are made for another suitably qualified colleague to take over your role" (Good Medical Practice, p17).

Therefore, Dr Neil **should** consider this factor as he must refer the patient to a colleague. However, the reason this factor is **not** very important is because it should not affect Theresa's clinical care. Therefore, this factor **should be** considered.

Question 55: A

Very Important – if you have a conscientious objection to a procedure, you **must** make sure the patient has access to another suitably qualified doctor. This is outlined in Good Medical Practice which states "You must explain to patients if you have a conscientious objection to a particular procedure. You must tell them about their right to see another doctor and make sure they have enough information to exercise that right. In providing this information you must not imply or express disapproval of the patient's lifestyle, choices or beliefs. If it is not practical for a patient to arrange to see another doctor, you must make sure that arrangements are made for another suitably qualified colleague to take over your role" (Good Medical Practice, p17). Therefore, this factor **should** be considered.

Question Set 13

Question 56: A

Very Important – if Dr Johnson is publishing false research about experimental drugs, it could cause patients to receive unsafe drugs which would jeopardise patient safety. Therefore Rishi **must act** in line with Good Medical Practice which states "[you must] Take prompt action if you think that patient safety, dignity or comfort is being compromised" (Good Medical Practice, p11). Therefore, this consideration is **very important**.

Top Tip: Regardless of the personal consequences to your career or grades, you must act if you have concerns about patient safety.

Question 57: D

Not important at all – your primary concern must always be patient safety. This is outlined in Good Medical Practice which states "[you must] Take prompt action if you think that patient safety, dignity or comfort is being compromised" (Good Medical Practice, p11). Therefore, regardless of whether Dr Johnson is marking his SSC, Rishi has a responsibility to protect patient safety and so **must** take action. Therefore this consideration is **not important at all**.

Question 58: A

Very Important – part of the pillar of Justice is that doctors must comply with the law. This is principle is also outlined in Good Medical Practice which states "Patients need good doctors. Good doctors... act with integrity and within the law." (Good Medical Practice, p4). Dr Johnson is breaking the law by committing fraud therefore, Rishi **must** raise his concerns. Therefore, this consideration is **very important**.

Question 59: A

Very Important – maintaining public trust is a key principle in Good Medical Practice which states "Never abuse your patients' trust in you or the public's trust in the profession." (Good Medical Practice, p1). Therefore, if public trust is being undermined Rishi **must** consider this factor. Therefore, this consideration is **very important**.

Question Set 14

Question 60: A

Very Important – a doctor's decision to accept a gift from a patient depends on several factors. Doctors have a responsibility to maintain a good doctor-patient relationship with all their patients. This principle is outlined in Good Medical Practice which states "Patients need good doctors. Good doctors make the care of their patients their first concern... [they] establish and maintain good relationships with patients" (Good Medical Practice, p4). Therefore, Dr Connell must consider how his decision will affect his relationship with Melania, so this consideration is **very important**.

Top Tip: Remember, you are not ranking factors by importance. Multiple factors can be important or very important.

Question 61: D

Not Important at All – regardless of Dr Connell's wine taste, this should not influence his decision. Dr Connell's decision **must** only be based on how the gift affects his care for Melania. Therefore, this consideration is **not important at all**.

Question 62: A

Very Important – a doctor's decision to accept a gift from a patient depends on several factors. The value of a gift **must** influence a decision regarding whether to accept it for example, it would usually be appropriate to accept a cake but inappropriate to accept an expensive watch because you **must not** accept any gift which would affect your decision making.

A more valuable gift is more likely to influence your clinical decisions or give the appearance of influencing your clinical decisions. This principle is outlined in Good Medical Practice which states "You must not ask for or accept – from patients, colleagues or others – any inducement, gift or hospitality that may affect or be seen to affect the way you prescribe for, treat or refer patients or commission services for patients. You must not offer these inducements" (Good Medical Practice, p24). Therefore, Dr Connell **must** consider the value of the wine, so this consideration is **very important.**

Question 63: B

Important – a doctor's decision to accept a gift from a patient depends on several factors. The fact Dr Connell prescribes strong painkillers (which are controlled drugs) **should** affect whether Dr Connell's accepts the gift from Melania. If Dr Connell accepts the gift it could be or could be seen as an inducement which would violate Good Medical Practice which states "You must not ask for or accept – from patients, colleagues or others – any inducement, gift or hospitality that may affect or be seen to affect the way you prescribe for, treat or refer patients or commission services for patients. You must not offer these inducements" (Good Medical Practice, p24). The reason, this consideration is **not** very important is because this factor will **not always** warrant consideration, it will **only** be important in some specific circumstances. Therefore, Dr Connell **should** consider this factor so, this consideration is **important.**

Question 64: B

Important – a doctor's decision to accept a gift from a patient depends on several factors. The contents of the consultation may affect Dr Connell's decision on whether to accept the gift. For example, if Melania had just requested additional controlled drugs e.g. strong pain killers the gift could be or could be seen as an inducement which would violate Good Medical Practice which states "You must not ask for or accept – from patients, colleagues or others – any inducement, gift or hospitality that may affect or be seen to affect the way you prescribe for, treat or refer patients or commission services for patients. You must not offer these inducements" (Good Medical Practice, p24). The reason, this consideration is **not** very important is because the contents of the consultation will **not always** be important, it will **only** be important in some specific circumstances. Therefore, Dr Connell **should** consider this factor. So this consideration is **important.**

Question Set 15

Question 65: D

The duty of candour is a key principle in medical ethics. The duty of candour requires doctors to inform patients if they have made a mistake. This is outlined in Good Medical Practice which states "You must be open and honest with patients if things go wrong. If a patient under your care has suffered harm or distress, you should: a) put matters right (if that is possible) b) offer an apology c) explain fully and promptly what has happened and the likely short-term and long-term effects" (Good Medical Practice, p18). Therefore, by failing to inform the patient about the mistake Jane is violating Good Medical Practice, so this action is very inappropriate.

Top Tip: The duty of candour is a key ethical principle. If you ever make a mistake, you must be honest and open about it, to lie or cover up mistakes is always very inappropriate.

Question 66: C

By failing to admit a mistake, you are not complying with the duty of candour. This is outlined in Good Medical Practice which states "You must be open and honest with patients if things go wrong. If a patient under your care has suffered harm or distress, you should: a) put matters right (if that is possible) b) offer an apology c) explain fully and promptly what has happened and the likely short-term and long-term effects" (Good Medical Practice, p18). However, you are offering an apology which is consistent with Good Medical Practice. Therefore, as you are only partially abiding by the principles of Good Medical Practice, this action is inappropriate but not awful.

Question 67

Most appropriate = C, Least appropriate = B

Option 1 is **neither** the most appropriate **nor** the least appropriate option. Doctors have an obligation to maintain confidentiality except in a few specific circumstances. One exception is when public safety is at risk for example, if someone is driving while medically unfit. This exception to confidentiality is outlined in the GMC guidelines which states "There are also important uses of patient information for purposes other than direct care... Other uses are not directly related to the provision of healthcare but serve wider public interests, such as disclosures for public protection reasons" (GMC Confidentiality Guidelines, p10). However, this option is **not** the most appropriate because it escalates the situation without first having another conversation with Fraser. Therefore, option 1 is **neither** the most appropriate **nor** the least appropriate option.

Option 2 is the least appropriate option. By doing nothing, Sarah is knowingly putting the public at risk but failing to comply with her obligation to make disclosures in the public interest. This is outlined in GMC guidelines which states "There are also important uses of patient information for purposes other than direct care… Other uses are not directly related to the provision of healthcare but serve wider public interests, such as disclosures for public protection reasons" (GMC Confidentiality Guidelines, p10). Therefore, option 2 is the **least** appropriate option.

Option 3 is the most appropriate option. By talking to Fraser before escalating her concerns, Sarah is complying with her obligation to make disclosures in the public interest without escalating her concerns inappropriately. Therefore, option 3 is the **most** appropriate option.

Top Tip: Remember, you should always try and address the issue directly with the patient before breaking confidentiality.

Question 68

Most Appropriate – Talk to the director of the performance

Least Appropriate – Do nothing

Option 2 is the most appropriate option. Brenda has a responsibility to be respectful to her fellow students as outlined in GMC Guidance which states "You must treat all peers and colleagues fairly and with respect" (Achieving Good Medical Practice: Guidance for Medical Students, p31). Therefore, by directly talking to the director, Brenda can rectify the situation. Therefore, option 2 is the **most appropriate** option.

Option 3 is neither the most nor least appropriate option. This action would comply with Brenda's responsibility to be respectful to her fellow students as outlined in GMC Guidance which states "You must treat all peers and colleagues fairly and with respect" (Achieving Good Medical Practice: Guidance for Medical Students, p31). However, as this factor does **not** directly address the issue with the director, it is not the most appropriate option. Therefore, option 3 is **neither** the most **nor** least appropriate option.

Option 1 is the least appropriate option. Brenda has a responsibility to be respectful to her fellow students as outlined in GMC Guidance which states "You must treat all peers and colleagues fairly and with respect" (Achieving Good Medical Practice: Guidance for Medical Students, p31). Therefore, by doing nothing and allowing an inappropriate joke to be said during the performance, Brenda is being disrespectful. Therefore, option 1 is the **least appropriate** option.

Top Tip: It is always more appropriate to address your concerns directly with the person responsible before taking any other action.

Question 69

Most Appropriate – Talk to the lecturer after the lecture and explain his concerns

Least Appropriate – Do nothing

Option 1 is the most appropriate option. The lecturer has a responsibility to be respectful to their students as outlined in GMC Guidance which states "You must treat all peers and colleagues fairly and with respect" (Achieving Good Medical Practice: Guidance for Medical Students, p31). Therefore, by directly raising his concerns with the lecturer, Colin is upholding the GMC guidelines. Therefore, option 1 is the **most appropriate** option.

Option 3 is neither the most nor least appropriate option. This option unnecessarily escalates Colin's concerns before addressing them with the lecturer first. However, as this is still taking action, it is **not** the least appropriate option. Therefore, option 3 is **neither** the most **nor** least appropriate option.

Option 2 is the least appropriate option. This action would not address Colin's concerns and therefore is **inappropriate**. Therefore, option 2 is the **least appropriate** option.

Top Tip: If you have concerns about a colleague or fellow student, you must act.

45255046R00275